TOTAL REVISION:
EMQs FOR MEDICAL STUDENTS

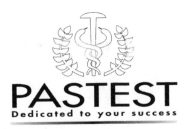

PASTEST
Dedicated to your success

TOTAL REVISION: EMQs FOR MEDICAL STUDENTS

Richard Bellamy
BMedSci(Hons) MBBS(Hons) MRCP DpPhil DipMgmt MSc DLSHT
DipMedEd MMedEd
ObaapaVitA Trial Director
Kintampo Health Research Centre
Ghana

Muzlifah Haniffa
BSc (Hons) MBBCh (Hons) MRCP
Specialist Registrar in Dermatology
Royal Victoria Infirmary
Newcastle-Upon-Tyne

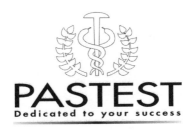

PASTEST
Dedicated to your success

© 2004 PasTest Ltd
Egerton Court
Parkgate Estate
Knutsford
Cheshire, WA16 8DX

Telephone: 01565 752000

First edition 2004

ISBN: 1 904627 226

A catalogue record for this book is available from the British Library.

The information contained within this book was obtained by the authors from reliable sources. However, while every effort has been made to ensure its accuracy, no responsibility for loss, damage or injury occasioned to any person acting or refraining from action as a result of information contained herein can be accepted by the publisher or the authors.

PasTest Revision Books and Intensive Courses

PasTest has been established in the field of postgraduate medical education since 1972, providing revision books and intensive study courses for doctors preparing for their professional examinations. Books and courses are available for the following specialties:

MRCP Part 1 and Part 2, MRCPCH Part 1 and Part 2, MRCOG, DRCOG, MRCGP, MRCPsych, DCH, FRCA, MRCS and PLAB.

For further details contact:

Tel: 01565 752000   Fax: 01565 650264
Email: enquiries@pastest.co.uk   **Web site: www. pastest.co.uk**

Typeset by Saxon Graphics Ltd, Derby
Printed and bound in Great Britain by the Alden Group

CONTENTS

Introduction   vii

Normal Values   ix

Glossary   xi

Paper 1 Questions   1

Paper 1 Answers   17

Paper 2 Questions   43

Paper 2 Answers   59

Paper 3 Questions   87

Paper 3 Answers   105

Paper 4 Questions   133

Paper 4 Answers   149

Paper 5 Questions   177

Paper 5 Answers   195

Index   223

INTRODUCTION

Extended matched questions (EMQs) are increasingly being used as the core test of knowledge in undergraduate and postgraduate examinations. Unfortunately for candidates the majority of practice examination books currently available use the traditional multiple choice question true/false answer format. The EMQ books that have been published to date have generally concentrated on the needs of candidates from overseas who are sitting the Professional and Linguistics Assessment Board (PLAB) examination and ask the candidate to match a diagnosis to the description of a clinical case. This style does not match that of many medical schools' undergraduate exams because the final MBBS needs to test a broad knowledge base. The EMQs in this book attempt to cover the knowledge that is likely to be tested in undergraduate medical examinations. The exact format of EMQs will vary between medical schools. The number of questions under each topic may differ, as may the number of answers between which the candidate must choose. To avoid confusing the reader we have chosen a single question style with five questions and six answers to choose between for each topic.

Some of our questions are much harder than others so do not despair if you find them difficult. We have done this for two reasons. Firstly, medical schools often use a combination of difficult and more straightforward questions. The difficult questions are useful to identify the best candidates, who deserve a distinction, and the easier questions are used to identify those who have not reached the required standard to pass. The second reason is that the reader learns something every time they encounter a question they cannot answer. If all of the questions were straightforward, the more able candidate would learn nothing from reading this book. To assist the reader we have graded the difficulty of the answers. Grade 1 (indicated by ☆) indicates a question that the majority of competent final year students will know the answer to. Grade 2 (☆☆) indicates a question which approximately 50% of final year students will be able to answer correctly. Grade 3 (☆☆☆) indicates a question that only the better students will usually know the answer to. This classification is somewhat arbitrary, as a question that is straightforward overall may still contain one or two difficult matches.

We have made the answers to the questions more detailed than occurs in most examination books. This is because many students prefer to answer questions without the distraction of frequently referring to reference texts. We hope that most students will find the amount of information we have provided about right, but we would still recommend consulting textbooks for additional information when needed.

The questions have been divided into five papers, each consisting of 60 topics covering 300 questions. Candidates wishing to complete the papers in mock examination conditions should allow themselves around three hours to complete each exam. This book covers all of the major medical specialties. Although it does not specifically aim to test surgical, obstetric or paediatric knowledge, these topics do arise within each of the systems-based subjects.

The papers each include the following number of questions by subject:

- Cellular and molecular biology — 2
- Statistics and epidemiology — 1
- Immunology — 2
- Clinical genetics — 2
- Neuroanatomy — 2
- Physiology, biochemistry and metabolism — 5
- Renal medicine — 4
- Endocrinology and diabetes — 4
- Gastroenterology — 4
- Neurology — 4
- Respiratory medicine — 4
- Rheumatology — 2
- Dermatology — 2
- Haematology — 3
- Infectious diseases and tropical medicine — 4
- Genitourinary medicine including HIV — 1
- Clinical pharmacology — 6
- Cardiovascular medicine — 4
- Psychiatry — 3
- Miscellaneous — 1

This breakdown is somewhat arbitrary as some questions could belong to more than one specialty. Each paper follows the same sequence of subjects and these are highlighted so that students revising a particular specialty can easily identify the relevant questions. The number of questions per specialty is designed to match that of the Member of the Royal College of Physicians (MRCP) exam and is not intended to reflect any perceived ranking of importance. Breakdown per specialty is likely to vary between medical schools but should be generally similar to that contained in this book. The first 14 questions in each paper cover 'basic science' subjects. Students sitting exams that do not cover these areas may wish to omit these questions if pressed for time. However, be aware that vertical integration of the curriculum in many medical schools has meant that many exams in the clinical part of the course will include clinically important, basic science questions.

We wish you every success and hope that you find this book useful and enjoyable. If you have any comments or suggestions for future editions we would be very pleased to hear from you.

Richard Bellamy
Muzlifah Haniffa

All royalties from this book will be donated to Médecins Sans Frontières

NORMAL VALUES

Haematology
Haemoglobin
   Males   13.5–17.5 g/dl
   Females   11.5–15.5 g/dl

Haemoglobin	
Males	13.5–17.5 g/dl
Females	11.5–15.5 g/dl
MCV	76–98 fl
PCV	35–55%
WCC	$4–11 \times 10^9$/l
Neut.	$2.5–7.58 \times 10^9$/l
Lymph.	$1.5–3.5 \times 10^9$/l
Platelets	$150–400 \times 10^9$/l
ESR	0–10 mm in the 1st hour
PT	10.6–14.9 s
PTT	23.0–35.0 s
TT	10.5–15.5 s
Fib	125–300 mg/dl
Vitamin B_{12}	160–900 pmol/l
Folate	1.5–10.0 μg/l
Ferritin	
Males	20–250 μg/l
Females	10–120 μg/l

Immunoglobulins
IgM	0.5–2.0 g/l
IgG	5–16 g/l
IgA	1.0–4.0 g/l

Biochemistry
Na^+	135–145 mmol/l
K^+	3.5–5.0 mmol/l
U	2.5–6.5 mmol/l
Cr	50–120 μmol/l
ALT	5–30 iu/l
AST	10–40 iu/l
Bili.	2–17 μmol/l
Alk P	30–130 iu/l
Alb.	35–55 g/l
γGT	5–30 iu/l
αFP	<10 ku/l
CCa	2.20–2.60 mmol/l
PO_4^{2-}	0.70–1.40 mmol/l
CK	23–175 iu/l

LDH	100–190 iu/l
Amylase	<200 u/l
Lactate	0.5–2.2 mmol/l
Mg^{2+}	0.75–1.00 mmol/l
Urate	0.1–0.4 mol/l
CRP	0–10 mg/l

Diabetes

Glucose	
Random	3.5–5.5 mmol/l*
Fasting	<7 mol/l
HbA_{1c}	<7.0%

Endocrinology

TSH	0.17–3.2 mu/l
T_4	11–22 pmol/l
Cortisol	
0900	140–500 nmol/l
2400	50–300 nmol/l
Growth Hormone	<10 ng/ml
Cholesterol	<5.2 mmol/l
Triglycerides	0–1.5 mmol/l
LDL	< 3.5 mmol/l
HDL	> 1.0 mmol/l
Total/HDL	< 5.0

Blood Gases

pH	7.35–7.45
pCO_2	4.6–6.0 kPa
pO_2	10.5–13.5 kPa
HCO_3	24–30 mmol/l
BE	−2–2.0 mmol/l

CSF

Protein	<0.45 g/l
Glucose	2.5–3.9 mmol/l (two-thirds plasma)
Cells	< 5mm³ (WCC)
Opening Pressure	6–20 cmH$_2$O

GLOSSARY

ABeAg	Hepatitis B envelope antigen
ACE	Angiotensin converting enzyme
ACTH	Adrenocorticotrophic hormone
ADH	Antidiuretic hormone
AIP	Acute intermittent porphyria
ALL	Acute lymphoblastic leukaemia
ALP	Serum alkaline phosphatase
ALT	Serum alanine aminotransferase
AML	Acute myeloid leukaemia
AP	Anteroposterior
APTT	Activated partial thromboplastin time
ASD	Atrial septal defect
BBB	Bundle Branch Block
BIPAP	Biphasic positive airway pressure
BPV	Benign positional vertigo
CAPD	Continuous ambulatory peritoneal dialysis
cGMP	Cyclic Guanosine monophosphate
CJD	Creutzfeldt-Jakob disease
CML	Chronic myeloid leukaemia
CML	Chronic myeloid leukaemia
CN	Cranial nerve
CNS	Central nervous system
COLD	Chronic obstructive lung disease
CPAP	Continuous positive airway pressure
CR	Complement receptor
CRH	Corticotrophin releasing hormone
DI	Diabetes insipidus
DMD	Duchenne muscular dystrophy
ESM	Ejection systolic murmur
FEV	Forced expiratory volume
FGFR	Fibroblast growth factor receptor
FSH	Follicle stimulating hormone
FVC	Forced vital capacity
GCS	Glasgow coma scale
GCSF	Granulocyte colony stimulating factor
GFR	Gromerular filtration rate
GHRH	Growth hormone releasing hormone
GIP	Glucose-dependent insulinotrophic peptide
GnRH	Gonadotrophin releasing hormone
HBsAg	Hepatitis B surface antigen
HBV	Hepatitis B Virus
HDL	High density lipoproteins
HFJV	High frequency jet ventilation
HLA	Human leukocyte antigen

CONTENTS

HMSN	Hereditary motor and sensory neuropathy
HONK	Hyperosmolar non-ketoacidotic coma
HRCT	High-resolution computed tomography
HSP	Henoch-Schönlein purpura
HUS	Haemolytic uraemic syndrome
ICAM	Intercellular adhesion molecules
INR	International normalized ratio
ITT	Insulin tolerance test
KUB	Kidneys, ureters, bladder
LDL	Low density lipoproteins
LH	Luteinising hormone
LSD	Lysergic acid diethylamide
MAP	Mitogen activated pathway
MDMA	Methylenedioxymethamphetamine
MGUS	Monoclonal gammopathy of undetermined significance
MODY	Maturity onset diabetes of young
MRI	Magnetic resonance imaging
NBV	Negative predictive value
NO	Nitric oxide
OHL	Oral hairy leukoplakia
PA	Posteroanterior
pANCA	Perinuclear antineutrophil cytoplasmic antibodies
PAS	Para-amino salicylic acid
PCR	Polymerase chain reaction
PPV	Positive predictive value
PSV	Pressure support ventilation
PT	Prothrombin time
PTH	Parathyroid hormone
RBC	Red blood cell
RPGN	Rapidly progressive glomerulonephritis
RTA	Renal tubular acidosis
SIADH	Syndrome of inappropriate antidiuretic hormone secretion
SIMV	Simultaneous intermittent mandatory ventilation
SLE	Systemic lupus erythematosus
SLE	Systemic lupus erythematosus
SSRI	Selective serotonin reuptake inhibitor
TBG	Thyroxine binding globulin
TNF	Tumour necrosis factor
TPHA	Treponema pallidum haemagglutination assay
TRH	Thyrotrophin releasing hormone
TSH	Thyroid stimulating hormone
TTP	Thrombotic thrombocytopaenic purpura
UDPGT	Uridine diphosphate glucuronyl transferase
UDPGT	Uridine diphosphate glucuronyl transferase
VIP	Vasoactive intestinal polypeptide
VLDL	Very low density lipoproteins
WBC	White blood cell
WDHA	Watery diarrhoea hypokalaemia achlorhydria
WPW	Wolff-Parkinson-White

PAPER 1 QUESTIONS

CELLULAR AND MOLECULAR BIOLOGY

1. THEME: ENZYMES

A Bacterial enzyme which cleaves foreign DNA at a specific recognition site
B Enzyme responsible for DNA transcription
C Enzyme which breaks down DNA without a specific recognition site
D Enzyme used in the polymerase chain reaction
E Enzyme responsible for DNA replication
F Enzyme producing cDNA

For each of the following enzymes select the best description from the above list. The items may be used once or not at all.

☐ 1. *Taq* polymerase
☐ 2. RNA polymerase
☐ 3. Reverse transcriptase
☐ 4. DNA polymerase
☐ 5. Restriction endonuclease

2. THEME: REGIONS OF DNA

A Splice donor
B 3′-flanking region
C 5′-flanking region
D Exon
E Intron
F Promoter

For each of the following regions of DNA select the best description from the above list. The items may be used once or not at all.

☐ 1. Intragenic region between coding DNA sequences
☐ 2. Region upstream of the coding DNA sequence
☐ 3. Region downstream of the coding DNA sequence
☐ 4. Region to which RNA polymerase binds
☐ 5. Coding DNA sequence

STATISTICS AND EPIDEMIOLOGY

3. THEME: REDUCING ERROR

A Placebo effect
B Type 2 error
C Type 1 error
D Failure of subjects to complete study
E Observer bias
F Confounding by unidentified risk factors

For each of the methods listed below select the most useful for reducing the source of error listed above. The items may be used once or not at all.

☐ 1. Use stricter probability value to declare a statistically significant difference between groups
☐ 2. Increase sample size of study
☐ 3. Blinding of investigators to individual subject's treatment group
☐ 4. Randomisation of study subjects to different treatment groups
☐ 5. Use of intention-to-treat analysis

IMMUNOLOGY

4. THEME: HUMAN LEUKOCYTE ANTIGENS

A   HLA-A3
B   HLA-B27
C   HLA-DR2
D   HLA-DR1
E   HLA-DR3
F   HLA-DR4

For each of the following diseases select the human leukocyte antigen (HLA) molecule that is associated with it from the above list. The items may be used once or not at all.

☐ 1. Narcolepsy
☐ 2. Reiter's syndrome
☐ 3. Dermatitis herpetiformis
☐ 4. Rheumatoid arthritis
☐ 5. Haemochromatosis

5. THEME: T CELL DIFFERENTIATION ANTIGENS

A   CD25
B   CD4
C   CD3
D   CD8
E   CD45RO
F   CD35

For each of the following descriptions select the best T cell differentiation antigen from the above list. The items may be used once or not at all.

☐ 1. Found on all T cells in association with the T cell receptor
☐ 2. Found on T helper cells, binds to antigens presented by HLA class II
☐ 3. Found on cytotoxic T cells, binds to antigens presented by HLA class I
☐ 4. Found on memory T cells
☐ 5. Found on activated T cells, binds to interleukin 2

CLINICAL GENETICS

6. THEME: SYNDROMES AND GENETIC MUTATIONS

A   Type I collagen gene
B   Type III collagen gene
C   Fibrillin gene
D   Cystic fibrosis transmembrane conductance regulator *CFTR* gene
E   Fibroblast growth factor receptor III *FGFR-III* gene
F   Cystathionine β-synthase gene

For each of the following syndromes select the gene in which a mutation may cause that syndrome from the above list. The items may be used once or not at all.

☐ 1. Marfan syndrome
☐ 2. Achondroplasia
☐ 3. Ehlers-Danlos type IV
☐ 4. Homocystinuria
☐ 5. Osteogenesis imperfecta type I

7. THEME: GENETIC INHERITANCE PATTERNS

A   Autosomal dominant
B   Non-hereditary
C   Autosomal recessive
D   Mitochondrial
E   X-linked dominant
F   X-linked recessive

For each of the following findings in the study of a familial disease select the gene inheritance pattern from the above list. The items may be used once or not at all.

☐ 1. Females virtually never affected
☐ 2. Multiple generations affected in most families
☐ 3. Inheritance is always from the mother
☐ 4. Markedly increased incidence in offspring of a consanguineous marriage
☐ 5. All daughters of an affected male inherit the disease susceptibility

NEUROANATOMY

8. THEME: CRANIAL NERVES

A Vagus nerve
B Oculomotor nerve
C Facial nerve
D Hypoglossal nerve
E Trigeminal nerve
F Glossopharyngeal nerve

For each of the following functions select the appropriate cranial nerve from the above list. The items may be used once or not at all.

- ☐ 1. Parasympathetic supply to lacrimal gland
- ☐ 2. Constriction of the pupil
- ☐ 3. Motor supply to laryngeal muscles
- ☐ 4. Sensory supply to the carotid sinus baroreceptor
- ☐ 5. Motor supply to pterygoid muscles

9. THEME: NERVE INJURY AND SIGNS

A Radial nerve compression against the shaft of the humerus
B Ulnar nerve compression against the olecranon
C Ulnar nerve damage at the wrist
D Avulsion of the lower roots of the brachial plexus
E Avulsion of the upper roots of the brachial plexus
F Axillary nerve compression in the axilla

For each of the following abnormalities select the appropriate nerve injury from the above list. The items may be used once or not at all.

- ☐ 1. Arm hangs with the shoulder internally rotated, elbow extended and the forearm pronated (waiter's tip position)
- ☐ 2. Claw hand deformity affecting all fingers and sensory loss on medial aspect of forearm and hand
- ☐ 3. Weakness of forearm supination and finger extension and sensory loss on dorsum of hand

- ☐ 4. Inability to abduct the arm at the shoulder
- ☐ 5. Claw hand deformity predominantly affecting the little and ring fingers and sensory loss on the medial aspect of the hand but not forearm

PHYSIOLOGY, BIOCHEMISTRY AND METABOLISM

10. THEME: HORMONE PRODUCTION

A Adrenaline
B Insulin
C Calcitonin
D Glucagon
E Cortisol
F Somatostatin

For each of the following structures select the hormone it produces from the above list. The items may be used once or not at all.

- ☐ 1. Pancreatic β cells
- ☐ 2. Pancreatic D cells
- ☐ 3. Pancreatic α cells
- ☐ 4. Adrenal medulla
- ☐ 5. Adrenal cortex

11. THEME: SERUM PROTEINS

A   Group-specific component
B   Haptoglobin
C   Albumin
D α_1-antitrypsin
E γ-globulin
F α_2-macroglobulin

For each of the following descriptions select the appropriate serum protein from the above list. The items may be used once or not at all.

☐ 1. A major inhibitor of proteolytic activity for which congenital deficiency is well recognised
☐ 2. A serum protease inhibitor of large molecular size
☐ 3. A polymorphic protein which binds haemoglobin
☐ 4. An abundant plasma protein which binds bilirubin
☐ 5. A protein which carries vitamin D

12. THEME: SERUM ELECTROPHORESIS PATTERN

A   Nephrotic syndrome
B   Chronic liver disease
C   Diabetes mellitus
D   Protein-losing enteropathy
E α_1-antitrypsin deficiency
F   Dysproteinaemia

For each of the following abnormal serum electrophoresis patterns select the appropriate disease from the above list. The items may be used once or not at all.

☐ 1. Diffuse elevation of γ-globulin
☐ 2. Sharply increased spike in γ-globulin
☐ 3. Low albumin and high β-globulin
☐ 4. Low albumin and moderately high α_2-globulin
☐ 5. Flat where α_1-globulin band should be

13. THEME: LIPIDS

A   High-density lipoproteins
B   Low-density lipoproteins
C   Chylomicrons
D   Very low density lipoproteins
E   Lipoprotein (a)
F   Fat globule within adipocyte

For each of the following descriptions select the appropriate lipid particle from the above list. The items may be used once or not at all.

☐ 1. Consists of 85–95% triglyceride and only 1–2% protein
☐ 2. Consists of 60–70% triglyceride, 10–15% cholesterol and 10% protein
☐ 3. Consists of 45% cholesterol, 20–30% phospholipids and 15–25% protein
☐ 4. Consists of 20% cholesterol, 30% phospholipids and 50% protein
☐ 5. A low-density lipoprotein-like particle found in atherosclerotic plaques

14. THEME: MEASURES OF LUNG VOLUME

A   Expiratory reserve volume
B   Vital capacity
C   Residual volume
D   Inspiratory capacity
E   Inspiratory reserve volume
F   Functional residual capacity

For each of the following descriptions select the appropriate measurement from the above list. The items may be used once or not at all.

☐ 1. Maximum volume of air that can be inhaled at the end of normal expiration
☐ 2. Maximum volume of air that can be inhaled at the end of inspiration
☐ 3. Maximum volume of air that can be exhaled after maximal inspiration
☐ 4. Maximum volume of air that can be exhaled at the end of expiration
☐ 5. Volume of air in lungs at the end of normal expiration

RENAL MEDICINE

15. THEME: RENAL TRACT INVESTIGATIONS

A Intravenous urogram
B Renal angiography
C Micturating cystourethrogram
D Abdominal X-ray
E Renal ultrasound
F Retrograde ureteropyelography

For each of the following select the most useful investigation from the above list. The items may be used once or not at all.

☐ 1. To identify/exclude renal tract obstruction in acute renal failure
☐ 2. To identify ureteric stones when the kidney is functioning
☐ 3. To identify the site of ureteric obstruction when the kidney is not functioning
☐ 4. To show ureteric reflux
☐ 5. To demonstrate nephrocalcinosis

16. THEME: GLOMERULONEPHRITIS

A Membranous glomerulonephritis
B Minimal change glomerulonephritis
C Rapidly progressive glomerulonephritis
D Mesangiocapillary glomerulonephritis
E Focal segmental glomerulosclerosis
F Berger's disease

For each of the following select the most appropriate condition from the above list. The items may be used once or not at all.

☐ 1. Commonest cause of nephrotic syndrome in children
☐ 2. Common cause of nephrotic syndrome associated with malignancy, heroin use and HIV infection
☐ 3. Common cause of haematuria with immunoglobulin A deposits seen on immunofluorescence microscopy
☐ 4. May present with acute renal failure and glomerular crescent formation on histology
☐ 5. Affected patients may have lipodystrophy and the presence of C3 nephritic factor

17. THEME: TREATMENT OF GLOMERULONEPHRITIDES

A Cyclophosphamide + methylprednisolone + plasmapheresis
B Cyclophosphamide + methylprednisolone
C Prednisolone
D Angiotensin-converting enzyme inhibitor + anticoagulants
E No treatment indicated
F Ciclosporin A

For each of the following situations select the most appropriate treatment from the above list. The items may be used once or not at all.

☐ 1. First-line treatment of nephrotic syndrome due to minimal change nephropathy
☐ 2. Frequently relapsing, steroid-dependent minimal change nephropathy
☐ 3. IgA nephropathy with haematuria but no proteinuria
☐ 4. IgA nephropathy with haematuria and proteinuria exceeding 1 g per day
☐ 5. Rapidly progressive glomerulonephritis due to Wegener's granulomatosis

18. THEME: DISEASE CAUSED BY RENAL TRANSPORT DEFECTS

A   Fanconi syndrome
B   Cystinuria
C   Alport's syndrome
D   Type 1 renal tubular acidosis
E   Type 2 renal tubular acidosis
F   Type 4 renal tubular acidosis

For each of the following select the most appropriate condition from the above list. The items may be used once or not at all.

☐ 1. Causes hypokalaemic acidosis due to failure of proximal convoluted tubule to secrete hydrogen ions and reabsorb bicarbonate
☐ 2. Causes hypokalaemic acidosis due to failure of distal nephron to generate hydrogen ion gradient
☐ 3. Hyperkalaemic acidosis associated with aldosterone deficiency
☐ 4. Syndrome of multiple tubular transport defects causing glycosuria, aminoaciduria, phosphaturia and renal tubular acidosis
☐ 5. Commonest inherited cause of aminoaciduria

ENDOCRINOLOGY AND DIABETES

19. THEME: TREATMENT OF ENDOCRINE CONDITIONS

A   Metyrapone
B   Finasteride
C   Demeclocycline
D   Prednisolone
E   Somatropin
F   Cabergoline

For each of the following conditions select the most appropriate treatment from the above list. The items may be used once or not at all.

☐ 1. Benign prostatic hypertrophy
☐ 2. Short stature
☐ 3. Syndrome of inappropriate antidiuretic hormone (SIADH)
☐ 4. Prolactinoma
☐ 5. Cushing's syndrome

20. THEME: AETIOLOGY OF DIABETES

A   Type I diabetes mellitus
B   Type II diabetes mellitus
C   Maturity-onset diabetes of the young
D   Type III (tropical) diabetes mellitus
E   Insulin receptor abnormalities
F   Glucagonoma-induced diabetes mellitus

For each of the following aetiological risk factors associations select the type of diabetes from the above list. The items may be used once or not at all.

☐ 1. Obesity and increased age
☐ 2. Necrolytic migratory erythema
☐ 3. Pancreatic fibrocalculous disease
☐ 4. Lipodystrophy and acanthosis nigricans
☐ 5. Autoimmune destruction of pancreatic islet cells

21. THEME: THYROID FUNCTION TEST

A   Raised thyroglobulin
B   Low T_4
C   Raised T_3
D   Raised T_4
E   Raised thyroid-stimulating hormone (TSH)
F   Low TSH

For each of the following descriptions select the appropriate thyroid function test result from the above list. The items may be used once or not at all.

☐ 1. Suggests tumour recurrence in a patient with previous thyroid cancer
☐ 2. Most commonly used test to diagnose hypothyroidism
☐ 3. Can be caused by Grave's disease or hypopituitarism
☐ 4. Most sensitive test of hyperthyroidism
☐ 5. Suggestive of hypothyroidism but affected by thyroxine-binding globulin levels

22. THEME: AMENORRHOEA

A   Polycystic ovary syndrome
B   Hyperprolactinaemia
C   Turner's syndrome
D   Adrenogenital syndrome
E   Hypopituitarism
F   Menopause

For each of the following test results select the most likely cause of amenorrhoea from the above list. The items may be used once or not at all.

☐ 1. High serum luteinising hormone (LH) and follicle-stimulating hormone (FSH), low urine 17-ketosteroids
☐ 2. Low serum LH and FSH, normal urine 17-ketosteroids
☐ 3. High serum LH and FSH, high urine 17-ketosteroids
☐ 4. High serum LH and low FSH, high urine 17-ketosteroids
☐ 5. Normal serum LH and FSH, normal urine 17-ketosteroids

GASTROENTEROLOGY

23. THEME: GASTROINTESTINAL HORMONES

A   Glucose-dependent insulinotrophic peptide
B   Secretin
C   Vasoactive intestinal polypeptide
D   Pancreatic polypeptide
E   Gastrin
F   Cholecystokinin

For each of the following actions select the stimulating hormone from the above list. The items may be used once or not at all.

☐ 1. Gastric acid secretion
☐ 2. Gallbladder contraction
☐ 3. Secretion of watery, alkaline pancreatic fluid
☐ 4. Insulin release
☐ 5. Secretion of water and electrolytes by colonic and small intestinal enterocytes

24. THEME: DYSPHAGIA

A   Pharyngeal pouch
B   Retrosternal goitre
C   Achalasia
D   Oesophagitis
E   Bulbar palsy
F   Oesophageal carcinoma

For each of the following presentations select the cause of dysphagia from the above list. The items may be used once or not at all.

☐ 1. Dysphagia initially worse for solid food items but eventually progressing to involve liquids
☐ 2. Chronic dysphagia accompanied by gurgling and neck swelling
☐ 3. Chronic dysphagia accompanied by coughing
☐ 4. Chronic painful dysphagia accompanied by pain on lying flat
☐ 5. Chronic dysphagia for liquids and solids with chest X-ray showing an air-fluid level behind the heart

25. THEME: BLOOD TESTS FOR HEPATITIS B VIRUS

A   HBsAg
B   Anti-HBc
C   HBV DNA
D   Anti-HBe
E   Anti-HBs
F   HBeAg

For each of the following descriptions select the appropriate hepatitis B blood test from the above list. The items may be used once or not at all.

☐ 1. Positive following vaccination or previous infection
☐ 2. Positive in all hepatitis B carriers
☐ 3. An antigen test which is positive in hepatitis B carriers with high infectivity
☐ 4. Positive following previous infection but not following vaccination
☐ 5. Useful to quantify replicating hepatitis B virus

26. THEME: ORAL LESIONS

A   HIV infection
B   Lichen planus
C   Pemphigus vulgaris
D   Bullous pemphigoid
E   Crohn's disease
F   Behçet's disease

For each of the following oral lesions select the appropriate associated condition from the above list. The items may be used once or not at all.

☐ 1. Recurrent oral ulcers in a patient with perianal fistulae
☐ 2. Vertical white streaks on the edge of the tongue
☐ 3. Lacy white lesions on the oral mucosa
☐ 4. Oral blisters in a patient with widespread superficial cutaneous blisters
☐ 5. Oral ulcers in a patient with genital ulcers and previous iritis

NEUROLOGY

27. THEME: NEUROLOGICAL DEFICITS CAUSED BY CRANIAL ARTERY OCCLUSIONS

A   Left middle cerebral artery
B   Right middle cerebral artery
C   Right anterior cerebral artery
D   Left posterior inferior cerebellar artery
E   Right posterior inferior cerebellar artery
F   Right posterior cerebral artery

For each of the following signs of neurological deficit in a right-handed patient select the appropriate artery from the above list. The items may be used once or not at all.

☐ 1. Weakness of left lower limb
☐ 2. Weakness and sensory loss of left upper limb
☐ 3. Receptive dysphasia
☐ 4. Left-sided homonymous hemianopia
☐ 5. Loss of pin-prick of left limbs and vibration sense of right limbs

28. THEME: VERTIGO

A   Acoustic neuroma
B   Vestibular neuronitis
C   Ramsay Hunt syndrome
D   Ménière's disease
E   Benign positional vertigo
F   Brainstem infarction

For each of the following findings select the most appropriate cause of vertigo from the above list. The items may be used once or not at all.

☐ 1. Vertigo associated with rapid head movements, with nystagmus which demonstrates fatigability on Hallpike's manoeuvre
☐ 2. Recurrent attacks of severe vertigo in a patient with progressive hearing loss and tinnitus
☐ 3. Progressive unilateral hearing loss and vertigo with subsequent development of fifth, seventh, ninth and tenth nerve palsies
☐ 4. Abrupt onset of severe vertigo and vomiting in the absence of tinnitus and deafness without other cranial nerve signs
☐ 5. Abrupt onset of severe vertigo, vomiting and nystagmus with a bulbar palsy but normal hearing

29. THEME: DISORDERS OF HIGHER CEREBRAL VISUAL FUNCTION

A   Visual agnosia
B   Visual inattention
C   Prosopagnosia
D   Visual disorientation
E   Gaze apraxia
F   Topographical disorientation

For each of the following select the most appropriate term from the above list. The items may be used once or not at all.

☐ 1. Inability to recognise faces by sight
☐ 2. Inability to locate the position of objects in space

☐ 3. Inability to orientate eyes and maintain visual fixation

☐ 4. Inability to perceive more than one visual stimulus simultaneously

☐ 5. Inability to recognise objects by sight

30. THEME: LOSS OF CONSCIOUSNESS

A   Seizure(s)
B   Stokes-Adams attack(s)
C   Vasovagal attack(s)
D   Transient ischaemic attack(s)
E   Stroke(s)
F   Orthostatic hypotension

For each of the following descriptions select the appropriate cause from the above list. The items may be used once or not at all.

☐ 1. Single episode preceded briefly by pallor and sweating; loss of consciousness for two minutes; full and rapid recovery

☐ 2. Several episodes often preceded by an aura; loss of consciousness for 30 minutes followed by drowsiness lasting several hours

☐ 3. Multiple episodes with no warning; loss of consciousness accompanied by pallor and bradycardia; recovery within seconds accompanied by facial flushing and speeding up of pulse

☐ 4. Single episode with no warning; loss of consciousness for 30 minutes followed by hemiparesis for 12 hours and then complete recovery

☐ 5. Multiple episodes occurring while urinating during the night; loss of consciousness for two minutes; full and rapid recovery

RESPIRATORY MEDICINE

31. THEME: X-RAY FINDINGS

A   Pectus excavatum
B   Enlarged left atrium
C   Left upper lobe lung pathology
D   Right middle lobe collapse
E   Right lower lobe collapse
F   Left lower lobe pathology

For each of the following chest X-ray abnormalities select the appropriate cause from the above list. The items may be used once or not at all.

☐ 1. Splaying of the carina

☐ 2. Blurring of the left heart border

☐ 3. Enlargement of the heart shadow on the left side

☐ 4. Blurring of the right heart border

☐ 5. Blurring of the medial aspect of the right hemidiaphragm

32. THEME: UPPER AIRWAY OBSTRUCTION

A   Epiglottitis
B   Tracheal stenosis
C   Tracheomalacia
D   Laryngeal nerve palsy
E   Bronchial carcinoma
F   Angioneurotic oedema

For each of the following presentations select the appropriate cause of upper airway obstruction from the above list. The items may be used once or not at all.

☐ 1. Acute stridor in a patient with previous recurrent episodes of severe colicky abdominal pain

☐ 2. One-day history of drooling, hoarse voice, sore throat and difficulty breathing in a young adult

☐ 3. Stridor, breathlessness and paroxysms of coughing one week after thyroidectomy

☐ 4. Chronic stridor and breathing difficulties in a patient who was on a mechanical ventilator for six weeks

☐ 5. Chronic voice change, nocturnal stridor and obstructive sleep apnoea in a patient who had a thyroidectomy five years previously

33. THEME: BRONCHIAL CARCINOMA STAGING

A $T_3 N_1 M_0$
B $T_4 N_3 M_0$
C $T_1 N_1 M_0$
D $T_1 N_3 M_0$
E $T_1 N_2 M_0$
F $T_3 N_3 M_0$

For each of the following descriptions of bronchial carcinoma select the appropriate stage from the above list. The items may be used once or not at all.

☐ 1. Tumour less than 3 cm diameter in a lobar bronchus with ipsilateral hilar lymph node involvement and no metastases
☐ 2. Tumour involving the chest wall with ipsilateral hilar lymph node involvement and no metastases
☐ 3. Tumour less than 3 cm diameter in a lobar bronchus with ipsilateral subcarinal lymph node involvement and no metastases
☐ 4. Tumour involving the chest wall with supraclavicular lymph node involvement and no metastases
☐ 5. Tumour involving the mediastinum with contralateral lymph node involvement and no metastases

34. THEME: LUNG FUNCTION TESTS

A Transfer factor for carbon monoxide
B Helium diffusion
C Spirometry
D Methacholine test
E Peak flow
F Flow-volume loop

For each of the following select the lung function test which is used to obtain this measurement from the above list. The items may be used once or not at all.

☐ 1. Airway responsiveness
☐ 2. Diffusion capacity
☐ 3. Solely a measure of maximal expiratory airflow

☐ 4. Distinguishing extrathoracic and intrathoracic airway obstruction
☐ 5. Residual volume

RHEUMATOLOGY

35. THEME: RED EYE

A Subconjunctival haemorrhage
B Conjunctivitis
C Acute iritis
D Acute glaucoma
E Scleritis
F Chronic glaucoma

For each of the following findings select the appropriate cause of red eye from the above list. The items may be used once or not at all.

☐ 1. Injected conjuctival vessels which blanche on pressure; normal iris, pupil and cornea
☐ 2. Injected iris, fixed dilated pupil and hazy cornea
☐ 3. Injected iris, small fixed pupil and turbid anterior chamber fluid
☐ 4. Bright red sclera with white rim around limbus; normal iris, pupil and cornea
☐ 5. Painful red eye with boggy swelling of eye coat

36. THEME: BONE OR JOINT PROBLEMS

A Sjögren's syndrome
B Ankylosing spondylitis
C Rheumatoid arthritis
D Tuberculosis
E Syringomyelia
F Osteoarthritis

For each of the following bone or joint problems select the appropriate predisposing condition from the above list. The items may be used once or not at all.

☐ 1. Atlanto-axial subluxation
☐ 2. Sacroileitis
☐ 3. Distal interphalangeal joint arthritis
☐ 4. Pott's disease
☐ 5. Charcot's arthropathy

DERMATOLOGY

37. THEME: DESCRIBING SKIN LESIONS

A   Macule
B   Plaque
C   Vesicle
D   Nodule
E   Bulla
F   Patch

For each of the following descriptions select the appropriate term from the above list. The items may be used once or not at all.

☐ 1. Fluid-filled elevation with a diameter greater than 0.5 cm
☐ 2. Fluid-filled elevation with a diameter less than 0.5 cm
☐ 3. Palpable lesion up to 1 cm in diameter
☐ 4. Non-palpable discoloured area less than 1 cm in diameter
☐ 5. Non-palpable discoloured area greater than 1 cm in diameter

38. THEME: NAIL ABNORMALITY

A   Koilonychia
B   Melanonychia
C   Clubbing
D   Splinter haemorrhages
E   Blue nails
F   Yellow nails

For each of the following select the resulting nail abnormality from the above list. The items may be used once or not at all.

☐ 1. Cytotoxic drug use
☐ 2. Lymphoedema
☐ 3. Prolonged chloroquine use
☐ 4. Iron deficiency
☐ 5. Cirrhosis

HAEMATOLOGY

39. THEME: RED BLOOD CELL ABNORMALITY

A   Acanthocytosis
B   Reticulocytosis
C   Poikilocytosis
D   Howell-Jolly bodies
E   Anisocytosis
F   Heinz bodies

For each of the following descriptions select the appropriate red blood cell abnormality from the above list. The items may be used once or not at all.

☐ 1. Densely staining particles of nuclear DNA seen at the cell periphery
☐ 2. Masses of denatured haemoglobin
☐ 3. Variation in red blood cell size
☐ 4. Spiculated red blood cells
☐ 5. Variation in red cell shape

40. THEME: LEUKAEMIA

A   Myelodysplastic syndrome
B   Acute lymphoblastic leukaemia
C   B cell type primary chronic lymphoid leukaemia
D   T cell type primary chronic lymphoid leukaemia
E   Chronic myeloid leukaemia
F   Acute myeloid leukaemia

For each of the following select the appropriate group of leukaemia from the above list. The items may be used once or not at all.

☐ 1. Includes Sézary cell leukaemia
☐ 2. Includes hairy cell leukaemia
☐ 3. Includes erythroleukaemia
☐ 4. A disease which is associated with Down's syndrome
☐ 5. A disease which is strongly associated with the Philadelphia chromosome

41. THEME: BONE MARROW TRANSPLANTATION

A Xenotransplant
B Allogeneic transplant
C Autologous transplant
D Syngeneic transplant
E Peripheral blood stem cell harvesting
F Leukocyte depletion

For each of the following descriptions select the appropriate term from the above list. The items may be used once or not at all.

☐ 1. Patient receives own bone marrow
☐ 2. Patient receives bone marrow from identical twin
☐ 3. Patient receives bone marrow from an HLA-matched relative
☐ 4. Patient receives bone marrow from a member of another species
☐ 5. Patient receives own cells harvested after chemotherapy and granulocyte colony-stimulating factor (GCSF) administration

INFECTIOUS DISEASES AND TROPICAL MEDICINE

42. THEME: VECTORS OF INFECTIOUS DISEASE TRANSMISSION

A *Phlebotomus* sandflies
B Hard-bodied ticks
C Rat fleas
D *Aedes* mosquitoes
E Triatomid bugs
F *Simulium* blackflies

For each of the following infectious diseases select the appropriate insect vector from the above list. The items may be used once or not at all.

☐ 1. Onchocerciasis
☐ 2. Visceral leishmaniasis
☐ 3. South American trypanosomiasis
☐ 4. Ehrlichiosis
☐ 5. Endemic typhus

43. THEME: BACTERIA AND TOXINS

A *Clostridium botulinum*
B *Corynebacterium diphtheriae*
C *Escherichia coli*
D *Vibrio cholerae*
E *Clostridium tetani*
F *Staphylococcus aureus*

For each of the following descriptions of the effects of toxins select the bacterium producing the toxin from the above list. The items may be used once or not at all.

☐ 1. Common cause of food poisoning producing vomiting within six hours of ingestion
☐ 2. Blockade of acetylcholine transmission at neuromuscular junction producing paralysis
☐ 3. A cytotoxin causing colonic inflammation
☐ 4. A cytotoxin causing myocarditis and congestive cardiac failure
☐ 5. Blockade of inhibitory neurotransmitters in spinal cord and brainstem producing uninhibited discharge from motor neurones

44. THEME: FUNGI

A *Sporothrix schenckii*
B *Pseudoallescheria boydii*
C *Rhizopus oryzae*
D *Pneumocystis carinii*
E *Pityrosporum ovale*
F *Coccidioides immitis*

For each of the following illnesses select the appropriate fungus from the above list. The items may be used once or not at all.

☐ 1. Influenza-like illness in endemic arid regions
☐ 2. Multiple subcutaneous nodules spreading along a lymphatic channel
☐ 3. Chronic swelling and suppuration of the foot with multiple sinus tracts
☐ 4. Nasal infection with necrosis of soft tissues and bone
☐ 5. Facial dermatitis with scaling around nasolabial folds

45. THEME: COMPLICATIONS OF HELMINTH INFECTION

A   Trichuris trichiura
B   Enterobius vermicularis
C   Diphyllobothrium latum
D   Necator americanus
E   Opisthorchis sinensis
F   Ascaris lumbricoides

For each of the following complications select the appropriate helminth from the above list. The items may be used once or not at all.

1. Microcytic anaemia
2. Megaloblastic anaemia
3. Pancreatitis
4. Rectal prolapse
5. Cholangiocarcinoma

GENITOURINARY MEDICINE

46. THEME: SYPHILIS

A   Benzathine penicillin 2.4 mega units IM as a single dose
B   Benzathine penicillin 2.4 mega units IM weekly for three weeks
C   Benzylpenicillin 4 mega units every four hours IV for ten days
D   Doxycycline 100 mg bd per os (PO) for 28 days
E   Ceftriaxone 1 g daily for 14 days
F   Ciprofloxacin 750 mg bd PO for 28 days

For each of the following presentations of syphilis select the recommended antibiotic treatment regimen from the above list. The items may be used once or not at all.

1. Not recommended for syphilis
2. Secondary syphilis
3. Latent syphilis with positive CSF VDRL (venereal disease reference laboratory)
4. Latent syphilis in a patient with previous penicillin anaphylaxis
5. Latent syphilis acquired several years previously

CLINICAL PHARMACOLOGY

47. THEME: ACUTE POISONING

A   Acetylcysteine
B   Dicobalt edetate
C   Fuller's earth
D   Penicillamine
E   Pralidoxime mesylate
F   Glucagon

For each of the following cases of acute poisoning select the appropriate treatment from the above list. The items may be used once or not at all.

1. Organophosphorous insecticide
2. Paraquat
3. β-blocker
4. Paracetamol
5. Cyanide

48. THEME: DRUG INTERACTIONS

A   Itraconazole
B   Amiodarone
C   Lisinopril
D   Ganciclovir
E   Paracetamol
F   Intravenous verapamil

For each of the following drugs select the interacting drug from the above list that causes a serious increased risk of side-effects. The items may be used once or not at all.

1. Indomethacin
2. Digoxin
3. Ciclosporin
4. Propranolol
5. Imipenem

49. THEME: RECREATIONAL DRUGS

A Alcohol
B Cannabis
C Tobacco
D Cocaine
E 1-methyl 4-phenyl
   1,2,3,6-tetrahydropyridine (MPTP)
F Methylenedioxymethamphetamine (MDMA)

For each of the following descriptions select the appropriate recreational drug from the above list. The items may be used once or not at all.

☐ 1. A recognised cause of myocardial infarction in young persons
☐ 2. Excess ingestion may cause cardiac arrhythmias, seizures, severe hyperthermia and rhabdomyolysis
☐ 3. A not uncommon cause of central pontine myelinolysis
☐ 4. An illegal drug which has been found to be associated with many traffic accidents
☐ 5. May induce a Parkinsonian syndrome

50. THEME: ROUTE OF DRUG ADMINISTRATION

A Desmopressin
B Pentamidine
C Warfarin
D Methotrexate
E Fomivirsen
F Diazepam

For each of the following routes of administration select the drug that is licensed for that route from the above list. The items may be used once or not at all.

☐ 1. Intrathecal
☐ 2. Inhalation
☐ 3. Intranasal
☐ 4. Rectal
☐ 5. Intravitreal

51. THEME: ENZYMES AND DRUG METABOLISM

A Cytochrome P450-IIE1
B Alcohol dehydrogenase
C Cytochrome P450-IIC
D Cytochrome P450-IID6
E Pseudocholinesterase
F N-Acetyltransferase

For each of the following drugs select the enzyme that plays an important role in its metabolism from the above list. The items may be used once or not at all.

☐ 1. Isoniazid
☐ 2. Propafenone
☐ 3. Paracetamol
☐ 4. Proguanil
☐ 5. Succinylcholine

52. THEME: MECHANISM OF ANTIBIOTIC ACTION

A Affects cell wall formation by inhibiting assembly of peptidoglycan polymers
B Affects bacterial DNA synthesis by inhibiting topoisomerase enzymes
C Affects cell wall formation by inhibiting peptidoglycan crosslinking
D Affects metabolism by inhibiting folic acid metabolism
E Affects protein synthesis by interaction with ribosomal RNA
F Affects messenger RNA synthesis by inhibiting DNA-dependent RNA polymerase

For each of the following antibiotics select the appropriate mechanism of action from the above list. The items may be used once or not at all.

☐ 1. Penicillin
☐ 2. Vancomycin
☐ 3. Gentamicin
☐ 4. Rifampin
☐ 5. Ciprofloxacin

CARDIOVASCULAR MEDICINE

53. THEME: JUGULAR VENOUS PRESSURE

A   y descent
B   x descent
C   cv wave
D   v wave
E   a wave
F   c wave

For each of the following select the appropriate features of a JVP trace. The items may be used once or not at all.

☐ 1. Atrial contraction
☐ 2. Tricuspid valve closure
☐ 3. Tricuspid valve regurgitation
☐ 4. Atrial relaxation after contraction
☐ 5. Tricuspid valve opening

54. THEME: CARDIOVASCULAR CLINICAL SIGNS

A   Pulsus bigeminus
B   Pulsus alternans
C   Kussmaul's sign
D   Pulsus paradoxus
E   Slow-rising pulse
F   Collapsing pulse

For each of the following conditions select the characteristic clinical sign from the above list. The items may be used once or not at all.

☐ 1. Pericardial tamponade and asthma
☐ 2. Aortic stenosis
☐ 3. Pericardial tamponade but not asthma
☐ 4. Aortic regurgitation
☐ 5. Severe cardiac failure

55. THEME: CHEST PAIN

A   Tietze's syndrome
B   Pericarditis
C   Oesophageal dysmotility
D   Musculoskeletal chest pain
E   Cardiac angina
F   Aortic dissection

For each of the following characteristic findings select the appropriate cause of chest pain from the above list. The items may be used once or not at all.

☐ 1. Follows exercise rather than coincides with it
☐ 2. Local tenderness at costochondral junctions
☐ 3. Severe pain of abrupt onset radiating between scapulae
☐ 4. Sharp pain exacerbated by swallowing or sternal pressure
☐ 5. Occurs during exercise and is exacerbated by a heavy meal or stress

56. THEME: ECG

A   Lead I
B   Lead II
C   Lead III
D   Lead aVL
E   Lead aVR
F   Lead aVF

For each of the following axes select the appropriate electrocardiograph limb lead from the above list. The items may be used once or not at all.

☐ 1. $+120°$
☐ 2. $-150°$
☐ 3. $0°$
☐ 4. $60°$
☐ 5. $+90°$

PSYCHIATRY

57. THEME: CLASSIFICATION OF NEUROSES

A   Adjustment disorder
B   Generalised anxiety disorder
C   Phobic anxiety disorder
D   Post-traumatic stress disorder
E   Panic disorder
F   Obsessive-compulsive disorder

For each of the following descriptions select the appropriate disorder from the above list. The items may be used once or not at all.

☐ 1. Sudden episodes of anxiety brought on by a specific stimulus
☐ 2. Sudden episodes of anxiety not related to a specific stimulus
☐ 3. Episodes of anxiety decreased by specific, repetitive behaviour
☐ 4. Avoidance, denial and anxiety occur in response to prolonged stressful circumstances
☐ 5. Anxiety, flashbacks and emotional numbness occur in response to severe stress

58. THEME: MALADAPTIVE BEHAVIOURS

A   Hypochondriasis
B   Dysmorphophobia
C   Malingering
D   Factitious disorder
E   Somatisation disorder
F   Psychogenic pain

For each of the following descriptions select the appropriate condition from the above list. The items may be used once or not at all.

☐ 1. Multiple changing symptoms which do not have a physical cause
☐ 2. Extreme concern about the presence of disease triggered by normal bodily sensations
☐ 3. Inappropriate anxiety about body image
☐ 4. Deliberate production of physical symptoms without material gain

☐ 5. Deliberate production of symptoms for material gain

59. THEME: PERSONALITY DISORDERS

A   Schizoid
B   Paranoid
C   Affective
D   Psychopathic
E   Obsessional
F   Histrionic

For each of the following characteristic traits select the appropriate personality disorder from the above list. The items may be used once or not at all.

☐ 1. Holds rigid viewpoints and has inability to change
☐ 2. Shallow, self-centred and demanding
☐ 3. Suspicious and argumentative
☐ 4. Cold, introspective and self-sufficient
☐ 5. Acts impulsively and does not feel guilt

MISCELLANEOUS

60. THEME: HEARING LOSS

A   Strial (metabolic) presbyacusis
B   Acoustic neuroma
C   Internal auditory artery thrombosis
D   Sensorineural presbyacusis
E   Ménières disease
F   Vestibular neuronitis

For each of the following problems select the appropriate cause of hearing loss from the above list. The items may be used once or not at all.

☐ 1. Sudden-onset unilateral hearing loss
☐ 2. Progressive bilateral hearing loss producing severe impairment of speech discrimination
☐ 3. Progressive bilateral hearing loss with good preservation of speech discrimination
☐ 4. Fluctuating bilateral hearing loss with tinnitus and vertigo
☐ 5. Progressive unilateral hearing loss often associated with other cranial nerve palsies

ANSWERS TO PAPER 1

The approximate difficulty rating for the answer to each question is given in brackets.

☆ (the majority of competent final year students will know the answer)

☆☆ (approximately 50% of final year students will be able to answer correctly)

☆☆☆ (only the better students will usually know the answer)

Q1. ENZYMES (☆☆)

1. D   2. B   3. F   4. E   5. A

DNA polymerase produces DNA copies from a DNA template, a process known as replication. This is a necessary part of cell division. When a single strand of DNA is copied the new copy is complementary to the first one. This means that the sequence is in the reverse orientation and adenine is replaced by thymine, cytosine by guanine and vice versa. RNA polymerase makes messenger RNA (mRNA) copies from genomic DNA, a process known as transcription. This is the first stage in the decoding of DNA to produce a protein molecule. The mRNA copy is complementary to the original DNA strand except that thymine is replaced by uracil. *Taq* polymerase is a heat-stable DNA polymerase derived from the bacteria *Thermophilus aquaticus*, which has evolved to survive in hot springs. It is used in the polymerase chain reaction (PCR) because it can survive the rapid cycles of heating and cooling used in the denaturation and annealing stages of the process. Reverse transcriptase is an enzyme produced by retroviruses to make complementary DNA (cDNA) copies of an RNA template. It is useful in molecular biology for PCR amplification of mRNA to produce libraries of genes expressed in particular tissues. A restriction endonuclease is an enzyme produced by bacteria which cleaves foreign DNA. It does this by recognising a specific sequence of DNA of usually four to eight nucleotides in length. These sequences are often palindromes of the complementary sequence

(eg CCGG). The enzymes are named after the bacteria from which they originated, eg *Hinf*I comes from *Haemophilus influenzae* and *Taq*I comes from *Thermophilus aquaticus*. DNase breaks down DNA throughout its length. Human recombinant DNase can be used to break down tenacious mucus in cystic fibrosis patients.

Q2. REGIONS OF DNA (☆)

1. E   2. C   3. B   4. F   5. D

RNA polymerase binds to the gene promoter to initiate gene transcription. Promoter DNA sequences include CACCC, CCAAT and ATAAA. The promoter is usually located upstream of the coding region designated the 5′ end. The 3′-flanking region is downstream of the coding DNA. The coding sequence is made up of exons that are separated by intervening sequences called introns. The transcribed messenger RNA (mRNA) molecule includes DNA from the 5′- and 3′-flanking regions and introns as well as the coding DNA. The introns are removed during mRNA processing before translation takes place. Introns are recognised by their characteristic beginning and end sequences, respectively named the splice donor and splice acceptor. DNA is translated into amino acid sequences by a triplet code. Each sequence of three bases corresponds to one amino acid. As there are 64 possible triplets (ie 4^3) and only 20 amino acids, some amino acids are encoded by more than one triplet code. This is known as redundancy and means that a polymorphism can be present in coding DNA without any change occurring in the amino acid sequence of the encoded polypeptide. The DNA-encoded start site for translation of the mRNA molecule is AGG. There are also three sequences which cause termination of mRNA translation: TAA, TAG and TGA.

Q3. REDUCING ERROR (☆☆☆)

1. C   2. B   3. E   4. F   5. D

It is essential for all doctors to be able to understand how errors can occur in research studies. Without this skill it is not possible to judge the value of published research and determine whether it is sufficiently convincing to affect our practice. A type 1 error occurs when a study finds a statistically significant difference between groups (or treatments) when in reality there is no difference. If a probability or *P* value of 0.05 is set then this will occur on one in 20 occasions. If the stricter *P* value of 0.01 is used it will only occur in one in 100 occasions. A type 2 error occurs when a study does not find a statistically significant difference between groups when in reality there is one. The probability that a type 2 error will not occur in any given study is called the power of the study. Power is increased by increasing the sample size. The placebo effect occurs when a patient believes that treatment will help his or her condition. This effect is minimised by the use of a 'dummy' treatment (the placebo) and blinding of the patient to which treatment is taken. Blinding of investigators who are analysing outcome events (eg whether a patient is cured) is performed to minimise observer bias (and also cheating!). Bias can also occur if the subjects who fail to complete a study responded differently from those who completed it. This bias can be minimised by performing an intention-to-treat analysis, where all subjects are analysed according to treatment allocation regardless of whether they complete the study. This method may reduce the magnitude of the apparent treatment effect of those on treatment, which is best calculated by an on-treatment analysis. Confounding may occur if one factor is associated with the exposure (or intervention) and the outcome. For example, if alcohol (exposure) were found to be associated with lung cancer (outcome) it might be a spurious result caused by association of both factors with smoking (confounder). Randomisation is the best method of avoiding confounding by known and unknown risk factors.

Q4. HUMAN LEUKOCYTE ANTIGENS (☆☆☆)

1. C   2. B   3. E   4. F   5. A

The class I major histocompatibility complex (MHC) antigens in humans are designated as human leukocyte antigens (HLA) A, B and C. Class II antigens are designated by DP, DQ and DR. Many diseases have consistently been found to be associated with specific HLA types. This could be explained by the HLA molecule itself being involved in the pathogenesis of the disease or linkage disequilibrium between the HLA gene and another nearby gene on the same chromosome (6p). The latter explanation is responsible for the association between HLA-A3 and haemochromatosis, which is caused by mutations in the *HFE* gene. The two commonest mutations are designated C282Y and H63D. HLA molecules could be involved in the development of autoimmune diseases if part of the molecule resembles a bacterial or viral epitope. For example part of HLA-B27 and part of a protein expressed by *Klebsiella pneumoniae* are similar. This suggests this organism may be a trigger for the development of Reiter's syndrome and ankylosing spondylitis in those with HLA-B27. HLA-DR3 is associated with many autoimmune diseases including Addison's disease, dermatitis herpetiformis, coeliac disease and type I diabetes mellitus. This may be due to the HLA-DR3 molecule reacting with self antigens that exhibit similarity to foreign antigens on bacteria or viruses.

Q5. T CELL DIFFERENTIATION ANTIGENS (☆☆)

1. C   2. B   3. D   4. E   5. A

CD3 consists of three chains of 19, 20 and 29 kDa. It is present on all T cells in association with the T cell receptor. It is important in T cell differentiation and proliferation. CD4 is a marker for T helper cells, which is also found on macrophages and some dendritic cells. This 55-kDa glycoprotein interacts with antigens presented by HLA class II. It is therefore important in the stimulation of T helper cells by antigen-presenting cells. The gp120 antigen of HIV binds to CD4 enabling HIV to enter T cells. CD8 is a marker for cytotoxic T lymphocytes (CTL). This 33-kDa glycoprotein interacts with foreign antigens presented by HLA class I. HLA class I is found on all cell types in contrast to HLA class II, which is only expressed by the cells of the immune system. CD8 enables the recognition and killing of infected cells by CTL. CD45RO is found on memory T cells and binds to CD22. CD45RA is a marker for 'virgin' T cells, which have not yet undergone proliferation. CD25 is also known as the interleukin 2 receptor. This molecule is present on activated T lymphocytes. It binds to the α-chain of interleukin 2 stimulating rapid T cell division. In the rare HTLV I-associated T cell leukaemia there is increased CD25 expression, which is thought to contribute to T cell proliferation. CD35 is also known as complement receptor 1.

Q6. SYNDROMES AND GENETIC MUTATIONS (☆☆)

1. C   2. E   3. B   4. F   5. A

Patients with the Marfan syndrome are tall and their limbs are disproportionately long relative to the trunk. Typically they have arachnodactyly, hypermobility and a high arched palate. Fibrillin, the gene for which is on chromosome 15, is a component of the suspensory ligament of the lens and elastin-containing tissues such as the aorta. Patients frequently develop lens dislocations (upwards) and aortic dilatation, which may produce aortic valve incompetence

and aortic dissection. Marfan syndrome is inherited as an autosomal dominant trait as is achondroplasia, which is caused by mutations in the *FGFR-III* gene. Many cases of achondroplasia are due to new mutations, which are particularly associated with increased paternal age. Patients are of short stature and have disproportionately short limbs, a large skull with frontal bossing and a small face. Many variants of Ehlers-Danlos syndrome are described. In type IV, the ecchymotic variant, patients show gross bruising and are prone to develop rupture of the great vessels and spontaneous bowel perforations. Mutations that may be dominantly or recessively inherited are located in the collagen III gene. Homocystinuria is an autosomal recessive condition caused by abnormalities in the cystathionine β-synthase gene on chromosome 21. Patients have a Marfanoid appearance and suffer from ocular (downward lens dislocation), skeletal, central nervous system and vascular complications. There is a tendency for arterial and venous thrombosis. Pyridoxine (vitamin B_6) prevents thromboembolism in some cases. There is increasing interest that patients who develop ischaemic heart disease at a young age may be heterozygotes for this condition. Type I osteogenesis imperfecta is the mild variant of this group of conditions. The condition is dominantly inherited and is usually due to a null (non-expressed) allele of the type I collagen gene. Patients have decreased bone density, thin sclerae (which appear blue) and mitral valve prolapse and develop aortic dilatation. In the lethal form (type II), which is usually due to a new dominantly expressed mutation, there is a mutant collagen chain produced. Mutations in the *CFTR* gene cause cystic fibrosis.

Q7. GENETIC INHERITANCE PATTERNS (☆)

1. F   2. A   3. D   4. C   5. E

In an autosomal dominant disease cases will usually be observed in multiple generations of a single family. However, some carriers of the abnormal gene may not manifest symptoms if the disease-producing gene mutation has partial penetrance. In autosomal recessive diseases usually only members of a single generation are affected and there is a marked increase in incidence in the offspring of consanguineous marriages. The mitochondrial genome is only inherited from the mother and mitochondrial diseases are therefore always maternally inherited. Males have only one X chromosome, and they pass this chromosome to all of their daughters and none of their sons. If a male is affected with an X-linked dominant disease then all of his daughters will inherit the predisposition to the disease. However, if the gene is not fully penetrant then they may not all develop symptomatic disease. In X-linked recessive diseases females are not usually affected. However, a female may occasionally be affected due to random inactivation of the X chromosome, resulting in a predominance of abnormal genes being expressed. More rarely a female may be homozygous for the abnormal allele or carry a reciprocal translocation between the X chromosome and an autosome, where the breakpoint involves the gene. Females with Duchenne muscular dystrophy (DMD) and X-autosome translocations were used to identify the DMD gene.

Q8. CRANIAL NERVES (☆)

1. C   2. B   3. A   4. F   5. E

The vagus nerve (CN X) supplies the larynx via its recurrent laryngeal branch. The vagus nerve also supplies motor and sensory fibres to the abdominal and thoracic viscera. The oculomotor nerve (CN III) supplies all of the external ocular muscles except superior oblique (supplied by CN IV, the trochlear nerve) and lateral rectus (CN VI, the abducens nerve). It also carries parasympathetic fibres which constrict the pupil. The facial nerve (CN VII) is motor to the muscles of facial expression and stapedius, the posterior belly of digastric and stylohyoid. It also receives afferent fibres from the anterior two-thirds of the tongue (taste), the floor of the mouth and palate and supplies parasympathetic fibres to the lacrimal,

submandibular and sublingual glands. The glossopharyngeal nerve (CN IX) receives afferent fibres from the carotid sinus baroreceptor, the carotid body chemoreceptor and the posterior third of the tongue and the pharynx. It also supplies motor fibres to the stylopharyngeus and parasympathetic fibres to the parotid gland. The trigeminal nerve has three divisions: ophthalmic, maxillary and mandibular, each receiving sensory fibres from part of the face. The mandibular division also has motor fibres to the muscles of mastication (masseter, temporalis and the medial and lateral pterygoids) and mylohyoid, tensor veli palatini, tensor tympani and the anterior belly of digastric. The hypoglossal nerve (CN XII) supplies motor fibres to the tongue.

Q9. NERVE INJURY AND SIGNS (☆☆)

1. E   2. D   3. A   4. F   5. B

Avulsion injury of the upper roots of the brachial plexus occurs if the shoulder is forcibly displaced downwards. This can occur during breech delivery (Erb's palsy) or when the shoulder strikes an obstacle when a rider is thrown forwards from a fast moving vehicle. Paralysis of deltoid, biceps, brachialis, brachioradialis, supraspinatus, infraspinatus and subscapularis occurs. This results in the arm hanging with the shoulder internally rotated, the elbow extended and the forearm pronated. This is known as the waiter's tip position. When there is forcible traction with the arm extended, avulsion of the lower roots of the brachial plexus may occur. This can occur at birth (Klumpke's paralysis) or when a falling person tries to catch hold of a branch or ledge. All of the intrinsic hand muscles are affected producing a claw hand deformity with extension at the metacarpophalangeal joints and flexion at the interphalangeal joints. There is also weakness of wrist flexion and sensory loss on the medial aspect of the forearm, the hand and the medial two fingers. Compression of the axillary nerve in the axilla can be produced by badly fitting crutches. This results in paralysis of deltoid so that the arm cannot be raised at the shoulder. Compression of the radial nerve against the middle third of the humerus can occur if an intoxicated person falls asleep with the arm over the back of a chair, known as 'Saturday night paralysis'. This results in weakness of brachioradialis, supinator and all of the forearm extensors. Sensory impairment is restricted to the back of the hand. When the ulnar nerve is damaged by compression against the olecranon a claw hand deformity occurs. However as the lateral two lumbricals are not affected, only the little and ring fingers are markedly flexed. Weakness of flexion of these fingers and of abduction of the little finger also occurs. Sensory loss affects the medial aspect of the hand but not the forearm. If the ulnar nerve is damaged at the wrist there is no sensory loss.

Q10. HORMONE PRODUCTION (☆)

1. B   2. F   3. D   4. A   5. E

Insulin is produced by the pancreatic β cells in the islets of Langerhans. Insulin decreases blood glucose and breakdown of protein and fat, and increases glucose entry into cells, glycogen storage and synthesis of protein and fatty acids. Adrenaline, glucagon, cortisol and somatostatin all increase blood glucose. Somatostatin is produced by the pancreatic D cells. It exerts a local effect on pancreatic α cells causing a decrease in release of glucagon. It also decreases release of insulin, the pituitary tropic hormones and gastrin and secretin. Glucagon increases release of glucose from glycogen and increases synthesis of glucose from amino acids and fatty acids. The adrenal medulla produces epinephrine and norepinephrine (previously called adrenaline and noradrenaline) and the adrenal cortex produces glucocorticoids and mineralocorticoids. Adrenaline increases glucose release from glycogen and increases release of fatty acids from adipose tissue. Cortisol increases synthesis of glucose from amino acids and fatty acids and antagonises the effects of insulin. Calcitonin is produced by the C cells in the thyroid gland.

Q11. SERUM PROTEINS (☆☆)

1. D   2. F   3. B   4. C   5. A

α^1-antitrypsin is the major part of α^1-globulin. This protein inactivates trypsin and other proteolytic enzymes. Three gene variants are recognised: 'M', which exhibits normal activity, 'Z', which exhibits very low activity and 'S', which is intermediate. Congenital α^1-antitrypsin deficiency is inherited as an autosomal recessive trait as MZ heterozygotes are clinically normal. ZZ homozygotes suffer from premature emphysema and cirrhosis of the liver. α^1-antitrypsin deficiency is also associated with a rare form of steroid-resistant panniculitis. α^2-macroglobulin is the major component of α^2-globulin and is an important serum protease inhibitor. Congenital deficiency of this enzyme has not been described, suggesting deficiency may be incompatible with survival. α^2-macroglobulin is a large molecule with a molecular weight of 800,000 Da. Haptoglobin binds haemoglobin from lysed erythrocytes and in intravascular haemolysis haptoglobin levels fall. This is used as a test for monitoring haemolytic activity. Haptoglobin consists of two light chains and two heavy chains. It is polymorphic in humans, with two alleles designated 1 and 2. Albumin is the most abundant plasma protein and binds a wide variety of small ions/molecules including drugs, hormones and metabolites. Bilirubin in serum is mostly bound to albumin. Group-specific component (gc) globulin binds the fat-soluble vitamin D, enabling it to be transported in blood. α^1-antitrypsin and haptoglobin are acute phase reactants and their levels will rise during inflammatory disorders. Other acute phase proteins include α^1-acid glycoprotein, caeruloplasmin, fibrinogen and C-reactive protein. γ-globulin consists of immunoglobulins.

Q12. SERUM ELECTROPHORESIS PATTERN (☆☆☆)

1. B 2. F 3. A 4. D 5. E

Serum protein electrophoresis separates proteins by size and charge. From anode to cathode the bands produced are albumin (52–68% of total protein), α^1-globulin (2.4–5.3%), α^2-globulin (6.6–13.5%), β-globulin (8.5–14.5%) and γ-globulin (10.7–20.0%). In different diseases characteristic abnormalities in serum protein electrophoresis patterns are seen. In chronic liver disease there is a diffuse and large elevation of the γ-globulin band (predominantly due to IgA in alcoholic hepatitis, IgG in autoimmune hepatitis and IgM in primary biliary cirrhosis). In chronic inflammatory diseases there is a diffuse but small increase in γ-globulin. In contrast, in dysproteinaemia the production of a monoclonal immunoglobulin results in a single sharp peak in the γ-globulin band. In hypogammaglobulinaemia there is a flat curve where the γ-globulin band should be. In both nephrotic syndrome and protein-losing enteropathy, the preferential loss of low molecular weight proteins results in a flatter albumin band. In the nephrotic syndrome this is compensated by a high β-globulin band whereas in protein-losing enteropathy there is moderately high α^2-globulin. α^1-antitrypsin is the major component of α^1-globulin and in deficiency of this enzyme there is a flat curve where the α-1-globulin band should be. Diabetes mellitus does not usually produce any abnormality on serum protein electrophoresis unless complicated by nephropathy.

Q13. LIPIDS (☆☆)

1. C 2. D 3. B 4. A 5. E

Lipids are hydrophobic and are carried through the circulation in particles containing triglycerides, cholesterol, phospholipids and proteins. Chylomicrons are produced in the intestines and carried to the liver which repackages the contents into very low density lipoproteins (VLDL), which circulate throughout the body and their contents are delivered to the tissues. Low-density lipoproteins (LDL) are then formed. High-density lipoproteins (HDL) are scavengers which return cholesterol to the liver. LDL-cholesterol and HDL-cholesterol are respectively positively and negatively correlated with risk of cardiovascular disease. Chylomicrons are low molecular weight particles containing a large amount of triglyceride and a small amount of cholesterol. Their levels rise after a fatty meal. Serum triglycerides are therefore markedly affected by recent food intake and should be measured fasting. Total cholesterol is little affected by recent food intake and levels can be measured in the non-fasting state but if the HDL:LDL cholesterol ratio is to be measured this should be performed fasting. VLDLs contain a large amount of triglycerides and a moderate amount of cholesterol, phospholipids and protein. They contain α^2-lipoprotein and pre-β-lipoprotein, as detected by electrophoresis. LDLs contain a small amount of protein, a large amount of cholesterol and moderate amounts of phospholipids and protein, and contain β-lipoprotein. HDLs contain a moderate amount of cholesterol and phospholipid, high levels of protein and very little triglyceride. HDL contains α^1-lipoprotein. Lipoprotein (a) is LDL linked to apolipoprotein (a). High levels in the circulation are associated with cardiovascular disease and stroke. Lipoprotein (a) has been found in atherosclerotic plaques and is believed to be involved in their pathogenesis. The fat globules stored within adipocytes consist almost entirely of hydrophobic triglyceride.

Q14. MEASURES OF LUNG VOLUME (☆)

1. D 2. E 3. B 4. A 5. F

Definitions of lung volume can be confusing. The most frequently measured value in clinical practice is the vital capacity, which can be performed with a simple spirometer. Vital capacity is the maximum volume of air that can be slowly exhaled after maximal inspiration. Forced vital capacity is the maximum volume that can be exhaled when the subject exhales as rapidly as possible. These values are usually similar, but in obstructive airways disease collapse of airways during forceful expiration may result in air-trapping so that the forced vital capacity is lower than the vital capacity. Vital capacity is reduced by an increase in residual volume or a decrease in total lung capacity. Measuring the sub compartments of the total lung capacity helps to distinguish between these possibilities. Expiratory reserve volume is the maximum volume of air that can be exhaled after expiration. The functional residual capacity equals the expiratory reserve volume plus the residual volume (air in lungs after maximal expiration). The functional residual capacity and the residual volume can be measured by helium dilution techniques. Residual volume is increased in emphysema due to air-trapping. The inspiratory capacity is the maximum volume of air that can be inhaled at the end of normal expiration. This is equivalent to the tidal volume (volume of air inhaled/exhaled with each breath) plus the inspiratory reserve volume. The inspiratory reserve volume can be defined as the maximum volume of air that can be inhaled at the end of inspiration. During exercise the tidal volume increases and the inspiratory reserve volume decreases.

Q15. RENAL TRACT INVESTIGATIONS (☆)

1. E   2. A   3. F   4. C   5. D

Renal ultrasound is a useful test to identify urinary tract obstruction in acute renal failure. This will show whether there is ureteric dilatation and hydronephrosis. If there is obstruction an ultrasound-guided, antegrade nephrostomy may be required to relieve it. Renal ultrasound is also useful to identify mass lesions, perinephric abscesses and to indicate renal size. An intravenous urogram is used to identify the site of ureteric stones. It is only successful if the kidney is functioning. If there is complete obstruction the patient needs an antegrade nephrostomy or retrograde ureteropyelography. In the latter investigation a catheter is inserted into the ureter via a cystoscope. A micturating cystourethrogram is useful to demonstrate

suspected ureteric reflux in patients with chronic pyelonephritis. It can also be used to show the presence of bladder diverticuli. A plain abdominal X-ray will show nephrocalcinosis and calcified renal stones. It should always be performed before an intravenous urogram. A KUB film (kidneys, ureters, bladder) should be requested to ensure the correct level of X-ray penetration is performed. Renal arteriography is used to define renal tumour circulation, identify bleeding following renal trauma and diagnose renal artery stenosis in patients with uncontrolled hypertension.

Q16. GLOMERULONEPHRITIS (☆☆)

1. B   2. E   3. F   4. C   5. D

Minimal change glomerulonephritis causes around 90% of cases of nephrotic syndrome in children and 30% in adults. On light microscopy and immunofluorescence microscopy no abnormalities are seen. Electron microscopy shows fusion of podocytes. There is usually a good response to steroids although many cases relapse. Focal segmental glomerulosclerosis presents with proteinuria and nephrotic syndrome. Light microscopy shows sclerosis and hyaline deposits affecting foci of glomeruli with other glomeruli appearing normal. Immunofluorescence shows deposition of immunoglobulin M and C3. This condition is associated with HIV infection, heroin use, malignancy and vesicoureteric reflux. Over 50% of patients will eventually develop chronic renal failure. Berger's disease is a common cause of haematuria in young men. There is sometimes associated proteinuria, though mild cases have haematuria alone. On immunofluorescence deposits of IgA and C3 are seen and this condition is also known as IgA nephropathy. The prognosis is usually good but patients with proteinuria may eventually develop chronic renal failure. Rapidly progressive glomerulonephritis (RPGN) is also known as crescentic glomerulonephritis as histology shows glomerular hypercellularity with crescent formation. Immunofluorescence often shows subepithelial deposits of IgG and C3, though the findings do vary with the underlying cause. Wegener's granulomatosis, anti glomerular basement membrane antibody syndrome, microscopic polyangiitis and Henoch-Schönlein purpura may all cause RPGN. Mesangiocapillary glomerulonephritis is also known as membranoproliferative disease. Light microscopy shows a split in the basement membrane producing a characteristic 'tram-line' appearance. The condition is associated with shunt nephritis, endocarditis, lipodystrophy and the presence of C3-nephritic factor. Membranous glomerulonephritis is a common cause of adult nephrotic syndrome with a thickened basement membrane on histology.

Q17. TREATMENT OF GLOMERULONEPHRITIDES(☆☆☆)

1. C   2. F   3. E   4. D   5. B

Patients with an acute presentation of the nephrotic syndrome due to minimal change nephropathy, focal segmental glomerulosclerosis, immunoglobulin A nephropathy or membranous nephropathy are initially treated with high-dose oral prednisolone. If the patient develops steroid dependency and suffers from frequent relapses of nephrotic syndrome when the steroid dose is reduced, treatment with ciclosporin A or cyclophosphamide is usually commenced. These agents are also used if the patient fails to respond to steroid treatment. Patients with immunoglobulin A nephropathy should be periodically monitored for the development of proteinuria. If there is no proteinuria or less than 1 g every 24 hours then no treatment is required. If proteinuria exceeds this threshold then the patient should be treated with an angiotensin-converting enzyme inhibitor, dipyridamole and low-dose warfarin. For persistent proteinuria a combination of an angiotensin-converting enzyme inhibitor and an angiotensin II receptor antagonist is sometimes used. Patients with immunoglobulin A nephropathy and hypertension should also receive an angiotensin-converting enzyme inhibitor regardless of whether they have proteinuria. Rapidly progressive glomerulonephritis needs aggressive

management to prevent further renal damage. Patients with antiglomerular basement membrane antibody disease (Goodpasture's syndrome) should be given a combination of cyclophosphamide, pulsed intravenous methylprednisolone and plasmapharesis. There is no evidence that plasmapharesis is beneficial in Wegener's granulomatosis and this condition is therefore treated with the first two agents alone.

Q18. DISEASE CAUSED BY RENAL TRANSPORT DEFECTS (☆☆☆)

1. E   2. D   3. F   4. A   5. B

Type 1 renal tubular acidosis (RTA) is also called classical or distal-type RTA. There is failure of the distal nephron to generate an adequate hydrogen ion concentration between the distal nephron and the blood. This condition is associated with amphotericin B treatment, Sjögren's syndrome, primary biliary cirrhosis, fibrosing alveolitis, medullary sponge kidney and sickle cell disease. Patients develop hypokalaemic acidosis, osteomalacia, nephrocalcinosis and renal calculi. Chronic renal failure may occur because of ureteric obstruction, recurrent urinary tract infections and progressive nephrocalcinosis. Type 2 or proximal-type RTA is due to decreased proximal tubule secretion of hydrogen ions and consequent failure to reabsorb bicarbonate. Nephrocalcinosis does not occur and the prognosis is better than in the classical type. Type 2 RTA rarely occurs as an isolated lesion and is usually seen as part of the Fanconi syndrome. In this condition there are multiple proximal renal tubular reabsorption defects. This results in glycosuria, phosphaturia, aminoaciduria and type 2 RTA. Fanconi syndrome is associated with vitamin D deficiency, myeloma, Wilson's disease, lead toxicity and drugs (eg out of date tetracycline). Type 4 RTA causes hyperkalaemic acidosis and is associated with aldosterone deficiency, diabetes mellitus, amyloidosis, obstructive uropathy, gout and drugs (eg amiloride). Cystinuria is the commonest inherited aminoaciduria. There is loss of cystine, ornithine, arginine and lysine in the urine. Patients develop cystine stones at a young age and must drink large volumes of water to prevent this. Penicillamine is also used in treatment. Alport's syndrome is an X-linked or autosomal recessive disease due to defects in the collagen genes (eg *COL4A5*). Patients suffer from nephritis, sensorineural deafness, lens abnormalities and platelet dysfunction.

Q19. TREATMENT OF ENDOCRINE CONDITIONS (☆☆)

1. B   2. E   3. C   4. F   5. A

Finasteride is a 5-α-reductase inhibitor which blocks the conversion of testosterone to its more active metabolite dihydrotestosterone. This is useful in reducing prostatic enlargement in benign prostatic hypertrophy. Somatropin is biosynthetic human growth hormone. In contrast to previous preparations of growth hormone derived from human tissue it does not carry a risk of Creutzfeldt-Jakob disease. Somatropin is effective in treating short stature in those with growth hormone insufficiency and in girls with Turner's syndrome. SIADH results in water retention leading to hyponatraemia. It can be caused by intracranial pathology or by ectopic production as occurs in small cell lung cancer. SIADH can be treated by the tetracycline antibiotic, demeclocycline, which blocks the effect of antidiuretic hormone (ADH) on the renal tubule. Cabergoline is a stimulant of dopamine receptors which reduces prolactin secretion and can shrink prolactinomas. It can also be used in growth-hormone-secreting tumours causing acromegaly. It is also licensed for prevention of lactation in the puerperium but it should generally not be used for this purpose. Metyrapone is a competitive inhibitor of 11β-hydroxylase and is occasionally used in tests of anterior pituitary function. Metyrapone is useful for symptom control in Cushing's syndrome due to adrenocorticotrophic hormone production by carcinoma of the bronchus. It is also useful for treatment of Cushing's syndrome due to other causes when preparing the patient for surgery. Prednisolone and other glucocorticoids can cause iatrogenic Cushing's.

Q20. AETIOLOGY OF DIABETES (☆☆)

1. B   2. F   3. D   4. E   5. A

Type I diabetes is also known as insulin-dependent diabetes because if insulin is discontinued the patient will become ketoacidotic. Type I diabetes is strongly associated with autoimmune destruction of the pancreatic cells and the human leukocyte antigens DR3 and DR4. Patients usually develop the disease at a young age and they are generally thin when first diagnosed. Type II diabetes mellitus becomes more common with increasing age and there is a strong association with obesity. The condition is due to insulin resistance and is improved (sometimes abolished) by weight loss. Insulin secretion is generally normal or high and therefore type II diabetics rarely (if ever) become ketoacidotic. Although they may require insulin treatment for blood glucose control, type II diabetics are not insulin-dependent. Maturity-onset diabetes of the young (MODY) is a form of non-insulin-dependent diabetes which presents in young persons who are not usually obese. These patients do not develop ketoacidosis on withdrawal of insulin but some patients may do so during episodes of severe infection. There is familial aggregation in MODY and some cases have been found to be due to defects in the glucokinase gene or production of abnormal insulin. Tropical diabetes is associated with pancreatic fibrocalculous disease and malnutrition. Insulin secretion is reduced and there is also peripheral insulin resistance. People with inherited abnormalities of the insulin receptor develop diabetes and often have lipodystrophy and acanthosis nigricans. Diseases resulting in excess production of certain hormones can produce secondary diabetes including thyrotoxicosis, acromegaly, Cushing's syndrome, phaeochromocytoma and glucagonoma. Glucagonoma produces a characteristic skin rash known as necrolytic migratory erythema. Pancreatic disease, drugs (eg corticosteroids, catecholamines) and genetic syndromes (eg glycogen storage diseases) can also produce secondary diabetes.

Q21. THYROID FUNCTION TEST (☆)

1. A   2. E   3. F   4. C   5. B

There are a large number of thyroid function tests and the results can be bewildering. The most frequently used are thyroid-stimulating hormone (TSH) and thyroxine (T_4). Raised TSH indicates hypothyroidism (eg due to autoimmune thyroid disease, surgery, radioiodine treatment, drugs, iodine deficiency, excess thyroxine treatment, dyshormonogenesis) because there is a lack of inhibitory feedback by thyroid hormones on the pituitary gland. Raised TSH due to a TSH-secreting pituitary tumour is extremely rare. Low TSH usually indicates hyperthyroidism (eg Grave's disease or toxic multinodular goitre) due to excess thyroid hormone inhibiting TSH secretion. However, it must be interpreted with T_4 levels. If T_4 levels are normal or high the patient has hyperthyroidism. If TSH and T_4 levels are both low the patient probably has hypothyroidism secondary to pituitary failure. T_4 is metabolised to triiodothyronine (T_3) which is five times more active than T_4. T_3 is therefore a more sensitive test for hyperthyroidism and is useful when the diagnosis is uncertain. T_4 and T_3 are transported in serum bound to a protein called thyroxine-binding globulin (TBG). Total serum T_4 and T_3 levels are affected by levels of TBG, which are affected by pregnancy, oestrogens, steroid treatment and other factors. Free T_4 and T_3 levels can be measured to overcome this problem but these are more expensive. Following treatment of thyroid cancer thyroglobulin levels are used for monitoring purposes. Raised thyroglobulin is suggestive of tumour recurrence.

Q22. AMENORRHOEA (☆☆☆)

1. C   2. E   3. D   4. A   5. B

Amenorrhoea can be differentiated into primary (where the woman has never menstruated) and secondary (where amenorrhoea develops in a woman who had previously had normal menstruation). Primary amenorrhoea is generally due to congenital causes which may be anatomical (eg imperforate hymen) or physiological/hormonal (eg adrenogenital syndrome). Secondary amenorrhoea is usually due to pregnancy or an adult-onset disease such as polycystic ovary syndrome. In Turner's syndrome there is ovarian dysgenesis resulting in low oestradiol and progesterone levels. Lack of oestradiol inhibitory feedback to the pituitary results in high luteinising hormone (LH) and follicle-stimulating hormone (FSH) levels. In contrast, in hypopituitarism failure of LH and FSH production results in lack of ovarian stimulation resulting in low oestradiol and progesterone. In both conditions the affected woman will usually have underdevelopment of secondary sexual characteristics. In the adrenogenital syndrome, deficiency of 21-hydroxylase or other enzymes results in abnormal steroid hormone metabolism. This results in raised urine 17-ketosteroid levels and decreased circulating oestradiol and progesterone. Patients often have a masculinised appearance. Lack of pituitary inhibition results in high LH and FSH. In polycystic ovary syndrome the LH:FSH ratio is increased and urine 17-ketosteroid levels are high. Plasma and urine testosterone levels are also raised. Prolactin is secreted by the pituitary gland and this is inhibited by dopamine which travels down the pituitary stalk. Hyperprolactinaemia can be caused by a prolactinoma, compression of the pituitary stalk or dopamine antagonists. LH and FSH levels are usually normal in isolated hyperprolactinaemia. Oestradiol and progesterone levels are low because the prolactin exerts a suppressive effect on the ovaries. The patient may also experience galactorrhoea. During the menopause, LH and FSH will be high and urine 17-ketosteroids will be normal.

Q23. GASTROINTESTINAL HORMONES (☆☆)

1. E   2. F   3. B   4. A   5. C

Gastrin is synthesised in the G cells of the gastric antrum and the small intestine. Secretion of gastrin is stimulated by protein ingestion and gastric distension. Its principal action is the stimulation of gastric acid secretion. Cholecystokinin is produced by the I cells of the duodenal and jejunal mucosa. Secretion is stimulated by the ingestion of long-chain fatty acids. Cholecystokinin stimulates gallbladder contraction. Secretin is produced by the S cells of the duodenal and jejunal mucosa. Secretion is stimulated by an acid pH in the duodenum as may occur after stomach emptying following a meal. Secretin stimulates the secretion of watery, alkaline pancreatic fluid. Glucose-dependent insulinotrophic peptide (GIP) was formerly known as gastric inhibitory peptide. It is produced by the K cells in the upper small intestinal mucosa. Secretion of GIP is stimulated by ingestion of carbohydrates and long-chain fatty acids. Its principal actions are stimulation of insulin release and inhibition of gastric secretions. Vasoactive intestinal polypeptide (VIP) is a neurotransmitter found in the post ganglionic nerve fibres in the submucosa of the small intestine. VIP is a potent stimulator of water and electrolyte secretion by the enterocytes in the small and large intestines. Pancreatic polypeptide is produced by hormone-secreting cells in the pancreas. Secretion occurs after a meal. Pancreatic polypeptide inhibits pancreatic exocrine secretion.

Q24. DYSPHAGIA (☆)

1. F   2. A   3. E   4. D   5. C

When a patient complains of difficulty swallowing it is important to ascertain whether the problem is difficulty with initiating the swallowing movement, pain on swallowing (called odynophagia) or a feeling that food is becoming stuck. The duration of symptoms and whether the condition is intermittent or progressive must also be ascertained. Progressive dysphagia initially involving solid foods but eventually involving liquid is suggestive of an oesophageal carcinoma, particularly if accompanied by dramatic weight loss. There is often accompanying pain on swallowing. A pharyngeal pouch fills with food during eating and compresses the oesophagus, causing swallowing difficulties. There may be gurgling sounds during eating and swelling of the neck. The patient may also complain of halitosis. Neck swelling is also seen in a goitre with retrosternal extension but this does not enlarge during a meal. Bulbar palsy causes difficulty in making the swallowing movement. Attempts at swallowing are likely to be accompanied by coughing due to aspiration of food into the trachea. The patient may also have difficulty with speech. Oesophagitis is a common problem associated with regurgitation of acid from the stomach. Pain occurs on eating and also on lying flat. The patient may find relief by sleeping propped up by pillows to assist drainage of acid from the oesophagus. Achalasia is failure of relaxation of the oesophageal sphincter and contraction of the oesophageal muscles. This produces a dilated oesophagus and dysphagia of liquids and solids. There may be chest pain and frequent regurgitation of food. Chest X-ray shows an air-fluid level in the oesophagus behind the heart.

Q25. BLOOD TESTS FOR HEPATITIS B VIRUS (☆)

1. E   2. A   3. F   4. B   5. C

Anti-HBs antibodies (to hepatitis B surface antigen) are found in those who have previously been infected with hepatitis B virus (HBV) and in those who have been successfully vaccinated against it. A titre of greater than 100 indicates good immunity. Anti-HBc antibodies (to hepatitis B core antigen) are only found in those who have previously been infected. As the core antigen is not a component of the vaccine, anti-HBc antibodies are not found in those who have been vaccinated. HBsAg (hepatitis B surface antigen) is the screening test for hepatitis B carriers. However, many carriers do not have actively replicating virus and are of low infectivity. HBeAg (hepatitis B envelope antigen) indicates patients who have actively replicating virus and who are therefore of high infectious risk to others. Patients who are HBeAg positive are usually anti-HBe antibody negative and vice versa. There is a variant of HBV called the pre-core mutant which does not produce HBeAg. Patients with actively replicating pre-core mutant HBV will therefore be HBeAg negative. These patients can be identified by the presence of HBV DNA in the blood (usually not detectable in low infectivity HBeAg negative cases). HBV DNA is a quantitative assay and can also be used to measure the level of virus replication. This is useful in predicting those most likely to develop liver disease and in determining the response to treatment.

Q26. ORAL LESIONS (☆☆)

1. E   2. A   3. B   4. C   5. F

Recurrent oral ulcers and perianal fistulae are common problems in patients with Crohn's disease. Other perianal conditions which occur in Crohn's disease include skin tags and abscesses. Fistulae may also form between the gastrointestinal tract and the bladder, vagina or abdominal wall. Oral hairy leukoplakia (OHL) is the name given to vertical white streaks along the edge of the tongue. OHL is strongly suggestive of HIV infection and is seen in almost 50% of patients with advanced AIDS. OHL is caused by Epstein-Barr virus infection. Lichen planus is a cutaneous condition characterised by itchy, flat-topped violaceous papules covered by lines of white dots (Wickham's striae). In the mouth lichen planus produces a lacy white appearance on the buccal mucosa. These lesions can be distinguished from *candida* infection because they cannot be removed by scraping. Pemphigus vulgaris and bullous pemphigoid cause widespread cutaneous blistering. In pemphigus vulgaris the lesions are superficial and the blisters usually become deroofed. Pemphigus vulgaris frequently causes blistering of the oral mucosa but this rarely occurs in bullous pemphigoid. Behçet's disease is an autoimmune disease causing oral and genital ulceration in association with acute iritis. It is most commonly seen in those of Eastern Mediterranean origin.

Q27. NEUROLOGICAL DEFICITS CAUSED BY CRANIAL ARTERY OCCLUSION (☆☆)

1. C   2. B   3. A   4. F   5. E

The blood supply to the brain comes from the circle of Willis via the anterior, middle and posterior cerebral arteries. The blood vessels into the circle of Willis are the internal carotid arteries and the vertebrobasilar arteries. These form anastomoses via the anterior and posterior communicating arteries. Occlusion of one vessel may still allow some perfusion of the affected cerebral tissue via the other branches (depending on the site of occlusion). The anterior cerebral artery supplies the medial aspect of the hemisphere. The medial aspect of the hemisphere supplies the lower limbs so anterior cerebral artery occlusion results in contralateral lower limb weakness. The middle cerebral artery supplies motor and sensory innervation for the face and upper limb. Occlusion results in contralateral hemiplegia (upper limb more affected than lower) and sensory loss over the contralateral face and upper limb. If the dominant hemisphere is involved (the left side in right-handed people) there will be an additional receptive dysphasia due to the involvement of

Wernicke's area. The posterior cerebral artery supplies the occipital lobe. Occlusion results in a contralateral homonymous hemianopia. In some cases of cortical blindness there is macular sparing. The posterior inferior cerebellar arteries are branches of the basilar artery which is formed from the vertebral artery. They supply blood to the cerebellum and brainstem and contribute to the circle of Willis via the posterior communicating arteries. Occlusion results in the lateral medullary syndrome of ipsilateral loss of facial sensation and a dissociated sensory loss in the limbs. Dissociated sensory loss means contralateral loss of pain and temperature sensation (these fibres decussate on entering the spinal cord) and ipsilateral loss of fine touch, vibration and proprioception (these fibres decussate in the brainstem). There is also an ipsilateral Horner's syndrome, ataxia, nystagmus on looking to the side of the lesion, dysphagia and dysarthria.

Q28. VERTIGO (☆☆)

1. E   2. D   3. A   4. B   5. F

Patients often complain of feeling dizzy and it is essential to ascertain what they mean by this term to identify those with true vertigo. Benign positional vertigo (BPV) is the commonest cause and is associated with rapid head movements. In Hallpike's test the patient is slowly laid down from a sitting to a supine position with the neck extended over the couch. This procedure is then repeated with the head facing to one side and then the other. In BPV this movement will characteristically induce nystagmus which is unidirectional and fatigable (reduced on repeat testing). A central cause will produce nystagmus which is present in both directions of head turning and which is not fatigable. Ménière's disease is caused by endolymphatic hydrops of the semicircular canals. This produces progressive hearing loss and tinnitus and recurrent attacks of severe rotational vertigo lasting between 20 minutes and several hours. These attacks are frequently associated with nausea and vomiting. An acoustic neuroma causes unilateral hearing loss and vertigo. As

the tumour grows a cerebellopontine angle syndrome may develop with involvement of the fifth, seventh, ninth and tenth cranial nerves. Raised intracranial pressure may occur as a late feature. Acoustic neuroma is associated with neurofibromatosis (especially type 2). Vestibular neuronitis is believed to be caused by a viral infection. There is an abrupt onset of severe vertigo, nausea and vomiting without tinnitus or deafness. The severe vertigo subsides within a few days though it may take much longer for the patient to recover fully. Infarction of the vertebrobasilar circulation (eg the posterior inferior cerebellar artery) also causes abrupt onset of vertigo with nausea, vomiting and nystagmus. There are usually cranial nerve palsies and sensory and motor problems affecting the limbs. Ramsay Hunt syndrome is the association of facial palsy and vesicles at the external auditory meatus caused by herpes zoster virus. There is often associated deafness, tinnitus and vertigo.

Q29. DISORDERS OF HIGHER CEREBRAL VISUAL FUNCTION (☆☆)

1. C   2. D   3. E   4. B   5. A

Cerebral hemisphere damage can affect visual function even though control of eye movements, the visual pathways and the visual cortex are intact. These specific forms of visual dysfunction may cause apparently bizarre behaviour which is sometimes mistaken for dementia. Visual agnosia is the failure to recognise familiar objects by sight alone. This can markedly affect activities of daily living as even simple tasks, such as making tea, become impossible if the sufferer cannot recognise the items required. This condition is epitomised by Oliver Sachs' story *'The man who mistook his wife for a hat'*. One specific form of visual agnosia is prosopagnosia, the inability to recognise faces. This may result in the patient being unable to recognise a close relative until they hear his or her voice. Prosopagnosia is usually due to bilateral damage to the posterior part of the temporal lobes and inferior part of the parietal lobes. Gaze apraxia is the inability to orientate the eyes towards and maintain fixation on objects in space despite normal ocular muscle function and oculogyric reflexes. On testing the eye movements the patient will not be able to follow the examiner's moving finger. Visual disorientation is the inability to accurately identify the position of objects in space despite adequate visual acuity and fields. A patient with this defect may have difficulty in picking up a cup or other object. Visual inattention is the inability to perceive more than one stimulus simultaneously. If the examiner is testing visual fields by finger movements the patient will not realise if the fingers of both hands are waved at the same time. Visual inattention, visual disorientation and gaze apraxia may all be seen together, a condition known as Balint's syndrome. This occurs when there is parietal lobe damage. Topographical disorientation is the inability to remember routes which should be familiar (eg finding one's way around one's own house).

Q30. LOSS OF CONSCIOUSNESS (✫)

1. C   2. A   3. B   4. D   5. F

Blackouts are a common problem and the history is the key to the diagnosis. If possible interview witnesses to the event as well as the patient. Vasovagal attacks are provoked by emotion, pain or standing for long periods. They are caused by reflex bradycardia and peripheral vasodilatation. The onset occurs over a few seconds accompanied by pallor, sweating and a feeling that the visual fields are closing in. The patient is usually unconscious for around two minutes and a full recovery occurs rapidly. Be suspicious the blackouts are not due to a vasovagal attack if there is no obvious precipitating factor, if the patient is incontinent or if several attacks occur over a short period of time. Seizures are often preceded by an aura, a sensory warning which tells many epilepsy sufferers when an attack is about to occur. Blackouts due to many causes may be accompanied by limb-jerking but seizures should be suspected if there is a classic tonic-clonic progression. Other features

suggesting seizures are attacks occurring during sleep, urinary and/or faecal incontinence or tongue-biting. Drowsiness may last for several hours after an attack and paralysis may occur for up to 24 hours. Stokes-Adams attacks are caused by cardiac arrhythmias producing decreased cardiac output. There is frequently no warning and the patient is often pale and bradycardic during the attack. Recovery is rapid and is accompanied by facial flushing and a rapid increase in the pulse rate. The attacks are not related to posture and may occur with increasing frequency.

A transient ischaemic attack may cause loss of consciousness and focal neurological deficit for up to 24 hours. If there is a residual neurological impairment for more than 24 hours this is defined as a stroke. Orthostatic hypotension is a common problem in the elderly where there is loss of consciousness after standing from lying down. It can be caused by an inadequate vasomotor reflex in autonomic neuropathy or by diuretics or other medication. Orthostatic hypotension may be exacerbated by urination as the increase in abdominal pressure impairs venous return.

Q31. X-RAY FINDINGS (✫)

1. B   2. C   3. A   4. D   5. E

Splaying of the carina occurs if the left atrium is enlarged or if there is a large subcarinal mass. Left atrial enlargement also produces a double right heart border. The normally sharp mediastinal and diaphragmatic borders become blurred if there is disease in the adjacent lung. Blurring of the left heart border is caused by disease in the lingula, part of the left upper lobe. Left lower lobe pathology causes blurring of the medial aspect of the left hemidiaphragm. Enlargement of the heart shadow on the left can be caused by left ventricular enlargement or displacement as occurs in pectus excavatum. Pectus excavatum also causes blurring of the right heart border; however this is more commonly seen in right middle lobe collapse. Additional features of right middle lobe collapse include inferior displacement of the horizontal fissure on the posteroanterior and lateral films and forward displacement of the lower half of the oblique fissure on the lateral. Right lower lobe collapse causes downward displacement of the hilum and blurring of the medial aspect of the right hemidiaphragm. On the lateral film the oblique fissure is displaced downwards and backwards.

Q32. UPPER AIRWAY OBSTRUCTION (☆☆)

1. F   2. A   3. C   4. B   5. D

Previous recurrent bouts of colicky abdominal pain in a patient presenting with acute stridor suggest a diagnosis of angioneurotic oedema. There may also be a history of cutaneous, non-itchy, urticaria-like skin lesions. This condition is autosomal dominantly inherited and there may therefore be a relevant family history. Acute epiglottitis can affect adults as well as children. In adults the most likely diagnoses are *Streptococcus pneumoniae* or *Staphylococcus aureus* whereas in young children *Haemophilus influenzae* type B is the commonest cause. Tracheomalacia can be caused by prolonged external pressure such as from a retrosternal goitre. After thyroidectomy stridor, breathlessness and paroxysms of coughing may develop. Insertion of a silicone endotracheal stent can prevent this condition. Tracheomalacia can also be a primary condition presenting in childhood. Tracheal stenosis can be caused by prolonged endotracheal intubation or scarring after closure of a tracheostomy. Laryngeal nerve palsies are a not uncommon late complication of thyroidectomy. Scarring at the site of the thyroidectomy scar probably leads to progressive worsening of operative damage to the nerve. The typical presentation is with voice change, nocturnal stridor, decreased exercise tolerance, obstructive sleep apnoea and eventual respiratory failure. Bronchial carcinoma is probably the commonest cause of tracheal obstruction, occurring when a tumour erodes into the tracheal lumen.

Q33. BRONCHIAL CARCINOMA STAGING (☆☆)

1. C   2. A   3. E   4. F   5. B

In the tumour (T), nodes (N), metastasis (M) classification the higher the number assigned to each factor the more advanced the disease. It is not necessary to memorise this classification. However, it is important to recognise which features indicate more advanced disease (which will enable you to answer this and other similar questions).

For tumour:
T_0 = no evidence of any tumour
T_{is} = carcinoma in situ
T_x = malignant cells in bronchial secretions but no other evidence of tumour
T_1 = tumour less than 3 cm diameter in a lobar or more distal bronchus
T_2 = tumour more than 3 cm diameter and more than 2 cm distal to the carina or pleural involvement
T_3 = tumour less than 2 cm from but not at the carina or involvement of chest wall, diaphragm, pericardium or mediastinal pleural involvement
T_4 = tumour involving the mediastinum, great vessels, heart, trachea, oesophagus, vertebral body, carina or presence of a malignant effusion

For lymph node involvement:

N_0 = no lymph node involvement (as proven on mediastinoscopy)
N_1 = peribronchial or ipsilateral hilar lymph nodes only
N_2 = ipsilateral mediastinal or subcarinal lymph nodes
N_3 = scalene, supraclavicular or contralateral mediastinal or hilar lymph nodes

For distant metastases:
M_0 = none
M_1 = distant metastases

Q34. LUNG FUNCTION TESTS (☆)

1. D   2. A   3. E   4. F   5. B

Peak flow is the simplest test of lung function and is a measure of the patient's maximal expiratory airflow. This bedside test is effort dependent and falsely low readings can be produced by poor patient technique. Spirometry measures the forced expiratory volume in one second (FEV_1) and the forced vital capacity (FVC). A normal ratio for these measures, FEV_1/FVC, is greater than 70%. The results are not effort dependent and obstructive and restrictive ventilatory defects can be distinguished. Flow-volume loops monitor airflow throughout inspiration and expiration and enable extrathoracic and intrathoracic airway obstructions to be distinguished. In intrathoracic small airway obstruction, the airways quickly collapse on expiration resulting in a rapid fall in airway flow and a prolongation of the expiratory time. In intrathoracic large airway obstruction the expiratory curve is markedly flattened. In contrast, in extrathoracic obstruction the inspiratory curve is flattened more than the expiratory one. The helium diffusion test is used to estimate the residual volume of air which remains in the lungs after maximal expiration. This is increased in diseases causing air-trapping such as emphysema. The methacholine test is used to measure airway responsiveness. An increasing dose of methacholine is given and the effect on airflow is measured. There is typically an increased response in chronic airflow obstruction and asthma. The transfer factor for carbon monoxide is used as a measure of the diffusing capacity of the lung. It is dependent on the area and the thickness of the alveolar-capillary membrane, any inhomogeneity in matching of ventilation and perfusion and on the cardiac output. It is usually markedly decreased in emphysema and fibrosing alveolitis and is increased by alveolar haemorrhage.

Q35. RED EYE (☆☆)

1. B   2. D   3. C   4. A   5. E

The red eye can be caused by a relatively minor condition or one which is an immediate threat to sight. It is therefore very important to be able to distinguish between the different causes of a red eye so that appropriate action can be taken

before damage occurs. Conjunctivitis presents as injection of conjunctival vessels which blanche on pressure. The pupil, iris, cornea, anterior chamber and intraocular pressure are all normal in this condition. Acute (closed-angle) glaucoma presents as an acutely painful red eye. The pupil is fixed, dilated and oval, the iris is injected, the cornea is hazy, the anterior chamber is shallow and the intraocular pressure is very high. If the eyeball is palpated through the eyelid it will feel stony-hard. In contrast the eye with chronic glaucoma is not usually red or painful and the anterior chamber is not shallow. In acute iritis the pupil is small and fixed, the iris is injected, the cornea is normal and there is turbid fluid in the anterior chamber. In acute iritis the eye is usually painful. The appearance of a subconjunctival haemorrhage is alarming but this condition resolves spontaneously and does not threaten vision. The bright red sclera leaves a white rim around the limbus. The iris, pupil, cornea and anterior chamber are all normal in appearance. In scleritis the eye is usually painful. Although the sclera is usually red and swollen with a boggy feel, it may appear normal if the disease affects the posterior aspect of the globe. This condition is most common in rheumatoid arthritis and should be suspected in any patient with this disease who presents with a red eye. Episcleritis is a commoner and more benign cause of a red eye in rheumatoid arthritis. This condition is not usually painful, though there may be some irritation or discomfort.

Q36. BONE OR JOINT PROBLEMS (☆☆)

1. C   2. B   3. F   4. D   5. E

Atlanto-axial subluxation occurs following erosion of the odontoid peg and/or rupture of its supporting ligaments. Greater than 4 mm separation between the arch of the atlas and the odontoid process is abnormal and causes a risk of spinal cord compression. This condition is associated with rheumatoid arthritis and patients with severe rheumatoid disease should therefore not have their necks vigorously extended (eg during intubation). Sacroileitis is a feature of the HLA-B27-associated seronegative arthropathy, ankylosing spondylitis. It is best viewed with anteroposterior pelvic radiography. Arthritis of the distal interphalangeal joints of the hands is a typical feature of osteoarthritis. In contrast the proximal interphalangeal joints are usually affected by rheumatoid arthritis. Pott's disease refers to a crush fracture of the thoracic spine caused by tuberculous osteomyelitis. This condition causes a marked spinal flexion deformity. Charcot's joints are severely deformed joints which result from neuropathic injury. Syringomyelia and tabes dorsalis (a form of neurosyphilis) are the classical causes but in the Western world these joints are now more commonly caused by diabetic neuropathy.

Q37. DESCRIBING SKIN LESIONS (☆)

1. E   2. C   3. D   4. A   5. F

Understanding dermatological terminology is essential to be able to describe cutaneous lesions accurately. Bullae are fluid-filled elevations of the skin which are greater than 0.5 cm in diameter. They are seen in pemphigus, pemphigoid and epidermolysis bullosa. Vesicles are fluid-filled elevations which are less than 0.5 cm. They are commonly seen in herpes virus infections and dermatitis herpetiformis. Non-palpable discoloured areas of skin are called macules and patches. A macule is less than 1 cm diameter and a patch is greater than 1 cm. Palpable lesions are called papules, nodules and plaques. A papule is a superficial elevation up to 0.5 cm in diameter. A nodule is a well-defined, solid lesion of up to 1 cm diameter. Coalescence of papules and/or nodules can produce larger disc-like lesions. When greater than 2 cm diameter they are called plaques.

Q38. NAIL ABNORMALITY (☆☆)

1. B   2. F   3. E   4. A   5. C

Dark linear nail pigmentation is known as melanonychia. This is seen in Addison's disease, pituitary tumours, cytotoxic chemotherapy and treatment with anti-HIV drugs such as zidovudine. It is also seen in normal subjects who are non-Caucasian. Yellow nails have a generalised yellow discoloration with increased curvature, loss of the cuticle and paronychia. Yellow nail syndrome is associated with peripheral lymphoedema. Blue nails are most evident by looking at the lunulae. They occur in those with Wilson's disease and in people receiving prolonged treatment with amodiaquine, chloroquine or mepacrine. Spoon-shaped nails or koilonychia are a common feature of iron deficiency. Clubbing refers to the appearance of nails with increased lateral and transverse curvature, sponginess of the nail bed and loss of the angle of the nail. Clubbing is associated with a large number of conditions including subacute bacterial endocarditis, cyanotic congenital heart disease, fibrosing alveolitis, bronchiectasis, empyema, lung abscess, bronchial carcinoma, tuberculosis, cystic fibrosis, asbestosis, mesothelioma, cirrhosis, inflammatory bowel disease and thyroid acropathy. Splinter haemorrhages are caused by disruption of capillaries along the dermal ridges. They occur in trauma, bacterial endocarditis, Raynaud's disease and the systemic vasculitides.

Q39. RED BLOOD CELL ABNORMALITY (☆☆)

1. D   2. F   3. E   4. A   5. C

Howell-Jolly bodies are densely stained purple particles seen at the periphery of red cells due to fragments of nuclear DNA. They are present after splenectomy and are also seen when there is ineffective erythropoiesis or intense erythrocyte production, as occurs during haemolysis. Heinz bodies are masses of denatured haemoglobin which can be seen on phase-contrast microscopy. They occur during oxidative stress, eg in glucose-6-phosphate dehydrogenase deficiency, and when there is excess globin chain production, eg in thalassaemia and following splenectomy. Anisocytosis is variation in red cell size and is seen in reticulocytosis or combined microcytic/macrocytic anaemia. Anisocytosis also occurs after transfusion of normocytic packed red cells in a patient with microcytic or macrocytic anaemia. Acanthocytosis is the presence of irregular, spiculated red cells which have an abnormal membrane lipid content. This occurs in liver disease and in abetalipoproteinaemia. Poikilocytosis is variation in red cell shape. This is seen in sickle cell disease, microangiopathic haemolysis, leukaemia, extramedullary haematopoiesis and bone marrow stress due to any cause. Reticulocytosis is the presence of increased numbers of immature, nucleated red blood cells in the peripheral circulation.

Q40. LEUKAEMIA (☆☆)

1. D   2. C   3. F   4. B   5. E

Leukaemia can be classified as acute or chronic and by cell type of origin (myeloid lineage or lymphocyte lineage). T cell subtypes of primary chronic lymphoid leukaemia include large granular lymphocyte leukaemia, prolymphocytic leukaemia and Sézary cell leukaemia (Sézary syndrome includes these cells plus cutaneous erythroderma with Pautrier microabscesses on histology). B cell subtypes of chronic lymphoid leukaemia include chronic lymphocytic leukaemia, prolymphocytic leukaemia, hairy cell leukaemia and hairy cell variant. Acute myeloid leukaemia (AML) is classified as M0 (undifferentiated), M1 (undifferentiated myeloid), M2 (myeloid with granulocytic differentiation), M3 (promyelocytic), M4 (myelomonocytic), M5 (monocytic), M6 (erythroleukaemia) and M7 (megakaryoblastic). M3 and M4 have a better prognosis than other subtypes of AML. Acute lymphoblastic leukaemia (ALL) is the most common form of leukaemia in children. Risk factors include Down's syndrome, achondroplasia, xeroderma pigmentosum, X-linked agammaglobulinaemia, ataxia telangiectasia, radiation exposure and HTLV1 infection. The Philadelphia chromosome is a translocation with breakpoints between 9q34 and 22q11 resulting in the expression of the *bcr-abl* fusion gene. This translocation is occasionally present in ALL but is much more strongly associated with chronic myeloid leukaemia (CML). Subtypes of CML include chronic granulocytic, atypical chronic myeloid,

chronic neutrophilic, chronic myelomonocytic, juvenile chronic myelomonocytic and chronic eosinophilic. The myelodysplastic syndrome is a preleukaemic condition that may eventually progress to CML or AML.

Q41. BONE MARROW TRANSPLANTATION (☆)

1. C   2. D   3. B   4. A   5. E

Bone marrow transplantation is used in the attempt to cure several haematological malignancies and some inherited conditions. Indications include acute myeloid leukaemia following first (or later) remission, acute lymphoblastic leukaemia in second remission (first if adverse prognostic features), chronic myeloid leukaemia, inborn errors of metabolism, severe combined immunodeficiency, thalassaemia major and sickle cell disease. In autologous transplant the patient's own bone marrow is used. This is performed in leukaemia so that high-dose chemotherapy can be given to achieve total marrow ablation. There is a risk that the marrow harvested may contain leukaemic cells so that the disease is not always eradicated. Peripheral blood stem cell harvesting aims to reduce the risk of taking leukaemic cells. In this procedure the patient is given cytotoxic chemotherapy followed by GCSF. It is expected that normal stem cells will appear in the peripheral blood before malignant cells. These are harvested using a cell separator and then used in place of bone marrow for transfusion following total marrow ablation with further chemotherapy. In an allogeneic transplant the donor marrow comes from an HLA-matched sibling or a matched unrelated donor. The resultant graft-versus-leukaemia effect is believed to increase the probability of cure. However, the patient is also at risk of graft-versus-host disease which is particularly unpredictable with matched unrelated donors. A syngeneic transplant comes from an identical twin and there is therefore no graft-versus-host or graft-versus-leukaemia effect. This is immunologically equivalent to an autologous transplant but there is no risk of transfusing malignant cells. Xenotransplants come from other species. These are not used clinically because of difficulties in achieving adequate immune suppression and concerns over the theoretical risk of enabling viruses to cross the species barrier. There are fears that xenotransplants could select for novel pathogenic viruses which could then cause major epidemics among the human population. Any future programme of xenotransplants will need very careful regulation. Leukocyte depletion is the removal of white cells from red blood cell concentrates before transfusion. This helps reduce post-transfusion thrombocytopenia, risk of cytomegalovirus transmission (and theoretically prions) and helps prevent HLA sensitisation.

Q42. VECTORS OF INFECTIOUS DISEASE TRANSMISSION (☆☆☆)

1. F   2. A   3. E   4. B   5. C

Onchocerciasis is caused by *Onchocerca volvulus*, a tissue-dwelling nematode and is spread by the blackfly vector *Simulium*. Visceral leishmaniasis and Old World cutaneous leishmaniasis are transmitted by phlebotomine sandflies, whereas in the New World *Lutzomyia* sandflies are the vectors. South American trypansomiasis (Chagas disease) is caused by *Trypanosoma cruzi*, a blood- and tissue-dwelling protozoon. It is spread by reduviid bugs, also known as kissing bugs as they bite their victims around the lips. Human monocytic ehrlichiosis and human granulocytic ehrlichiosis are caused by *Ehrlichia chaffeensis* and *E. phagocytophila/ equi* respectively. *Amblyomma* and *Ixodes* ticks are the vectors which transmit these bacteria. Endemic or murine typhus is caused by infection with *Rickettsia typhi* and is spread to humans by the bite of infected rat fleas. *Aedes* mosquitoes spread dengue and yellow fever and other viral infections.

Q43. BACTERIA AND TOXINS (☆)

1. F   2. A   3. C   4. B   5. E

Ingestion of *Staphylococcus. aureus* enterotoxins is a common cause of food poisoning. Botulism is also usually acquired by ingestion of pre-formed toxin, though less commonly toxin can be produced by bacteria in the gut. It leads to muscle weakness and eventual paralysis which is often mistaken for Guillain-Barré, syndrome, myasthenia gravis or even psychogenic illness. Botulinum toxin (by inhalation) is feared as a potential biological weapon. *Escherichia. coli* O157 produces a toxin which is identical to that produced by *Shigella dysenteriae*. This can cause dysentery due to severe colitis and is associated with haemolytic uraemic syndrome. *Corynebacterium diphtheriae* primarily infects the mucus membranes of the tonsils, pharynx, larynx and nose. Strains which harbour the bacteriophage expressing the *tox* gene produce diphtheria toxin causing myocarditis, heart block and progressive cardiac failure. Subsequently neuropathy resembling Guillain-Barré, syndrome can occur. *Clostridium tetani* is commonly acquired in wounds and also occurs in neonates if non-sterile instruments are used to cut the umbilical cord. The tetanus toxin inhibits the neurotransmitters glycine and gamma amino butyric acid at inhibitory neurones. This results in uninhibited discharge of motor neurones producing muscle spasms, opisthotonos, lock-jaw and risus sardonicus. Anti toxins are available for botulinum, diphtheria and tetanus toxins. The toxin produced by *Vibrio cholerae* produces secretory diarrhoea.

Q44. FUNGI (☆☆☆)

1. F   2. A   3. B   4. C   5. E

Coccidioides immitis is a dimorphic fungus (exhibits yeast and mould forms) that grows in arid regions of the Western hemisphere. Following dust-storms multiple cases of pulmonary infection occur producing respiratory symptoms and non-specific malaise and fatigue resembling influenza. Primary disease in immunocompetent subjects does not usually require treatment but in the immunocompromised, severe disseminated infection may occur. *Sporothrix schenckii* initially causes a single subcutaneous nodule which then spreads along lines of lymphatic drainage. Bone, lung and disseminated infections may occur in sporotrichosis but are rare. Madura foot is the name given to chronic subcutaneous infection with multiple sinus tracts. It can be caused by several species of *Nocardia* or *Actinomyces* bacteria (called actinomycetoma) or by fungi (called eumycetoma). Fungal species causing Madura foot include *Pseudoallescheria boydii*, *Madurella mycetomatis*, *M. grisea*, *Exophiala jeanselmei*, *Acremonium recifei* and many other species. *Pseudoallescheria boydii* is the hyphal form of a dimorphic fungus which in its yeast form is known as *Scediosporum apiospermum*. This can cause fungal brain abscesses in the immunocompromised host. Craniofacial mucormycosis is an extremely destructive condition which begins as nasal or sinus infection and may result in destruction of the hard palate and cheek, orbital cellulitis, internal carotid artery involvement and cerebral infarction. It has extremely high mortality. *Rhizopus oryzae* is the most common causative organism but it can also be due to other *Rhizopus* species, *Mucor*, *Rhizomucor* and *Cunninghamella*. The facial eczematous condition known as seborrhoeic dermatitis is caused by the host response to the yeast *Pityrosporum ovale*. This yeast is also the cause of pityriasis versicolor, a widespread depigmenting skin disease. *Pneumocystis carinii* is a common cause of interstitial pneumonia in patients with AIDS. Although previously classified as a protozoon it is now known to be a yeast.

Q45. COMPLICATIONS OF HELMINTH INFECTION (☆☆)

1. D   2. C   3. F   4. A   5. E

Necator americanus and *Ankylostoma duodenale* are hookworms which cause gastrointestinal bleeding at the site of attachment of their mouthparts. Heavy infestations can result in iron deficiency and microcytic anaemia. Over one billion people are infected with hookworms worldwide and this is the commonest global cause of iron-deficiency anaemia. *Diphyllobothrium latum*, the fish tapeworm, is an uncommon cause of vitamin B_{12} deficiency and megaloblastic anaemia. It was previously a recognised problem in Scandinavia, where infection was acquired by eating uncooked freshwater fish. *Ascaris lumbricoides* is an extremely common roundworm which can grow up to 20 cm in length. It infrequently causes serious problems in adults although in children it may contribute to malnutrition by causing indigestion and decreased appetite. Adult worms can cause complications such as appendicitis, cholangitis or pancreatitis by migrating into the appendix, common bile duct or pancreatic duct. *Trichuris trichiura*, also known as the whipworm, infects the caecum and colon, sometimes producing abdominal discomfort and tenesmus. In extremely heavy infestations it can cause rectal prolapse. *Opisthorchis sinensis* (also known as *Clonorchis sinensis*) is a trematode which is acquired by eating undercooked freshwater fish in South East Asia. This flatworm infects the biliary tract and is the cause of oriental cholangitis. Chronic infections can lead to bile duct fibrosis and cholangiocarcinoma. The threadworm *Enterobius vermicularis* is a common parasite of young children, which causes perianal itching.

Q46. SYPHILIS (☆☆☆)

1. F   2. A   3. C   4. D   5. B

Primary, secondary and latent syphilis of less than one year duration can be treated with a single dose of intramuscular benzathine penicillin. If latent syphilis is believed to have been acquired more than a year previously three doses are given at weekly intervals. In primary and secondary disease the serum VDRL should be monitored after treatment to ensure that treatment has been effective. Patients with neurological symptoms, those who are HIV positive, those with a VDRL titre greater than or equal to 1:32, those with gumma or other active disease and those for whom penicillin cannot be used should have a lumbar puncture. If the CSF VDRL is positive the patient should be treated for neurosyphilis with ten to 14 days of high-dose intravenous penicillin. If the patient reports a history of adverse reaction to penicillin it is important to identify whether this was an allergic reaction. In many cases desensitisation to penicillin may be indicated, particularly if the patient has neurological involvement. If the patient cannot be given penicillin then doxycycline or ceftriaxone are suitable but if the patient has a severe penicillin allergy then doxycycline would be preferred. Ciprofloxacin is not a recommended treatment for syphilis.

Q47. ACUTE POISONING (☆☆)

1. E   2. C   3. F   4. A   5. B

Organophosphorous insecticides inhibit cholinesterase activity causing anxiety, sweating, vomiting, flaccid paralysis and eventually convulsions, coma and pulmonary oedema. Absorption can occur by inhalation, ingestion and through intact skin. Atropine and the cholinesterase reactivator pralidoxime mesylate are used to reverse the effects of excess acetylcholine. Concentrated paraquat is available only to farmers. Ingestion results in acute vomiting and diarrhoea, followed by ulceration of the oral and pharyngeal mucosa, renal failure and pulmonary fibrosis. Oral administration of large quantities of Fuller's earth adsorbs paraquat and reduces absorption. Oral magnesium sulphate or mannitol is also given to promote diarrhoea. In acute overdose β-blockers cause bradycardia and hypotension leading to cardiogenic shock. If this remains unresponsive to atropine, intravenous glucagon is given. Deliberate self-poisoning with as few as 20 to 30 tablets of paracetamol can lead to hepatocellular necrosis and less commonly renal tubular necrosis. Plasma paracetamol concentration is measured four or more hours after ingestion and if found

to be above the normal treatment line, acetylcysteine is administered. If patients are on enzyme-inducing drugs, including carbamazepine, phenobarbitone, phenytoin, rifampin and alcohol, a level above half the normal treatment line requires treatment. If a large number of tablets have been ingested treatment should be commenced before results are available. Cyanide poisoning has caused an estimated 400 deaths in the past 20 twenty years, mostly by suicide or homicide. Symptoms include headache, ataxia, convulsions, paralysis, coma and eventually cardiopulmonary arrest. The patient may have a classic brick red complexion and the breath may smell of bitter almonds. Specific antidotes include dicobalt edetate alone or sodium nitrite followed by sodium thiosulphate. Penicillamine is used to treat poisoning with lead and other heavy metals.

Q48. DRUG INTERACTIONS (☆☆)

1. C   2. B   3. A   4. F   5. D

Many of the drugs listed above may interact with each other. The interactions listed are those which are the most hazardous. Administration of an angiotensin-converting enzyme inhibitor to a patient taking indomethacin can cause hyperkalaemia and renal failure. Amiodarone increases the plasma concentration of digoxin. If the two are given together the concentration of digoxin should be halved. Itraconazole and other hepatic enzyme inhibitors such as erythromycin increase plasma ciclosporin concentrations, causing increased risk of renal and hepatic dysfunction. If intravenous verapamil is given to patients receiving a β-blocker there is a serious risk of cardiac failure, severe hypotension and heart block. The carbapenem antibiotic imipenem lowers the seizure threshold and co-administration of ganciclovir should be avoided due to the resulting increased risk of convulsions.

Q49. RECREATIONAL DRUGS (☆☆)

1. D   2. F   3. A   4. B   5. E

Cocaine inhibits norepinephrine (noradrenaline) reuptake in peripheral sympathetic nerve terminals and stimulates central sympathetic outflow. In overdose cocaine can cause prolonged convulsions, metabolic acidosis, aortic dissection, subarachnoid haemorrhage, cerebral haemorrhage and myocardial infarction. It has been estimated that cocaine is associated with 25% of myocardial infarcts in 18- to 45-year-olds in the USA. MDMA is more commonly known as 'ecstasy', a drug used increasingly commonly at raves and clubs. MDMA causes norepinephrine, dopamine and serotonin release from the peripheral autonomic and central nervous systems. Although believed by many users to be safe it can lead to dehydration, electrolyte abnormalities, renal failure, hyperthermia, rhabdomyolysis, cardiac arrhythmias and seizures. Alcohol can cause a large number of central nervous system problems the best known of which are Wernicke's encephalopathy and Korsakoff's psychosis. Central pontine myelinolysis is also well described in both the presence and absence of hyponatraemia. Hypokalaemia, hypophosphataemia, hypoxaemia and vitamin B deficiencies may also be contributing factors. Extrapontine demyelination may also occur, for example of the central white matter including the corpus callosum, optic chiasma and cerebellar peduncles, a condition known as Marchiafava-Bignami syndrome. Alcohol is frequently associated with road traffic accidents, as is cannabis. A study in Scotland found that 39% of blood samples from drivers suspected of drug or alcohol use following an accident contained cannabis. MPTP is converted by the enzyme monoamine oxidase B to 1-methyl 4-phenylpyridine (MPP+), a potent dopamine-releasing agent. Investigation of an outbreak of Parkinsonian symptoms among intravenous drug users led to the elucidation of the pathology of Parkinson's disease and the development of a mouse model.

Q50. ROUTE OF DRUG ADMINISTRATION (☆☆)

1. D   2. B   3. A   4. F   5. E

Methotrexate is administered intrathecally for the treatment of CNS lymphoma and for CNS prophylaxis in childhood acute lymphoblastic leukaemia. Pentamidine is given monthly by inhalation for *Pneumocystis carinii* pneumonia prophylaxis for those intolerant of sulphur drugs. When used in treatment it must be given intravenously. Desmopressin is a synthetic antidiuretic hormone given intranasally or orally as replacement therapy in cranial diabetes insipidus. Rectal diazepam is a useful treatment for those in status epilepticus when the intravenous route is unavailable or resuscitation facilities are not immediately available. Fomivirsen is antisense RNA against cytomegalovirus. It is administered by intravitreal injection for treatment of cytomegalovirus retinitis.

Q51. ENZYMES AND DRUG METABOLISM (☆☆☆)

1. F   2. D   3. A   4. C   5. E

Isoniazid is metabolised by *N*-acetyltransferase. Acetylator status shows genetic variation and those classified as slow acetylators have increased risk of peripheral neuropathy with isoniazid. It is controversial whether slow acetylators are at increased risk of isoniazid-induced hepatotoxicity or not. Propafenone is oxidised by cytochrome P450-IID6, as are metoprolol, captopril and flecainide. Nine per cent of the Caucasian population show slow metabolism by this enzyme. Quinidine inhibits the activity of cytochrome P450-IID6 thus increasing propafenone concentrations. When consumed in moderate amounts by normal people alcohol is predominantly metabolised by alcohol dehydrogenase. In chronic drinkers induction of microsomal oxidising enzymes occurs, particularly cytochrome P450-IIE1. This enzyme is also responsible for converting paracetamol to toxic metabolites, accounting for the increased susceptibility of alcoholics to paracetamol-related hepatotoxicity. Proguanil is metabolised by cytochrome P450-IIC. Poor metabolisers do not convert this drug to the active compound cycloguanil and may therefore be at increased risk of failure of malaria prophylaxis. Pseudocholinesterase deficiency may occur in as many as one in 1000 of the population. In normal subjects succinylcholine produces transient muscle depolarisation, but in those with pseudocholinesterase deficiency it can produce prolonged paralysis.

Q52. MECHANISM OF ANTIBIOTIC ACTION (☆☆☆)

1. C   2. A   3. E   4. F   5. B

Penicillins and glycopeptides such as vancomycin are bactericidal antibiotics which act by inhibition of bacterial cell wall synthesis. Glycopeptides act on the second stage of this process by inhibiting the assembly of peptidoglycan polymers. Penicillins act on the third stage by inhibiting transpeptidases which crosslink proteoglycans. Gentamicin and other aminoglycosides have a complex mechanism of action. These antibiotics bind to the bacterial outer membrane and cause rearrangement of lipopolysaccharide, disrupting cell permeability. Aminoglycosides become irreversibly trapped within the bacterial cytoplasm and the intracellular concentration becomes much higher than the extracellular one. Interaction with ribosomal RNA causes misreading of messenger RNA, causing miscoding and premature termination of protein synthesis. Rifampin is a naturally occurring antibiotic produced by the mould *Streptomyces mediterranei*. It inhibits DNA-dependent RNA polymerase, preventing chain initiation, so that messenger RNA synthesis cannot occur. 4-quinolones, such as ciprofloxacin, inhibit the topoisomerase enzymes DNA gyrase and topoisomerase IV. This inhibits bacterial DNA synthesis and repair mechanisms. Trimethoprim and sulphonamides inhibit folic acid metabolism.

Q53. JUGULAR VENOUS PRESSURE (☆)

1. E   2. F   3. C   4. B   5. A

The jugular venous pressure is examined clinically with the patient lying at 45° If the maximum height is greater than 4 cm vertically above the manubriosternal angle it is said to be elevated. Venous pressure can be monitored more accurately by placement of a central venous catheter. The 'a' wave represents atrial contraction filling the right ventricle. The tricuspid valve should be open at this stage. If the atrium contracts against a closed tricuspid valve this produces a giant (or 'cannon') 'a' wave. This occurs regularly in junctional rhythms and irregularly in the atrioventricular dissociation of complete heart block. The 'a' wave is followed by the 'x' descent which represents atrial relaxation after contraction. The 'c' wave is a small wave occurring during the 'x' descent, caused by ballooning backwards of the tricuspid valve as it closes. The 'v' wave follows the 'x' descent and represents the phase of venous filling with the right atrium becoming more tense. During this phase ventricular systole is occurring and the tricuspid valve is closed. If there is tricuspid incompetence, the backward jet of blood causes the pressure in the right atrium to rise and the 'c' and 'v' waves merge producing a 'cv' wave. The 'y' descent follows the v wave and is caused by opening of the tricuspid valve releasing pressure in the right atrium. On inspiration the jugular venous pressure falls and on expiration it rises. However, in constrictive pericarditis and pericardial tamponade this pattern is reversed, a phenomenon called Kussmaul's sign. In addition the 'x' and 'y' descents are said to be steeper than usual though this is difficult to recognise. A raised jugular venous pressure which does not vary with respiration occurs in superior vena cava obstruction.

Q54. CARDIOVASCULAR CLINICAL SIGNS (☆☆)

1. D   2. E   3. C   4. F   5. B

In normal subjects the arterial blood pressure drops slightly during inspiration and rises during expiration due to changes in intrathoracic pressure. If this pressure difference is greater than 10 mmHg this is called pulsus paradoxus (though it is an exaggeration of the normal response not a paradoxical difference). Pulsus paradoxus occurs in asthma due to the large changes in intrathoracic pressure which occur during respiration. It is also seen in pericardial tamponade probably because pericardial pressure rises on inspiration, impeding left ventricular filling. The central venous pressure usually falls during inspiration and this is exaggerated in asthma. In pericardial tamponade right ventricular filling is impeded by inspiration and this causes central venous pressure to rise, a finding known as Kussmaul's sign. The character of a slow-rising pulse is best palpated over the carotid artery. This pulse has reduced amplitude with an early notch in the upstroke and it is followed by a thrill. Measuring the blood pressure reveals a narrow pulse pressure. A slow-rising pulse is a feature of aortic stenosis. A collapsing pulse has a large amplitude and a rapid upstroke. If the palm of the hand is placed over the radial artery and the arm is elevated, the pulse is felt as a <u>tapping</u> impulse. A collapsing pulse is a feature of aortic regurgitation. This sign may be accompanied by a visible carotid artery pulsation (Corrigan's sign), nail bed pulsations (Quincke's sign), head-nodding (de Musset's sign) and a diastolic flow murmur over the femoral artery when it is partially occluded (Durosiez's sign). Pulsus alternans occurs in severe cardiac failure when the left ventricle is unable to fully contract during each systole. The heart rhythm is regular but the pulse amplitude alternates between a smaller and a larger pulsation. Pulsus alternans should be distinguished from bigeminy. Pulsus bigeminus is due to a ventricular ectopic beat alternating with each sinus beat. There is alternation in both the pulse volume and its timing (shorter interval then longer one).

Q55. CHEST PAIN (☆☆)

1. C   2. A   3. F   4. B   5. E

Diagnosis of the cause of chest pain is often difficult. Severity of chest pain is not a useful guide as angina may cause only a dull ache and musculoskeletal pain and oesophageal spasm may be severe. All causes of pain may cause pallor and sweating because of the autonomic response and these are not reliable signs of pain of cardiac origin. In stable angina the chest pain is produced by a predictable level of exercise and relieved by rest. The pain tends to come on more easily in the mornings, in cold weather, after a heavy meal or during any cause of tachycardia (eg fever, stress). Angina radiates to different locations (jaw, left arm, left hand, etc) in different patients depending on their somatic nerve supply distribution. However, the pain usually radiates to the same location each time in an individual patient. The pain of oesophageal dysmotility/spasm may be induced by exercise, making it difficult to distinguish from angina. In addition this pain may be reduced by smooth muscle relaxants such as nitrates and calcium channel blockers. However, oesophageal dysmotility typically follows exercise rather than occurring during exertion. The pain may be briefly relieved by swallowing, which can be a useful bedside test. Tietze's costochondritis produces local tenderness over the costochondral junctions and is not usually related to exercise. Aortic dissection produces sudden onset, severe chest pain which radiates to the interscapular region. A detectable difference in blood pressure between the upper limbs may be found. In pericarditis there is a sharp pain which is exacerbated by deep inspiration, swallowing, twisting or sternal pressure. The pain is relieved by sitting up and leaning forwards. Musculoskeletal chest pain is usually related to movement and posture. When it is exacerbated by breathing the patient may complain of being 'short of breath' causing confusion with angina.

In some patients this pain can be reproduced by forced rotation of the chest.

Q56. ECG (☆)

1. C   2. E   3. A   4. B   5. F

The limb leads look at the frontal (coronal) plane of the heart, whereas the chest leads look at the horizontal plane. Leads I, II and III are bipolar leads. Lead I is produced by connecting the negative electrode to the right arm and the positive electrode to the left arm. The net vector of electrical movement is horizontally towards the left, the direction labelled as 0°. Lead II is produced by connecting the positive electrode to the left foot and the negative electrode to the right arm, giving a net vector of +60°. Lead III is produced by connecting the positive electrode to the left foot and the negative electrode to the right arm, giving a net vector of +120°. The augmented leads aVL, aVR and aVF are unipolar leads. These measure the direction of electrical movement towards a single electrode from the heart, the position of which is based on a modification of the central electrode of Wilson. aVL, aVR and aVF respectively measure current movement towards the left arm (–30°), the right arm (–150°) and the left foot (90°).

Q57. CLASSIFICATION OF NEUROSES (☆☆)

1. C   2. E   3. F   4. A   5. D

Symptoms of anxiety include fearful anticipation, restlessness, irritability, palpitations, chest discomfort, hyperventilation, dyspnoea, dry mouth, difficulty swallowing, loose motions and the urgent need to pass urine. In phobic anxiety disorder symptoms are brought on by a specific situation or feared object. Symptoms may be elicited by social contact (social phobia), leaving the house (agoraphobia), confined spaces (claustrophobia), spiders (arachnophobia) or many other stimuli. In panic disorder similar episodes of severe anxiety occur but there is no consistent, provoking, external stimulus. In generalised anxiety disorder frequent and prolonged episodes of anxiety occur and this may become an almost continuous state. In obsessive-compulsive disorder patients suffer repeated intrusive thoughts. Common themes include thoughts about disease and cleanliness, imagining performing embarrassing acts and internal debates. The obsessive thoughts are accompanied by a compulsion to perform a specific behaviour repetitively (eg handwashing) and resisting this causes anxiety. Performing the behaviour provides relief of anxiety but this creates reinforcement of the compulsion. Adjustment disorder is an emotional response to a prolonged stressful situation. Common responses include denial, avoidance, depression, anger, poor sleep and anxiety. Post-traumatic stress disorder occurs as a reaction to a severely stressful event such as a road traffic accident, violent attack, fire, war, etc. The main features of this condition are anxiety, daytime images of the event (flashbacks), nightmares and an inability to feel normal emotions.

Q58. MALADAPTIVE BEHAVIOURS (☆☆)

1. E   2. A   3. B   4. D   5. C

Somatisation disorder is recurrent episodes of multiple symptoms without an underlying physical cause. Common complaints include itching, nausea, indigestion, abdominal pains and headaches. The symptoms change over time and the patient is not reassured by normal investigations. In hypochondriasis there is extreme concern about the presence of disease arising from awareness of common bodily sensations such as forceful heart beats, joint pains, aching muscles and constipation. There is an association with depression, anxiety and obsessional disorders, but hypochondriasis is sometimes the primary problem. Dysmorphophobia is an inappropriate concern over the body image, ie the distress is out of proportion to the actual appearance of the 'abnormal' part. Patients may be concerned about the shape of the nose, ears, breast size, etc and they often seek help from plastic surgeons. Factitious disorder is the deliberate production of symptoms or signs without there being any real material gain in doing this. The patient's motivation is not clear but many sufferers appear to obtain psychological benefit from their condition. Dermatitis artefacta and Münchausen's syndrome are both examples of factitious disorders. Malingering is the deliberate production of symptoms for some material gain. This may relate to compensation or other benefits such as time off work. Psychogenic pain is the sensation of pain for which there is no physical stimulus. The description of the pain is often bizarre and the patient claims it is totally incapacitating.

Q59. PERSONALITY DISORDERS (☆☆)

1. E   2. F   3. B   4. A   5. D

Each individual has his or her own personality traits. These should only be regarded as personality disorders when they are extreme and cause problems for that person or others. Those with personality disorders display persistently abnormal behaviour from childhood. This contrasts with most other forms of psychiatric problem where there is usually a preceding history of normal social functioning. The obsessional personality is characterised by the holding of rigid views and an inability to change. These persons are often moralistic and expect high standards of themselves and others. The histrionic or hysterical subject is shallow, self-centred, inconsiderate and often demanding. The tendency to swing from one extreme of emotion to the other is common. Persons with a paranoid personality disorder are suspicious and argumentative and are usually ungrateful for things done for them. There is usually distrust of and hostility towards others. The schizoid personality is characterised by emotional coldness and introspection. These persons appear not to need others, tend not to confide even in those closest to them and often underplay their medical complaints. The psychopath acts impulsively, lacks guilt for his or her actions, appears heartless, cruel, aggressive and is sometimes violent. These persons fail to make loving relationships and are said not to learn from experience. The affective personality disorder is one of abnormal mood. This may be abnormally high or low or swing between the two extremes (cyclothymia).

Q60. HEARING LOSS (☆☆☆)

1. C   2. D   3. A   4. E   5. B

Presbyacusis is slowly progressive, bilateral, age-related hearing loss. There are several types of presbyacusis but these often occur together. Sensory presbyacusis resembles the hearing loss that occurs due to noise-induced damage. The problem is caused by damage to the hair cells and organ of Corti. In neural presbyacusis high-tone frequencies are less affected than lower tones resulting in severe loss of speech discrimination. There is loss of cochlear neurones from the whole of the cochlear apparatus. In strial (or metabolic) presbyacusis there is a flat pure tone audiogram and good speech discrimination. This condition is due to atrophy of the stria vascularis causing impairment of endolymph function. Ménière's disease is the triad of episodic vertigo, tinnitus and fluctuating hearing loss. Initially low frequencies are affected, but severe hearing loss affecting all frequencies may eventually occur. Nystagmus is invariably seen during an acute attack. Vestibular neuronitis also causes severe vertigo but hearing is usually unaffected. Acoustic neuroma is a schwannoma of the eighth cranial nerve. This produces progressive, unilateral hearing loss, tinnitus, disequilibrium and vertigo. Palsies affecting the fifth and seventh cranial nerves also occur. Sudden onset of unilateral hearing loss can be caused by trauma or internal auditory artery occlusion from thrombosis or autoimmune vasculitis. Steroids may be beneficial in the latter condition.

PAPER 2 QUESTIONS

CELLULAR AND MOLECULAR BIOLOGY

1. THEME: ONCOGENES

A   *c-myc*
B   *p53*
C   *PML-RARα*
D   *bcr-abl*
E   *Rb1*
F   *K-ras*

For each of the following descriptions select the appropriate oncogene from the list above. The items may be used once or not at all.

☐ 1. Encodes a cytoplasmic protein where disruption is associated with pancreatic cancer
☐ 2. Encodes a fusion protein associated with chronic myeloid leukaemia
☐ 3. Encodes a nuclear protein where over-expression is associated with breast cancer
☐ 4. Encodes a tumour suppressor gene which is believed to have a key role in cell cycle control
☐ 5. Encodes a fusion protein associated with acute promyelocytic leukaemia

2. THEME: INTRACELLULAR ORGANELLES

A   Endoplasmic reticulum
B   Nucleus
C   Lysosome
D   Mitochondria
E   Golgi apparatus
F   Ribosome

For each of the following descriptions select the appropriate intracellular organelle from the list above. The items may be used once or not at all.

☐ 1. Site of main oxidative reaction to produce energy for cell
☐ 2. Site of protein synthesis
☐ 3. Site of majority of cytoplasmic enzyme reactions
☐ 4. Site of storage for cellular genetic information
☐ 5. Membrane-bound vesicles storing enzymes

STATISTICS AND EPIDEMIOLOGY

3. THEME: STATISTICAL DEFINITIONS

A   Standard deviation
B   Median
C   Range
D   Standard error
E   Mode
F   Mean

For each of the following definitions select the appropriate statistical term from the list above. The items may be used once or not at all.

☐ 1. Central value when the values are listed in ascending order of magnitude
☐ 2. Sum of all the values divided by the number of values
☐ 3. Measure of spread of values around the mean
☐ 4. Most frequent value
☐ 5. Spread of estimates of sample means around the true population mean

IMMUNOLOGY

4. THEME: IMMUNOGLOBULIN ISOTYPES

A   IgA
B   IgB
C   IgD
D   IgE
E   IgG
F   IgM

For each of the following descriptions select the appropriate immunoglobulin isotype from the list above. The items may be used once or not at all.

☐ 1. The major immunoglobulin in serum
☐ 2. The initial immunoglobulin produced in response to infection
☐ 3. A dimeric secreted immunoglobulin involved in mucosal protection
☐ 4. An immunoglobulin which binds to B cells in lymphoid follicles, found in very low concentrations in serum
☐ 5. An immunoglobulin which causes mast cell degranulation

5. THEME: CYTOKINES

A   Interferon γ
B   Interleukin 2
C   Interleukin 4
D   Interleukin 8
E   Interferon α
F   Tumour necrosis factor α

For each of the following descriptions select the appropriate cytokine from the list above. The items may be used once or not at all.

☐ 1. Produced by T helper 1 (Th$_1$) cells, stimulates T cell activation
☐ 2. Produced by Th$_2$ cells, promotes IgE production
☐ 3. Produced by Th$_1$ and cytotoxic T lymphocytes, stimulates HLA class I and II expression
☐ 4. Produced by T cells and macrophages, produces fever and shock
☐ 5. Chemokine that attracts neutrophils

CLINICAL GENETICS

6. THEME: PATTERNS OF INHERITANCE

A   Autosomal dominant
B   Autosomal recessive
C   Mitochondrial
D   X-linked dominant
E   Pseudoautosomal
F   X-linked recessive

For each of the following familial diseases select the appropriate pattern of inheritance from the list above. The items may be used once or not at all.

☐ 1. Duchenne muscular dystrophy
☐ 2. Huntington's chorea
☐ 3. Vitamin-D-resistant (hypophosphataemic) rickets
☐ 4. Leber's hereditary optic neuropathy
☐ 5. Cystic fibrosis

7. THEME: GENETIC ABNORMALITIES

A   Turner's syndrome
B   Schizophrenia
C   Prader-Willi syndrome
D α^0-thalassaemia
E   Sickle cell anaemia
F   Fragile X syndrome

For each of the following genetic abnormalities select the appropriate condition from the list above. The items may be used once or not at all.

☐ 1. Trinucleotide repeat expansion
☐ 2. Gene deletion
☐ 3. Point mutation
☐ 4. Abnormal karyotype
☐ 5. Genomic imprinting with expression of null allele

NEUROANATOMY

8. THEME: CRANIAL NERVES

A   Olfactory nerve
B   Maxillary division of the trigeminal nerve

C Glossopharyngeal nerve
D Facial nerve
E Mandibular division of the trigeminal nerve
F Hypoglossal nerve

For each of the following openings of the skull select the appropriate route of entry for the cranial nerves listed above. The items may be used once or not at all.

- [ ] 1. Foramen rotundum
- [ ] 2. Foramen ovale
- [ ] 3. Stylomastoid foramen
- [ ] 4. Jugular foramen
- [ ] 5. Cribriform plate

9. THEME: NERVE ROOTS

A C5-C6
B C6-C7
C C7-C8
D S4-S5
E L2-L4
F S1-S2

For each of the following tendon stretch reflexes select the appropriate nerve root from the list above. The items may be used once or not at all.

- [ ] 1. Finger (flexion) jerk
- [ ] 2. Triceps
- [ ] 3. Biceps
- [ ] 4. Ankle plantarflexion
- [ ] 5. Knee flexion

PHYSIOLOGY, BIOCHEMISTRY AND METABOLISM

10. THEME: TUMOUR MARKERS

A CA-125
B CA-19.9
C α-fetoprotein
D β-HCG
E PSA
F CA-15.3

For each of the following types of cancer select the appropriate tumour marker from the list above. The items may be used once or not at all.

- [ ] 1. Choriocarcinoma
- [ ] 2. Ovarian cancer
- [ ] 3. Breast cancer
- [ ] 4. Pancreatic cancer
- [ ] 5. Primary hepatocellular cancer

11. THEME: CRYSTALS IN SYNOVIAL FLUID

A Corticosteroid
B Monosodium urate
C Hydroxyapatite
D Cholesterol
E Cystine
F Calcium pyrophosphate

For each of the following descriptions select the appropriate crystal isolated from synovial fluid from the list above. The items may be used once or not at all.

- [ ] 1. Negatively birefringent, needle-shaped crystals
- [ ] 2. Positively birefringent rods, needles and rhomboid shapes
- [ ] 3. Negatively birefringent notched rhomboid shapes
- [ ] 4. Small needles which may require electron microscopy to be visualised
- [ ] 5. Positively and negatively birefringent, flat and variably shaped crystals

12. THEME: DIABETIC COMA

A Hyperosmolar non-ketoacidotic coma
B Ketoacidosis
C Metformin toxicity
D Hypoglycaemia
E Salicylate poisoning
F Severe sepsis

For each of the following findings in a diabetic patient select the most likely cause of coma from the list above. The items may be used once or not at all.

☐ 1. Raised blood glucose, blood pH of 7.10, increased anion gap, marked dehydration, normal lactate
☐ 2. Blood pH of 7.45, normal anion gap and no dehydration
☐ 3. Raised blood glucose, blood pH of 7.10, increased anion gap, marked dehydration, raised lactate
☐ 4. Raised blood glucose, blood pH of 7.45, normal anion gap and marked dehydration
☐ 5. Normal blood glucose, blood pH of 7.20, increased anion gap, no dehydration

13. THEME: THYROID HORMONE PRODUCTION

A Triiodothyronine
B Thyroid peroxidase
C Thyroglobulin
D Monoiodotyrosine
E Thyroxine
F Diiodotyrosine

For each of the following descriptions of substances involved in thyroid hormone production select the best match from the list above. The items may be used once or not at all.

☐ 1. Most hormonally active thyroid hormone
☐ 2. Hormonally inactive precursor that is used to make T_3 and T_4
☐ 3. Enzyme catalysing the iodination of tyrosyl residues
☐ 4. Hormonally inactive precursor that is used to make T_3 but not T_4

☐ 5. Large glycoprotein molecule that contains the thyroid hormone precursors

14. THEME: VITAMINS

A α-tocopherol
B Nicotinic acid
C Hydroxocobalamin
D Riboflavin
E Pyridoxine
F Thiamine

For each of the following descriptions select the appropriate vitamin from the list above. The items may be used once or not at all.

☐ 1. Has a key role in the glycolytic and pentose phosphate shunt pathways
☐ 2. Is a cofactor for conversion of tryptophan to nicotinic acid
☐ 3. Is involved in metabolism of short-chain fatty acids
☐ 4. Is a cofactor for nicotinamide adenine dinucleotide in cellular respiration
☐ 5. Is involved in the synthesis of nucleotide precursors for incorporation into DNA

RENAL MEDICINE

15. THEME: RENAL TRACT INVESTIGATIONS

A Acute glomerulonephritis
B Renal tuberculosis
C Contaminated specimen
D Chlamydial urethritis
E Bladder carcinoma
F Haemoglobinuria

For each of the following test results select the appropriate condition from the list above. The items may be used once or not at all.

☐ 1. Positive urine dipstick test for blood but no red blood cells seen on microscopy
☐ 2. Positive urine dipstick test for blood, dysmorphic red blood cells and red cell casts seen on microscopy

☐ 3. Positive urine dipstick test for blood, red blood cells seen on microscopy but no dysmorphic cells and no red cell casts

☐ 4. Numerous white blood cells and no squamous epithelial cells seen on microscopy but negative bacterial culture

☐ 5. Numerous white blood cells and no squamous epithelial cells seen on microscopy of first catch urine specimen but very few white blood cells seen in midstream urine sample

16. THEME: URINARY PROTEIN EXCRETION

A   Normal daily albumin excretion
B   Microalbuminuria
C   Tamm-Horsfall proteinuria
D   Tubular pattern of proteinuria
E   Highly selective proteinuria
F   Non-selective proteinuria

For each of the following definitions select the appropriate form of urinary protein excretion from the list above. The items may be used once or not at all.

☐ 1. Ratio of clearance of immunoglobulin to clearance of transferrin less than 0.10

☐ 2. Ratio of clearance of immunoglobulin to clearance of transferrin greater than 0.20

☐ 3. Between 50 mg and 200 mg of albumin excreted per day

☐ 4. A 200-kDa glycoprotein secreted by the thick limb of the loop of Henle

☐ 5. Excretion of low molecular weight proteins including α_1-microglobulin and β_2-microglobulin

17. THEME: RENAL DISEASE HISTOLOGY

A   Sarcoidosis
B   Sjögren's syndrome
C   Diabetes mellitus
D   Systemic lupus erythematosus
E   Hepatitis B infection
F   Amyloidosis

For each of the following histological findings select the appropriate renal disease from the list above. The items may be used once or not at all.

☐ 1. Glomerulosclerosis, interstitial fibrosis and Kimmelstiel-Wilson nodules

☐ 2. Membranous nephropathy with subepithelial, subendothelial and mesangial antigen complex deposits

☐ 3. Glomerular deposits of material with green birefringence on polarised light microscopy

☐ 4. Interstitial nephritis with granuloma formation

☐ 5. Diffuse mesangial aggregates containing immunoglobulins G, A and M and complement components C1q, C3 and C4

18. THEME: RENAL DISEASE CLASSIFICATION

A   Henoch-Schönlein purpura
B   Immunoglobulin A nephropathy
C   Antiglomerular basement membrane antibody disease
D   Membranous nephropathy
E   Minimal change nephropathy
F   Thin membrane nephropathy

For each of the following presentations select the most likely renal disease from the list above. The items may be used once or not at all.

☐ 1. Young adult male with recurrent episodes of pharyngitis and haematuria

☐ 2. Young adult with brief history of arthritis, palpable purpura, glomerulonephritis and abdominal pain

☐ 3. Young adult with longstanding, persistent, asymptomatic, microscopic haematuria with family history of the same condition

☐ 4. Four-year-old child with nephrotic syndrome and highly selective proteinuria

☐ 5. Young adult with acute history of haemoptysis, malaise, breathlessness, peripheral oedema and oliguria

ENDOCRINOLOGY AND DIABETES

19. THEME: INHERITED ABNORMALITY

A Gsα gene
B 21-hydroxylase gene
C 11β-hydroxylase gene
D 5α-reductase gene
E 17α-hydroxylase gene
F 3β-hydroxysteroid dehydrogenase gene

For each of the following statements select the appropriate inherited abnormality for the gene in the list above. The items may be used once or not at all.

☐ 1. Commonest cause of congenital adrenal hyperplasia
☐ 2. Causes ambiguous genitalia in male infants but masculinisation occurs at puberty
☐ 3. Causes polyostotic fibrous dysplasia
☐ 4. Causes androgen deficiency and mineralocorticoid excess
☐ 5. Causes androgen and mineralocorticoid excess

20. THEME: CORTICOSTEROID PRODUCTION REGULATION

A Pro-opiomelanocortin
B Melanocyte-stimulating hormone
C Vasopressin
D β-lipotrophin
E Gonadotrophin-releasing hormone
F Cortisol

For each of the following descriptions select the appropriate substance from the list above. The items may be used once or not at all.

☐ 1. Stimulator of adrenocorticotrophic hormone (ACTH) secretion
☐ 2. Inhibitor of ACTH secretion
☐ 3. Precursor of ACTH
☐ 4. Produced with ACTH when precursor is broken down
☐ 5. Produced by cleavage of ACTH

21. THEME: PITUITARY FUNCTION TESTS

A Growth hormone assay
B Adrenocorticobrophic hormone (ACTH) assay
C Insulin tolerance test
D Metyrapone test
E Combined gonadotrophin-releasing hormone (GnRH), thyrotrophin-releasing hormone (TRH), corticotrophin-releasing hormone (CRH), growth hormone-releasing hormone (GHRH) stimulation test
F Oral glucose tolerance test

For each of the following situations select the appropriate test of pituitary function from the list above. The items may be used once or not at all.

☐ 1. Testing the adequacy of growth hormone and ACTH secretion
☐ 2. Diagnosis of suspected acromegaly
☐ 3. Investigation of Cushing's disease
☐ 4. Diagnosis of suspected ACTH deficiency
☐ 5. Testing anterior pituitary function after pituitary surgery

22. THEME: PITUITARY TUMOURS

A Thyrotroph adenoma
B Somatotroph adenoma
C Craniopharyngioma
D Glycoprotein-producing adenoma
E Lactotroph adenoma
F Corticotroph adenoma

For each of the following descriptions select the appropriate pituitary tumour from the list above. The items may be used once or not at all.

☐ 1. Commonest hormone-secreting tumour
☐ 2. Rare condition accounting for less than 1% of pituitary tumours
☐ 3. Cause of Nelson's syndrome
☐ 4. Cause of acromegaly
☐ 5. Tumour arising from embryological remnant of Rathke's pouch

GASTROENTEROLOGY

23. THEME: GASTROINTESTINAL DISEASE

A   Hirschsprung's disease
B   Coeliac disease
C   Pseudomembranous colitis
D   Crohn's disease
E   Ulcerative colitis
F   Ischaemic colitis

For each of the following findings select the appropriate condition from the list above. The items may be used once or not at all.

☐ 1. Iron-deficiency anaemia and positive anti-endomyseal antibodies
☐ 2. Chronic diarrhoea with rectal biopsy histology showing inflammation confined to the mucosa
☐ 3. Iron-deficiency anaemia with rectal biopsy histology showing transmural inflammation
☐ 4. Diarrhoea with thumbprinting of bowel wall on barium enema
☐ 5. Diarrhoea with *Clostridium difficile* toxin in stool

24. THEME: GASTROINTESTINAL DISEASE

A   Barrett's oesophagus
B   Schatzki ring
C   Plummer-Vinson syndrome
D   Rolling hiatus hernia
E   Sliding hiatus hernia
F   Achalasia

For each of the following descriptions select the appropriate condition from the list above. The items may be used once or not at all.

☐ 1. Incomplete relaxation of the gastro-oesophageal sphincter and impairment of oesophageal peristalsis
☐ 2. Presence of columnar epithelium in the oesophagus
☐ 3. Part of the stomach in the thorax with upward displacement of the gastro-oesophageal sphincter

☐ 4. Part of the stomach in the thorax with a normally positioned gastro-oesophageal sphincter
☐ 5. Luminal stenosis at the gastro-oesophageal junction

25. THEME: HORMONE-SECRETING TUMOURS

A   Insulinoma
B   VIPoma
C   Carcinoid tumour
D   Somatostatinoma
E   Glucagonoma
F   Gastrinoma

For each of the following problems select the appropriate type of hormone-secreting tumour from the list above. The items may be used once or not at all.

☐ 1. Necrolytic migratory erythema
☐ 2. Drowsiness and confusion on waking which is relieved by food
☐ 3. Recurrent peptic ulceration
☐ 4. Watery diarrhoea exceeding 3 litres per day, hypokalaemia and achlorhydria
☐ 5. Cholelithiasis, diabetes mellitus and steatorrhoea

26. THEME: INVESTIGATION OF GASTROINTESTINAL PROBLEMS

A   Glucose tolerance test
B   Faecal fat measurement
C   Bile acid breath test
D   Schilling test
E   Xylose absorption test
F   Small intestinal biopsy

For each of the following select the most appropriate investigation from the list above. The items may be used once or not at all.

☐ 1. Demonstration of malabsorption syndrome
☐ 2. Demonstration of carbohydrate malabsorption
☐ 3. Investigation of terminal ileal function
☐ 4. Demonstration of bacterial overgrowth of small intestine
☐ 5. Demonstration of alactasia

NEUROLOGY

27. THEME: NYSTAGMUS

A   Downbeat nystagmus
B   Pendular nystagmus
C   Nystagmus to the right on looking to the right, no nystagmus to the left
D   Nystagmus affecting only the right eye on looking to the right
E   Upbeat nystagmus
F   Horizontal nystagmus in the direction of gaze on looking to both right and left, but more marked when looking to the left

For each of the following select the form of nystagmus from the list above that is most likely to occur following damage to this area of the central nervous system. The items may be used once or not at all.

☐ 1. Floor of the fourth ventricle
☐ 2. Area around the foramen magnum
☐ 3. Left cerebellar hemisphere
☐ 4. Left medial longitudinal fasciculus
☐ 5. Left vestibular apparatus

28. THEME: PATHOLOGY

A   Parkinson's disease
B   Carbon monoxide poisoning
C   Multisystem atrophy
D   Progressive supranuclear palsy
E   Huntington's disease
F   Corticobasal degeneration

For each of the following pathological findings select the appropriate condition from the list above. The items may be used once or not at all.

☐ 1. Lewy body deposition and damage to the zona compacta of the substantia nigra
☐ 2. Neurofibrillary tangles and widespread damage to the basal ganglia and periaqueductal grey matter
☐ 3. Glial cytoplasmic inclusions and variable damage to the basal ganglia, Purkinje cells of the cerebellar cortex, inferior olives and the intermediolateral columns of the thoracic spinal cord
☐ 4. Damage to the frontal and parietal cortex and the basal ganglia
☐ 5. Bilateral necrosis of the striatum and globus pallidus

29. THEME: CRANIAL NERVE LESIONS

A   CN I alone
B   CN III alone
C   CN III, IV and VI
D   CN IX, X and XII
E   CN V, VII and VIII
F   CN V and VI

For each of the following conditions select the resulting cranial nerve (CN) lesion from the list above (in the absence of raised intracranial pressure). The items may be used once or not at all.

☐ 1. Posterior communicating artery aneurysm
☐ 2. Acoustic neuroma
☐ 3. Frontal lobe tumour
☐ 4. Infection in the petrous part of the temporal bone
☐ 5. Cavernous sinus thrombosis

30. THEME: GAIT ABNORMALITY

A   Cerebellar damage
B   Proximal myopathy
C   Peripheral motor neuropathy
D   Peripheral sensory neuropathy
E   Bilateral upper motor neurone damage
F   Extrapyramidal damage

For each of the following abnormalities of gait select the appropriate neurological problem from the list above. The items may be used once or not at all.

☐ 1. Scissoring gait
☐ 2. Waddling gait
☐ 3. High-stepping gait
☐ 4. Broad-based, ataxic gait
☐ 5. Shuffling gait

RESPIRATORY MEDICINE

31. THEME: HISTOLOGY OF RESTRICTIVE LUNG DISEASE

A Cryptogenic fibrosing alveolitis
B Extrinsic allergic alveolitis
C Histiocytosis X
D Lymphangioleiomyomatosis
E Bronchiolitis obliterans with organising pneumonia
F Asbestosis

For each of the following types of histological appearance select the appropriate type of restrictive lung disease from the list above. The items may be used once or not at all.

☐ 1. Granulation tissue within the alveoli and bronchioles
☐ 2. Fibrosis of alveolar walls with intra-alveolar macrophages
☐ 3. Interstitial eosinophilic granulomas and Langerhan's cells
☐ 4. Small non-necrotising granulomas around bronchioles and presence of mucosal ulceration
☐ 5. Presence of ferruginous bodies

32. THEME: INVESTIGATIONS

A Magnetic resonance imaging
B Bronchography
C Pulmonary arteriography
D Ventilation-perfusion scan
E High-resolution computed tomography
F Transthoracic ultrasound

For each of the following select the appropriate investigation from the list above. The items may be used once or not at all.

☐ 1. Imaging of interstitial lung disease
☐ 2. Diagnosis of thoracic aortic dissection
☐ 3. Non-invasive confirmation of suspected pulmonary embolism
☐ 4. Gold standard for diagnosis of pulmonary embolism
☐ 5. Identifying loculations within a pleural effusion

33. THEME: ASTHMA

A Hypersensitivity-induced occupational asthma
B Seasonal atopic asthma
C Byssinosis
D Churg-Strauss syndrome
E Continuous atopic asthma with nocturnal exacerbations
F Irritant-induced occupational asthma

For each of the following causative agents select the type of asthma most likely to occur from the list above. The items may be used once or not at all.

☐ 1. Chlorine gas
☐ 2. Isocyanates
☐ 3. Pollen from flowering plants
☐ 4. Cotton dust
☐ 5. *Dermatophagoides pteronyssinus*

34. THEME: INHALED DRUGS

A Salmeterol
B Ipratropium bromide
C Zafirlukast
D Sodium cromoglicate
E Beclomethasone diproprionate
F Salbutamol

For each of the following descriptions select the appropriate inhaled drug from the list above. The items may be used once or not at all.

☐ 1. Short-acting β^2-adrenoceptor agonist
☐ 2. Long-acting β^2-adrenoceptor agonist
☐ 3. Anticholinergic agent
☐ 4. Mast cell stabiliser
☐ 5. Corticosteroid

RHEUMATOLOGY

35. THEME: RHEUMATOLOGICAL DISEASE RISK FACTORS

A   Systemic lupus erythematosus
B   Gout
C   Reiter's syndrome
D   Fibromyalgia
E   Pyrophosphate arthropathy
F   Dermatomyositis

For each of the following risk factors select the appropriate rheumatological condition from the list above. The items may be used once or not at all.

☐ 1. Glucose-6-phosphatase deficiency
☐ 2. Haemochromatosis
☐ 3. Procainamide therapy
☐ 4. Bronchial carcinoma
☐ 5. *Campylobacter* gastroenteritis

36. THEME: LESIONS AND NODES

A   Bouchard's node
B   Aschoff nodule
C   Rheumatoid nodule
D   Gouty tophus
E   Heberden's node
F   Osler's node

For each of the following lesions select the appropriate node/nodule from the list above. The items may be used once or not at all.

☐ 1. Small, circumscribed, erythematous, tender cutaneous nodule on the pulp of a finger
☐ 2. Bony swelling at the distal interphalangeal joint
☐ 3. Bony swelling at the proximal interphalangeal joint
☐ 4. Irregular firm nodule on the cartilaginous helix of the ear
☐ 5. Perivascular lesion with a central core of necrotic material

DERMATOLOGY

37. THEME: FACIAL ERUPTIONS

A   Angular cheilitis
B   Erysipelas
C   Rosacea
D   Lupus erythematosus
E   Contact dermatitis
F   Seborrhoeic dermatitis

For each of the following statements select the appropriate facial eruption from the list above. The items may be used once or not at all.

☐ 1. Red papules and pustules occurring on the greasy skin of the forehead, cheeks, chin and nose
☐ 2. Often caused by *candida* infection
☐ 3. Usually caused by *Pityrosporum ovale* infection
☐ 4. Eyelid oedema is frequently seen
☐ 5. Generally exacerbated by sunlight

38. THEME: CUTANEOUS DRUG ERUPTIONS

A   Urticaria
B   Erythema multiforme
C   Psoriasiform eruption
D   Toxic erythema
E   Eczematous eruption
F   Fixed drug eruption

For each of the following select the appropriate cutaneous eruption from the list above. The items may be used once or not at all.

☐ 1. Widespread, erythematous, maculopapular rash more marked on the trunk than limbs
☐ 2. Immediate reaction caused by type I hypersensitivity
☐ 3. Erythematous lesions more numerous on extremities than trunk and often involving palms and soles
☐ 4. Type IV hypersensitivity often caused by previous sensitisation to topical agents
☐ 5. Discrete erythematous plaques occurring at the same site on repeated occasions

HAEMATOLOGY

39. THEME: CLOTTING

A   Disseminated intravascular coagulation
B   von Willebrand's disease
C   Haemophilia
D   Heparin
E   Vitamin K deficiency
F   Idiopathic thrombocytopenic purpura

For each of the following clotting results select the appropriate condition from the list above. The items may be used once or not at all.

(PT = prothrombin time, APTT = activated partial thromboplastin time)

☐ 1. Normal PT, platelet count and bleeding time; markedly prolonged APTT and thrombin time
☐ 2. Markedly prolonged PT, APTT and thrombin time; prolonged bleeding time; low platelet count
☐ 3. Normal PT, APTT and thrombin time; prolonged bleeding time; low platelet count
☐ 4. Normal thrombin time, platelet count and bleeding time; markedly prolonged PT; prolonged APTT
☐ 5. Normal PT, thrombin time, platelet count and bleeding time; markedly prolonged APTT

40. THEME: WHITE BLOOD CELL ABNORMALITIES

A   Dohle bodies
B   Pelger-Huët cells
C   Atypical lymphocytes
D   Drumstick appendage to nucleus
E   Hypersegmented neutrophils
F   Giant lysosomes

For each of the following conditions select the appropriate white blood cell abnormality from the list above. The items may be used once or not at all.

☐ 1. Myeloproliferative disease
☐ 2. Chediak-Higashi disease
☐ 3. Vitamin B_{12} deficiency
☐ 4. Severe burns
☐ 5. Acute Epstein-Barr virus infection

41. THEME: HAEMOLYSIS

A   Schumm's test
B   Reticulocyte count
C   Direct antiglobulin test
D   Haptoglobin
E   Indirect antiglobulin test
F   Blood film examination for helmet cells

For each of the following descriptions select the appropriate investigation of haemolysis from the list above. The items may be used once or not at all.

☐ 1. Detects antibody on patients' red blood cells
☐ 2. Detects antibody in patient's serum
☐ 3. Identifies methaemalbumin, a marker of intravascular haemolysis
☐ 4. Indicates level of red cell turnover
☐ 5. Indicates microangiopathic damage

INFECTIOUS DISEASES AND TROPICAL MEDICINE

42. THEME: DIAGNOSIS OF INFECTION

A   Falciparum malaria
B   Onchocerciasis
C   Syphilis
D   Neonatal HIV infection
E   Hookworm
F   Disseminated *Mycobacterium avium*

For each of the following diagnostic methods select the appropriate infection from the list above. The items may be used once or not at all.

☐ 1. Blood culture
☐ 2. Skin biopsy
☐ 3. Nucleic acid sequence binding assay
☐ 4. Specific antibody detection
☐ 5. Antigen detection test on blood

43. THEME: INFECTIOUS ORGANISM TRANSMISSION

A   Mosquito-borne
B   Water ingestion
C   Airborne
D   Direct contact with respiratory droplets
E   Sexual transmission
F   Water contact

For each of the following infectious organisms select the usual mode of transmission from the list above. The items may be used once or not at all.

☐ 1. *Haemophilus ducreyi*
☐ 2. *Dracunculus medinensis*
☐ 3. *Schistosoma haematobium*
☐ 4. *Neisseria meningitidis*
☐ 5. *Mycobacterium tuberculosis*

44. THEME: ANTIBIOTICS

A   No recommended treatment
B   Linezolid
C   Ceftazidime
D   Meropenem
E   Co-trimoxazole
F   Vancomycin

For each of the following bacterial infections select the recommended antibiotic treatment from the list above. The items may be used once or not at all.

☐ 1. *Burkholderia pseudomallei* septicaemia
☐ 2. *Stenotrophomonas maltophilia* pneumonia
☐ 3. Extended spectrum β-lactamase producing *Klebsiella pneumoniae* meningitis
☐ 4. Vancomycin-resistant *Enterococcus faecalis* bacteraemia
☐ 5. *Escherichia coli* O157:H7 colitis

45. THEME: MALIGNANCY ASSOCIATED WITH MICROORGANISMS

A   Adult T cell leukaemia
B   Kaposi's sarcoma
C   Hepatocellular carcinoma
D   Lymphoma of mucosa-associated lymphoid tissue
E   Nasopharyngeal carcinoma
F   Squamous cell carcinoma of anus

For each of the following microorganisms select the appropriate malignancy from the list above. The items may be used once or not at all.

☐ 1. Epstein-Barr virus
☐ 2. HTLV1
☐ 3. Human papilloma virus
☐ 4. Human herpes virus 8
☐ 5. *Helicobacter pylori*

GENITOURINARY MEDICINE

46. THEME: GENITOURINARY CONDITIONS

A   *Treponema pertenue*
B   *Gardnerella vaginalis*
C   *Treponema pallidum*
D   *Chlamydia trachomatis*
E   *Trichomonas vaginalis*
F   Herpes simplex virus

For each of the following genitourinary conditions select the appropriate causative organism from the list above. The items may be used once or not at all.

☐ 1. Vaginitis with a copious foamy discharge with pH >4.5
☐ 2. Vaginitis with malodorous vaginal discharge and 'clue cells' on a wet preparation
☐ 3. Single painless penile dry ulcer with no lymphadenopathy
☐ 4. Prostatitis in an 18-year-old man
☐ 5. Group of multiple painful ulcers with purulent exudate

CLINICAL PHARMACOLOGY

47. THEME: PRESCRIBING FOR INFECTIOUS DISEASES

A   Palivizumab
B   Lamivudine
C   Ribavirin
D   Zidovudine
E   Foscarnet
F   Zanamivir

For each of the following select the appropriate agent from the list above. The items may be used once or not at all.

☐ 1. Treatment of established hepatitis B
☐ 2. Adjunctive therapy for eradication of hepatitis C
☐ 3. Treatment of cytomegalovirus pneumonia
☐ 4. Treatment of established influenza A virus infection
☐ 5. Prophylaxis against respiratory syncytial virus

48. THEME: PHARMACOKINETIC INTERACTIONS

A   Warfarin and colestyramine
B   Oestrogens and rifampicin
C   Theophylline and erythromycin
D   Lithium and thiazide diuretics
E   Bezafibrate and simvastatin
F   Digoxin and amiodarone

For each of the following mechanisms of pharmacokinetic interactions select the appropriate drug pair from the list above. The items may be used once or not at all.

☐ 1. Increased drug metabolism
☐ 2. Decreased drug metabolism
☐ 3. Decreased renal tubular secretion
☐ 4. Increased renal tubular reabsorption
☐ 5. Decreased gastrointestinal absorption

49. THEME: CONDITIONS AND DRUGS TO BE AVOIDED

A   Glucose-6-phosphate dehydrogenase (G6PD) deficiency
B   Diabetes mellitus
C   Moderate renal impairment
D   Liver disease
E   Acute porphyria
F   None of the above

For each of the following drugs select the condition from the list above in which the drug should be avoided. The items may be used once or not at all.

☐ 1. Intravenous ceftriaxone
☐ 2. Oral ofloxacin
☐ 3. Oral tetracycline
☐ 4. Oral itraconazole
☐ 5. Intravenous quinine

50. THEME: ADVERSE DRUG REACTIONS

A   Fever with eosinophilia
B   Myositis
C   Systemic lupus erythematosus
D   Pulmonary alveolitis
E   Psoriasis
F   Colour blindness

For each of the following drugs select the adverse reaction from the list above that is associated with it. The items may be used once or not at all.

☐ 1. Phenytoin
☐ 2. Amiodarone
☐ 3. Ethambutol
☐ 4. Dapsone
☐ 5. Simvastatin

51. THEME: CYTOTOXIC DRUGS AND THEIR ADVERSE EFFECTS

A   Paclitaxel
B   Busulfan
C   Cyclophosphamide
D   Doxorubicin
E   Vinblastine
F   Vincristine

For each of the following adverse effects select the most likely cytotoxic drug from the list above. The items may be used once or not at all.

☐ 1. Haemorrhagic cystitis
☐ 2. Progressive pulmonary fibrosis
☐ 3. Cardiomyopathy
☐ 4. Peripheral and autonomic neuropathy
☐ 5. Severe hypersensitivity reactions

52. THEME: CORTICOSTEROID POTENCY

A   Betamethasone valerate 0.1%
B   Clobetasone butyrate 0.05%
C   Hydrocortisone 1%
D   Fludrocortisone
E   Clobetasol propionate 0.05%
F   Calcipotriol

For each of the following levels of relative corticosteroid potency select the appropriate topical steroid preparation from the list above. The items may be used once or not at all.

☐ 1. No corticosteroid activity
☐ 2. Mild corticosteroid
☐ 3. Moderately potent corticosteroid
☐ 4. Potent corticosteroid
☐ 5. Very potent corticosteroid

CARDIOVASCULAR MEDICINE

53. THEME: ECG

A   Left bundle branch block
B   Right bundle branch block
C   Acute anteroseptal myocardial infarct
D   Acute inferior myocardial infarct
E   Left ventricular hypertrophy
F   Right ventricular hypertrophy

For each of the following electrocardiographic patterns select the appropriate cardiac condition from the list above. The items may be used once or not at all.

☐ 1. S wave in lead V_6 greater than 30 mm and QRS width less than 100 ms
☐ 2. Absent R wave in lead V_1 and QRS width greater than 120 ms
☐ 3. Dominant R wave in lead V_1 and QRS width less than 100 ms
☐ 4. Dominant R wave in lead V_1 and QRS width greater than 120 ms
☐ 5. Q waves and greater than 2 mm ST elevation in leads V_1 to V_4 and QRS less than 100 ms

54. THEME: HEART MURMURS

A   Aortic stenosis
B   Ventricular septal defect
C   Mitral valve prolapse
D   Patent ductus arteriosus
E   Pulmonary regurgitation
F   Mitral stenosis

For each of the following heart murmurs select the appropriate cardiac abnormality from the list above. The items may be used once or not at all.

☐ 1. Late systolic murmur
☐ 2. Early diastolic murmur
☐ 3. Mid-diastolic murmur
☐ 4. Pansystolic murmur
☐ 5. Ejection systolic murmur

55. THEME: BROAD COMPLEX TACHYARRHYTHMIA

A   Atrial fibrillation with an accessory pathway
B   Torsade de pointes
C   Ventricular tachycardia
D   Atrioventricular re-entry tachycardia plus functional left bundle branch block
E   Atrial fibrillation with left bundle branch block
F   Atrioventricular nodal re-entry tachycardia plus functional left bundle branch block

For each of the following findings select the appropriate type of broad complex tachyarrhythmia from the list above. The items may be used once or not at all.

- [ ] 1. Irregular rhythm, absent R in V_1, ST depression and T wave inversion in the left precordial leads
- [ ] 2. Irregular rhythm, previous resting ECG shows a short PR interval
- [ ] 3. Irregular rhythm with varying QRS axis, previous resting ECG shows long QT interval
- [ ] 4. Regular rhythm, atrioventricular dissociation and occasional capture beats
- [ ] 5. Regular rhythm, absent R in V_1, ST depression and T wave inversion in the left precordial leads, resting ECG shows a short PR interval

56. THEME: CARDIAC PROBLEMS ASSOCIATED WITH OTHER CONDITIONS

A Aortic stenosis
B Pulmonary stenosis
C Tricuspid regurgitation
D Coarctation of the aorta
E Mitral regurgitation
F Aortic regurgitation

For each of the following conditions select the associated cardiac problem from the list above. The items may be used once or not at all.

- [ ] 1. Myocardial infarction
- [ ] 2. Turner's syndrome
- [ ] 3. Syphilis
- [ ] 4. Endocarditis in an intravenous drug user
- [ ] 5. Fallot's tetralogy

PSYCHIATRY

57. THEME: CLASSIFICATION

A Bulimia nervosa
B Psychogenic vomiting
C Anorexia nervosa
D Pica
E Alcohol dependence syndrome
F Lysergic acid diethylamide (LSD) abuse

For each of the following statements select the appropriate condition from the list above. The items may be used once or not at all.

- [ ] 1. Weight is 15% less than that expected for age, sex and height
- [ ] 2. Withdrawal symptoms are a prominent feature
- [ ] 3. Episodic involuntary vomiting occurs
- [ ] 4. Associated with mental retardation
- [ ] 5. Synaesthesia is a frequent symptom

58. THEME: PSYCHIATRIC SYMPTOMS

A Autoscopic hallucination
B Delusional perception
C Delusional mood
D Third person auditory hallucination
E Elementary hallucination
F Second person auditory hallucination

For each of the following descriptions select the appropriate psychiatric symptom from the list above. The items may be used once or not at all.

- [ ] 1. Patient hears a running commentary describing his/her actions
- [ ] 2. Patient sees his/her own body projected into external space
- [ ] 3. Patient hears a voice give him/her a command
- [ ] 4. Patient sees a real traffic light change colour and interprets it as a message from God
- [ ] 5. Patient incorrectly thinks he/she is dying as a result of a change in affect

59. THEME: SCHIZOPHRENIA

A   Tic
B   Posturing
C   Mannerism
D   Stereotypy
E   Echolalia
F   Echopraxia

For each of the following descriptions select the appropriate feature of schizophrenia from the list above. The items may be used once or not at all.

☐ 1. Repeated regular movements without obvious significance
☐ 2. Repeated movements with obvious significance
☐ 3. Persistently repeating another person's words
☐ 4. Persistently repeating another person's movements
☐ 5. Adoption of an unusual position for a sustained period of time

MISCELLANEOUS

60. THEME: IMPAIRED DECISION-MAKING CAPACITY

A   Guardian
B   Caregiver
C   Surrogate decision-maker
D   Durable power of attorney for health care
E   Advance directive
F   Living will

For each of the following descriptions related to patients with impaired decision-making capacity select the appropriate term from the list above. The items may be used once or not at all.

☐ 1. An informal representative of the patient's premorbid wishes
☐ 2. A person who has been formally appointed by the courts to make decisions on the patient's behalf

☐ 3. A prior formal written statement by a competent patient directing when to withdraw and when to withhold life-sustaining treatment
☐ 4. Informal verbal or written communications by a competent patient indicating future wishes in the event of developing impaired decision-making capacity
☐ 5. An informal advisor on the patient's recent quality of life

ANSWERS TO PAPER 2

The approximate difficulty rating for the answer to each question is given in brackets.

☆ (the majority of competent final year students will know the answer)

☆☆ (approximately 50% of final year students will be able to answer correctly)

☆☆☆ (only the better students will usually know the answer)

Q1. ONCOGENES (☆☆☆)

1. F   2. D   3. A   4. B   5. C

Cancer is due to abnormal proliferation of cells. This can occur when a gene causing cell growth and replication is overexpressed or when the function of a tumour suppressor gene is disrupted. H-ras, K-ras and N-ras are GTP-binding proteins found in cytoplasm. Point mutations in the genes that encode these proteins result in loss of function and this is associated with the development of cancers. Mutations disrupting the *K-ras* gene occur in 75% of pancreatic cancers, 35% of colonic cancers and 30% of lung cancers. The *bcr-abl* fusion gene arises when a translocation occurs between chromosome 9p and the immunoglobulin region on 22q (the Philadelphia chromosome). Occasionally the chromosome 9 translocation is to the immunoglobulin regions on chromosomes 2 or 14. The protein product of this fusion gene has increased tyrosine kinase activity and stimulates unregulated cell proliferation causing the development of chronic myeloid leukaemia (CML). The *bcr-abl* gene rearrangement is present in 90% of cases of CML. *c-myc* encodes a nuclear protein. Overexpression of this gene follows chromosome translocation or gene amplification. This *c-myc* overexpression is often found in breast cancers. *p53* is a tumour suppressor gene which is important in cell cycle control. It is believed to halt the cell cycle before DNA replication occurs if chromosomal DNA is damaged. *p53* plays a key role in preventing many different cancers. Point mutations in *p53* resulting in gene dysfunction are associated with breast, colon and lung cancers. *Rb1* is also a tumour suppressor gene. A retinoblastoma develops if both copies of this gene are deleted. In hereditary retinoblastoma one mutant copy of the gene is inherited and the second mutation occurs in somatic cells. The retinoic acid receptor α (RARα) gene is located on chromosome 17q12-21. A translocation between chromosome 15q22 (where the PML locus occurs) and chromosome 17q12-21 produces a fusion gene called *PML-RARα*. The product of this fusion gene stimulates a growth factor receptor causing proliferation of promyelocytic cell lines. It is present in the great majority of cases of acute promyelocytic leukaemia. All-*trans*-retinoic acid can induce complete remission in this condition.

Q2. INTRACELLULAR ORGANELLES (☆)

1. D   2. F   3. A   4. B   5. C

Mitochondria are found only in eukaryotic organisms. They contain their own genetic information (which is inherited only from the mother) and are the site of the cell's energy production. Ribosomes are the site at which messenger RNA is converted into a polypeptide chain, a process known as translation. The nucleus stores the cell's genetic information and is the site of transcription, which is the conversion of DNA into messenger RNA. Most cytoplasmic reactions occur on the endoplasmic reticulum. Rough endoplasmic reticulum has ribosomes attached along its surface and smooth endoplasmic reticulum does not. Lysosomes are membrane-bound vesicles that can digest unwanted material. In the case of phagocytes, lysosomes fuse with phagosomes, which contain foreign material ingested from the cell surface. The resultant phagolysosome becomes acidified, enabling the destruction of potentially harmful bacteria. The Golgi apparatus is involved in the transport of proteins to the cell membrane.

Q3. STATISTICAL DEFINITIONS (☆)

1. B   2. F   3. A   4. E   5. D

The mean and standard deviation are respectively used to describe the location and spread of values in a normal distribution. The mean is the arithmetic average or the sum of all values divided by the number of values. The standard deviation describes the spread of individual values around the mean. In the normal distribution, 67% of all values are located within plus or minus one standard deviation of the mean and 95% are within two standard deviations. Often we do not know the true mean of a population and we take a sample to try to estimate it. The larger the sample size the more accurate the estimate is likely to be. If we take several samples of equal size the mean value of the sample means will be the same as the true population mean. However, the individual sample means may differ from the population mean due to chance. The spread of the sample means around the true population mean is called the standard error of the mean. This value is often confused with standard deviation. The difference is that the standard deviation is a measure of the spread of individual values and the standard error is a measure of the precision of the estimate of the mean. The term variance is also sometimes used and this is the square of the standard deviation. The range is the spread of the highest to lowest values. This is useful to examine whether a distribution is skewed rather than normal. Skewed distributions are not symmetrically distributed around the mean and are said to be positively skewed if there are unusually high values or negatively skewed if there are unusually low ones. In a skewed distribution, the median is a better estimate than the mean of the 'average' value, as it is less distorted by extreme outliers. The mode is the most frequently occurring value and may be useful to examine unusual distributions.

Q4. IMMUNOGLOBULIN ISOTYPES (☆)

1. E   2. F   3. A   4. C   5. D

There are four subtypes of immunoglobulin (IgG). IgG1 is the major subtype found in serum. IgG binds C1q, crosses the placenta and is important in the secondary response to infection. IgM is the initial immunoglobulin produced in the primary response to infection. It is found in serum as five IgM molecules bound together by a J chain. IgM can also bind C1q. Serological tests for IgM and IgG can be used to distinguish between recent and previous infections. In an acute infection, IgM will be positive, whereas if infection occurred in the past only IgG will be positive. IgA is secreted as a dimeric molecule joined by a J chain and attached to mucosa by a secretory piece. It is involved in mucosal immunity in the gut and the respiratory tract. IgD and IgE are present at very low concentrations in serum. IgD is found bound to B cells in lymphoid follicles. IgE is bound to mast cells via the Fc portion of its epsilon-chain. Crosslinking of IgE molecules by foreign antigens produces mast cell degranulation with release of histamine, kinins and leukotrienes. IgE is important in the host response to helminths and plays an important part in type I hypersensitivity reactions. IgB does not exist.

Q5. CYTOKINES (☆☆☆)

1. B   2. C   3. A   4. F   5. D

Cytokines are small polypeptides that act as signals between cells of the immune system. Interferon γ is a 20- to 24-kDa molecule produced by T helper (Th$_1$) and cytotoxic T lymphocytes, which binds to macrophages, monocytes, B cells, fibroblasts, epithelial and endothelial cells. It causes cell activation and proliferation and increases HLA class I and II antigen expression. Tumour necrosis factor α (TNFα) is so-named because it can lyse tumour cells in vitro. It is produced by T cells and macrophages and is responsible (with interleukins 1 and 6) for much of the fever, inflammation and shock that occur in infections. TNFα is important in the host response to infection but in excess quantities may cause harm. The TNFα-blocking antibody infliximab and the soluble TNFα receptor etanercept are used to suppress inflammation in treatment-resistant, highly active rheumatoid arthritis and Crohn's disease. Interleukin 2 is a 15- to 20-kDa molecule produced by Th_1 cells which binds to activated T cells via CD25, stimulating T cell activation and proliferation. Interleukin 4 is a 15- to 19-kDa molecule produced by Th_2 cells which binds to T and B cells, bone marrow cells, fibroblasts, epithelial and endothelial cells. It promotes IgE production and activates macrophages to produce proinflammatory cytokines. It also inhibits Th_1 cell activation. Interleukin 8 is a small cysteine-rich peptide that is chemoattractant for neutrophils. Other chemokines include macrophage inflammatory proteins and RANTES (**r**egulated on **a**ctivation, **n**ormal **T** cell **e**xpressed and **s**ecreted). Interferon α is produced by many cells and enhances natural cellular resistance to viral infections.

Q6. PATTERNS OF INHERITANCE (☆☆)

1. F   2. A   3. D   4. C   5. B

Becker and Duchenne muscular dystrophy are both caused by abnormalities of the very large dystrophin gene on the X chromosome. Becker is a clinically milder variant with later presentation. Severe, progressive muscular weakness and cardiomyopathy are characteristic. Huntington's chorea is an autosomal dominant condition caused by expansion of a triplet repeat sequence in a gene on chromosome 4, which encodes the

Huntington protein. Psychiatric symptoms may precede the development of chorea and progressive neurological deterioration by many years. There is much debate about the ethics of screening for this condition. Vitamin-D-resistant rickets is usually an X-linked dominant condition due to abnormalities in a gene designated *PHEX,* although there are also rare autosomal dominant and recessive forms. Leber's hereditary optic neuropathy is usually caused by point mutations in subunit 4 of respiratory chain 1 of the mitochondrial genome. Interaction with an X-linked gene may also be involved explaining the variable inheritance and penetrance patterns observed in this condition. Cystic fibrosis is an autosomal recessive condition due to mutations in the cystic fibrosis transmembrane conductance regulator *CFTR* gene on chromosome 7. Fifty-four per cent of European cystic fibrosis patients are homozygous for the ΔF508 mutation and 20% are heterozygotes. The ΔF508 nomenclature indicates that the mutation results in deletion of a phenylalanine amino acid from position 508 of the polypeptide chain. Patients who have one ΔF508 mutation and one other *CFTR* gene mutation (compound homozygotes) usually have less severe clinical disease and normal pancreatic function. The pseudoautosomal region is the part of the sex chromosomes common to the X and Y chromosomes.

Q7. GENETIC ABNORMALITIES (☆☆)

1. F   2. D   3. E   4. A   5. C

Trinucleotide repeat expansion is responsible for fragile X syndrome, Huntington's disease, myotonic dystrophy and several rarer diseases. In fragile X syndrome there is expansion of CGG repeats in the FMR1 gene at Xq27.3. Fewer than 50 copies of the repeat is believed to be normal; approximately 55 to 200 denotes a phenotypically normal 'pre-mutation' state. In fragile X patients there is instability of the region with massive expansion of the repeat and length variability between cells. In several trinucleotide repeat disorders, successive generations of affected individuals manifest progressively earlier and more severe disease. This process of 'genetic anticipation' was first described for myotonic dystrophy and is due to expansion of the unstable repeat between generations. There are two copies of the α-globin gene on each chromosome 16. α⁰-thalassaemia occurs when both copies of the gene are deleted and α⁺-thalassaemia is due to deletion of one copy. $\alpha^0\alpha^0$ homozygotes produce no α-globin chains, resulting in fatal hydrops fetalis. Most heterozygotes have mild disease unless they have another globin gene abnormality. The sickle cell mutation is a point mutation that results in a glutamic acid to valine amino acid substitution at position 6 of the β-globin chain. Only homozygotes suffer from sickling crises. The Turner's syndrome karyotype is 45X0. Affected subjects generally have short stature and poorly developed secondary sexual characteristics. Genomic imprinting refers to chromosomal regions where the genes inherited from one parental sex are always inactivated. If a gene abnormality exists but is inactivated it will exert no effect, but if the normal allele is inactivated then the abnormality will be expressed. For example, in Prader-Willi syndrome (gene on 15q12) only paternal transmission of the condition can occur as the maternal gene is inactivated. In contrast maternal transmission of the same region results in Angelman's syndrome, a phenotypically different condition. Despite extensive studies on schizophrenia, no conclusive evidence of an inherited defect has been identified.

Q8. CRANIAL NERVES (☆☆)

1. B   2. E   3. D   4. C   5. A

The olfactory nerve (CN I) enters the skull via openings in the cribriform plate of the ethmoid. Unilateral anosmia may be caused by a tumour such as a meningioma in the olfactory groove. The ophthalmic, maxillary and mandibular divisions of the trigeminal nerve (CN V) enter the skull through the superior orbital fissure, foramen rotundum and foramen ovale respectively. These then connect in the gasserian ganglion. The glossopharyngeal nerve (CN IX) enters the skull through the jugular foramen with the vagus (CN X) and accessory (CN XI) nerves. Tumours in this area may cause disruption of the function of all three nerves but sparing the function of the hypoglossal nerve (CN XII). The facial nerve (CN VII) enters the petrous part of the temporal bone through the stylomastoid foramen, passes along the facial canal and into the cranium through the internal acoustic meatus. It then passes though the cerebellopontine angle to its nucleus in the pons. Tumours in the cerebellopontine angle can cause ipsilateral fifth, seventh and eighth nerve palsies. The facial nerve gives off several branches along its course including the chorda tympani, parasympathetic supply to the lacrimal, submandibular, sublingual and salivary glands and the nerve to stapedius. Whether or not disruption of the function of these nerves has occurred is useful in identifying the likely anatomical site of a facial nerve lesion. The hypoglossal nerve leaves the skull through the hypoglossal foramen.

Q9. NERVE ROOTS (☆)

1. C   2. B   3. A   4. F   5. E

The tendon stretch reflexes are useful for localising pathology in the spinal cord or spinal nerve roots. It is also important to know the nerve root supply of the cutaneous reflexes: the superficial abdominal, the cremaster and the Babinski (plantar) reflexes. The biceps and supinator reflexes are both supplied by C5-C6, triceps by C6-C7, finger jerk by C7-C8, superficial abdominal by T7-T12, cremaster by L2, knee by L2-L4, ankle by S1-S2 and Babinski by S1. If the spinal cord is transected the effect of inhibitory neurones on the reflex arc is lost. Tendon stretch reflexes below that point will therefore be exaggerated or brisk. If there is nerve root damage preventing completion of the spinal reflex arc then the reflex will be absent. Reinforcement may be necessary to confirm a reflex is present if it cannot initially be demonstrated.

Q10. TUMOUR MARKERS (☆☆)

1. D   2. A   3. F   4. B   5. C

Tumour markers are blood assays that are frequently elevated in the presence of one or more types of cancer. They can be used as screening tests in the healthy population (eg the controversial use of prostate-specific antigen–psa–to screen for prostatic cancer) or to monitor response to therapy or relapse following remission. β-human chorionic gonadotrophin (β-HCG) is produced by trophoblastic tissue and is elevated in pregnancy, hydatidiform mole, choriocarcinoma and testicular germline tumours. CA stands for either carbohydrate antigen or cancer antigen. CA-125 is most frequently elevated in ovarian cancer but is also associated with cancers of the lung, gastrointestinal tract and cervix. CA-15.3 is two antigens detected by two monoclonal antibodies called 115D8 and DF3. 115D8 is an antibody against an antigen of milk fat globule membranes. DF3 is an antibody that detects an antigen from human breast cancer. The CA-15.3 test is a sandwich ELISA, which is only positive if both antigens are present. CA-19.9 is elevated in 80% of patients with pancreatic cancer. However, it can also be elevated in pancreatitis, cystic fibrosis and inflammatory bowel disease. α-fetoprotein is the major serum protein in the fetus. It is elevated in hepatocellular carcinoma and testicular and ovarian germline tumours. Other tumour markers include calcitonin produced by medullary thyroid cancer and carcino-embryonic antigen produced by colon, lung and breast cancer. PSA is elevated in prostate cancer and acute prostatitis.

Q11. CRYSTALS IN SYNOVIAL FLUID (☆☆)

1. B   2. F   3. D   4. C   5. A

Phase-contrast microscopy is useful for identifying crystals present in synovial fluid. Monosodium urate crystals are negatively birefringent, needle-shaped crystals located in intra- and extracellular locations. They occur in gout and are associated with a raised serum uric acid, though in an acute attack the serum level may fall, confusing the diagnosis. Calcium pyrophosphate crystals occur in pseudogout. They are positively birefringent rods, needles and rhomboid shapes, located intra- and extracellularly. Pseudogout is associated with hyperparathyroidism, haemochromatosis, hypophosphatasia and hypomagnesaemia. Chondrocalcinosis is often present with calcium pyrophosphate crystals. Cholesterol crystals occur extracellularly and are negatively birefringent, notched rhombic shapes. These crystals occur in hypercholesterolaemia and in chronic synovitis (eg in rheumatoid arthritis). Hydroxyapatite crystals are small intra- and extracellular needle-shaped crystals which may require electron microscopy to be seen. They are associated with osteoarthritis. Corticosteroid crystals are located intracellularly in those who have received intra-articular steroid injections. They are positively and negatively birefringent, flat and variably shaped crystals. Cystine crystals are deposited in tissues throughout the body in the rare condition of cystinosis.

Q12. DIABETIC COMA (☆☆)

1. B   2. D   3. F   4. A   5. E

Diabetics can present with coma for several different reasons. Diabetic ketoacidosis occurs only in type I diabetes. There is elevation of blood glucose and ketones and serum osmolality. Blood pH and serum bicarbonate are low and the patient is usually dehydrated. Anion gap is defined as the sum of serum sodium plus potassium ions minus bicarbonate and chloride (i.e. $Na^+ + K^+ - Cl^- - HCO_3^-$). The anion gap is increased when other anions such as ketones are present. In hypoglycaemia, there are low glucose, no ketones and osmolality, pH, bicarbonate and anion gap are usually normal. Hypoglycaemia can be caused by insulin or oral hypoglycaemic agents. Severe sepsis can cause lactic acidosis with a low pH and bicarbonate and usually a high blood glucose. The anion gap is markedly increased. Rarely lactic acidosis can be caused by metformin. In hyperosmolar non-ketoacidotic coma (HONK), blood glucose and serum osmolality are markedly elevated and the patient is usually very dehydrated. The pH, bicarbonate and anion gap are normal. HONK occurs in type II diabetics. In salicylate poisoning pH and bicarbonate are low and the anion gap is increased due to salicylic acid. The presence of ketones and dehydration are variable and the blood glucose and serum osmolality are usually normal.

Q13. THYROID HORMONE PRODUCTION (☆☆☆)

1. A   2. F   3. B   4. D   5. C

In the thyroid gland follicles, iodine is incorporated into the tyrosine residues of thyroglobulin to produce the hormonally inactive molecules monoiodotyrosine and diiodotyrosine. Thyroid peroxidase catalyses this reaction and couples the resultant iodotyrosyl residues together to form T_4 (thyroxine) and T_3 (triiodothyronine). T_4 consists of two diiodotyrosine molecules and T_3 consists of one molecule of monoiodotyrosine and one of diiodotyrosine. Thyroglobulin is a large glycoprotein molecule that is secreted into the follicular lumen colloid. The production of thyroglobulin is regulated by thyroid-stimulating hormone. Following the reactions catalysed by thyroid peroxidase, thyroglobulin undergoes proteolytic cleavage to release T_4 and T_3 into the systemic circulation. T_4 is produced in approximately 20 times the quantities of T_3 and is the predominant thyroid hormone found in the blood. However, T_3 is the most hormonally active thyroid hormone and T_4 therefore undergoes peripheral conversion to T_3.

Q14. VITAMINS (☆☆☆)

1. F   2. E   3. D   4. B   5. C

Vitamins A, D, E and K are fat soluble and the B group vitamins and vitamin C are water soluble. Thiamine (vitamin B_1) is involved in the glycolytic and pentose phosphate pathways of carbohydrate metabolism. Deficiency causes beriberi, a condition of high output cardiac failure or neurological degeneration causing demyelination, peripheral neuritis, Wernicke-Korsakoff syndrome and muscle atrophy. Riboflavin (vitamin B_2) is involved in the electron transport of oxidative metabolism and the metabolism of short-chain fatty acids. Deficiency causes dermatitis, angular stomatitis, cheilosis and glossitis. Nicotinic acid is a cofactor for nicotinamide adenine dinucleotide (NAD^+) and $NADP^+$, acting as an electron transporter for cellular respiration. Deficiency causes pellagra, the classic triad of photosensitive dermatitis, diarrhoea and dementia. Pyridoxine (vitamin B_6) is a cofactor for decarboxylases, deaminases and transaminases. Deficiency is often combined with other B group deficiencies, and symptoms resemble riboflavin deficiency. Pyridoxine is involved in the conversion of the amino acid tryptophan to nicotinic acid and deficiency can also lead to nicotinic acid deficiency and pellagra. Pyridoxal-5-phosphate is the active form of pyridoxine and the phosphorylation reaction can be blocked by isoniazid, hydralazine and penicillamine. Pyridoxine is therefore often given to those taking isoniazid, particularly if they are malnourished or have risk factors for the development of neuropathy (eg alcoholics and those infected with HIV). Hydroxycobalamine (vitamin B_{12}) is involved in the synthesis of nucleotide precursors for incorporation into DNA. Deficiency produces megaloblastic anaemia and neurological deterioration (eg subacute combined degeneration of the cord). Causes of hydroxocobalamin deficiency include terminal ileitis, pernicious anaemia, strict vegan diets and the fish tapeworm *Diphyllobothrium latum*. α-tocopherol (vitamin E) is an antioxidant that modulates free-radical damage. It is controversial whether high vitamin E intake may protect against cardiovascular disease.

Q15. RENAL TRACT INVESTIGATIONS (☆☆)

1. F   2. A   3. E   4. B   5. D

A positive dipstick test for blood can be caused by haematuria, haemoglobinuria or myoglobinuria. If there are no red blood cells seen on microscopy it is likely that the patient has haemoglobinuria due to intravascular haemolysis or myoglobinuria due to rhabdomyolysis. The presence of dysmorphic red blood cells (abnormal size and shape) in urine indicates that the source is from the kidney and not from lower down the urinary tract. Red cell casts are suggestive of a glomerular source of blood and are frequently seen in rapidly progressive glomerulonephritis. If a bladder tumour causes haemorrhage, red blood cells will be seen on microscopy but these will not be dysmorphic and there will not be red cell casts. The presence of numerous white blood cells in the urine with negative bacterial cultures is called sterile pyuria. Causes of this include renal tuberculosis, urinary tract infection due to a fastidious organism or with inhibition of growth by antibiotics, renal, ureteric or bladder calculi, analgesic nephropathy or drug-induced cystitis. A contaminated urine specimen is suggested by numerous squamous epithelial cells on microscopy. The significance of pyuria is then difficult to interpret and it is best to repeat the specimen. There may be a mixed bacterial growth from a contaminated specimen. Urethritis usually only causes pyuria in a first catch specimen. A midstream urine specimen contains few white blood cells. Bacterial culture will be negative but if the infection is due to *Chlamydia trachomatis* the chlamydial antigen test (on urethral swab) or the ligase chain reaction (on urine) will be positive.

Q16. URINARY PROTEIN EXCRETION (☆☆)

1. E   2. F   3. B   4. C   5. D

Daily albumin excretion by normal kidneys is less than approximately 50 mg per 24-hour period. Excretion of 50 to 200 mg per day is defined as microalbuminuria. This is below the level of detection of most urine dipsticks but it is important because in conditions such as diabetes it correlates with risk of later development of frank diabetic nephropathy. Tamm-Horsfall proteinuria is a normal finding. It refers to the urinary excretion of 20 to 30 mg per day of a 200-kDa glycoprotein by the thick limb of the loop of Henle. Urine dipsticks are sensitive for the detection of high molecular weight proteins such as albumin but are relatively insensitive to low molecular weight proteins. Dipstick tests are therefore generally negative in patients who have proteinuria due to damage to the proximal renal tubule (eg in cystinosis, heavy metal poisoning and connective tissue diseases). A tubular pattern of proteinuria is characterised by high levels of α_1-microglobulin, β_2-microglobulin, retinol binding protein, lysosome and immunoglobulins. In addition, immunoglobulin light chains may be found in the urine in patients with myeloma, a finding called Bence Jones proteinuria. Highly selective proteinuria indicates that there is much greater urinary excretion of the low molecular weight protein immunoglobulin G than there is of high molecular weight proteins such as albumin and transferrin. This is characteristic of minimal change nephropathy and carries a good prognosis in patients with the nephrotic syndrome. Non-selective proteinuria indicates that the ratio of immunoglobulin G to transferrin clearance is greater than 0.20. To measure this ratio, spot urine and plasma samples should be taken at the same time. A 24-hour collection is not necessary as the urine volumes are cancelled out in calculating the ratio $U_{IgG}. V/P_{IgG}:U_{transferrin}. V/P_{transferrin}.$

Q17. RENAL DISEASE HISTOLOGY (☆☆☆)

1. C   2. E   3. F   4. A   5. D

Diabetes mellitus causes glomerulosclerosis with nodule formation, an appearance known as the Kimmelstiel-Wilson lesion. There are also arteriolar hyalinosis and interstitial fibrosis. Patients initially develop microalbuminaemia and this progresses to proteinuria and in some cases eventual end-stage renal failure. The development of microalbuminuria is important because it is associated with increased risk of cardiac death. Chronic hepatitis B infection is associated with membranous nephropathy with subepithelial, subendothelial and mesangial deposits of antigen. There may also be a vasculitis and in some cases arteriolar microaneurysms occur. Amyloidosis of the immunoglobulin light chain type (AL) causes glomerular deposits, which appear as green birefringent material on polarised light microscopy. Later amyloid may be seen in tubules and in the interstitium. Immunofluorescence microscopy shows a peritubular pattern of monoclonal light chains along the tubular basement membrane. Sarcoidosis causes interstitial nephritis with the presence of non-caseating granulomas. This results in a tubular pattern of proteinuria and may lead to other features of Fanconi syndrome (eg glycosuria and phosphaturia). Hypercalcaemia may occur in sarcoidosis and this may also contribute to renal damage. Nephritis in systemic lupus erythematosus is characterised by diffuse mesangial aggregates that contain immunoglobulins G, A, M and the complement components C1q, C3 and C4. There may also be capillary thickening and/or glomerular crescent formation. Sjögren's syndrome causes a diffuse tubulointerstitial nephritis with infiltrates of lymphocytes, tubular atrophy and aggregates of immunoglobulin G and complement. Sjögren's syndrome is strongly associated with the development of the distal type of renal tubular acidosis.

Q18. RENAL DISEASE CLASSIFICATION (☆☆)

1. B   2. A   3. F   4. E   5. C

Immunoglobulin A nephropathy (Berger's disease) usually affects young adults and there is a predominance of male patients. The typical presentation is with recurrent episodes of pharyngitis, muscle pains, loin pains, high fever, lethargy and frank haematuria. These episodes each last around one to five days and there is then a rapid recovery. There is usually no hypertension or oedema. Henoch-Schönlein purpura affects the skin, kidneys, gut and joints. There is typically a flitting polyarthritis, colicky abdominal pain, palpable purpuric lesions on the extensor surfaces of the buttocks, ankles and elbows and acute glomerulonephritis. Diagnosis can be made by skin biopsy, which reveals immunoglobulin A and C3 in skin lesions. Thin membrane nephropathy is an autosomal dominant condition that causes persistent, asymptomatic, microscopic haematuria. Electron microscopy shows decreased width of the glomerular capillary basement membrane. The condition is believed to be benign and does not progress to renal failure. Minimal change nephropathy is the commonest cause of nephrotic syndrome in children aged one to six years. It also causes around a third of cases of nephrotic syndrome in adults. There is a highly selective proteinuria (immunoglobulin G clearance much greater than transferrin) without haematuria, hypertension or elevation of urea or creatinine. Remission can be rapidly induced with steroids in 90% of cases. Antiglomerular basement membrane antibody disease (Goodpasture's syndrome) affects the kidneys and lungs. It causes alveolar haemorrhage and rapidly progressive glomerulonephritis. Patients present with a short history of oliguria, peripheral oedema, breathlessness, malaise, myalgia, haemoptysis and fever. Haemoptysis typically occurs in smokers and is usually absent in non-smokers. Membranous nephropathy is an uncommon cause of nephrotic syndrome in children and causes around 30% of adult cases of this condition. There is often an underlying cause such as diabetes mellitus, drugs (eg penicillamine), systemic lupus erythematosus, rheumatoid arthritis, chronic hepatitis B or *Plasmodium malariae* infection.

Q19. INHERITED ABNORMALITY (☆☆☆)

1. B   2. D   3. A   4. E   5. C

Inherited enzyme deficiencies of the sex steroid, corticosteroid and mineralocorticoid metabolic pathways produce different forms of congenital adrenal hyperplasia. Hormones that are positioned after the enzyme block will be deficient and enzymes produced before the enzyme block will be found in excess. This is because of the lack of cortisol inhibitory feedback on the pituitary gland, resulting in excessive production of adrenocorticotrophic hormone. 21-hydroxylase deficiency is the commonest cause of congenital adrenal hyperplasia. Both this enzyme deficiency and the rarer 3β-hydroxysteroid dehydrogenase deficiency cause androgen excess and mineralocorticoid deficiency. Female infants have virilisation but male infants may not present until they develop severe salt wasting disease. 3β-hydroxysteroid dehydrogenase deficiency is often fatal. 17α-hydroxylase deficiency causes androgen deficiency and mineralocorticoid excess. This leads to hypertension and hyperkalaemia. 11β-hydroxylase deficiency leads to androgen excess and mineralocorticoid excess. Female fetuses are virilised, and hypertension and hyperkalaemia occur in both sexes. 5α-reductase converts testosterone to dihydrotestosterone. Deficiency of this enzyme results in males having ambiguous genitalia at birth. However, when testosterone production increases at puberty masculinisation occurs. Mutations of the Gsα cell signalling protein produce McCune-Albright's syndrome. This condition is characterised by polyostotic fibrous dysplasia, café-au-lait spots and endocrine dysfunction.

Q20. CORTICOSTEROID PRODUCTION REGULATION (☆)

1. C   2. F   3. A   4. D   5. B

Corticotrophin releasing hormone (CRH) is the main stimulator of adrenocorticotrophic hormone (ACTH) secretion by the anterior pituitary gland. Vasopressin alone has only a weak stimulatory action. However, it is important because it acts synergistically with CRH to augment ACTH release. Cortisol is produced by the adrenal gland in response to ACTH stimulation. It exerts direct negative feedback on ACTH secretion and indirect negative feedback by inhibition of vasopressin and CRH release. Pro-opiomelanocortin is a precursor molecule which is broken down to ACTH and β-lipotrophin. ACTH is subsequently broken down to corticotrophin-like peptide and melanocyte-stimulating hormone. β-lipotrophin is broken down to lipotrophin and β-endorphin. Gonadotrophin-releasing hormone regulates release of follicle-stimulating hormone and luteinising hormone. It does not influence secretion of ACTH.

Q21. PITUITARY FUNCTION TESTS (☆☆)

1. C   2. F   3. B   4. D   5. E

Tests of pituitary function fall into three categories:

1. Tests of baseline hormone levels [eg ACTH, follicle-stimulating hormone (FSH), luteinising hormone (LH), prolactin or thyroid-stimulating hormone (TSH) assays]
2. Tests of hormone secretion after stimulation (e.g. insulin tolerance test, metyrapone test, glucagon stimulation test, combined anterior pituitary test, TRH test)
3. Tests of hormone secretion after administration of specific inhibitors (oral glucose tolerance test, dexamethasone suppression test)

Baseline growth hormone levels vary widely and are therefore of little use in diagnosing growth hormone deficiency or acromegaly. The insulin tolerance test (ITT) is a good test of the adequacy of growth hormone secretion. This test also reveals the adequacy of ACTH secretion. Following the administration of insulin there is a peak of growth hormone and ACTH release after 45 to 60 minutes. The ITT requires supervision by a doctor because of the danger of hypoglycaemia and should generally not be used in those with ischaemic heart disease or epilepsy. Alternatives for investigating possible failure of growth hormone production include stimulation by levodopa, glucagon or arginine hydrochloride. An alternative for investigating suspected ACTH deficiency is the metyrapone test. This suppresses the negative feedback effect of cortisol on the pituitary and should stimulate ACTH release. In ACTH deficiency, the serum ACTH level does not rise. Baseline ACTH levels are useful for investigating adrenal failure and Cushing's disease. In both conditions the ACTH level will be high. In adrenal failure simultaneously measured cortisol will be low and in Cushing's disease it will be inappropriately high. The dexamethasone suppression test is also used in the diagnosis of Cushing's syndrome. The oral glucose tolerance test can be used to diagnose suspected acromegaly (and/or diabetes). In normal subjects serum growth hormone levels should be suppressed to less than 2 mU/l after this test, but they are not suppressed in acromegaly. The definitive diagnosis of acromegaly is now established by finding raised insulin-like growth factor 1 levels. The combined anterior pituitary test is a screening test of global pituitary function performed after pituitary surgery or irradiation. GnRH, TRH, CRH and GHRH are given simultaneously and sequential measurements of ACTH, TSH, LH, FSH, growth hormone and prolactin are subsequently performed.

Q22. PITUITARY TUMOURS (☆☆)

1. E 2. A 3. F 4. B 5. C

Pituitary tumours are now classified by their immunocytochemistry rather than simply as acidophilic, basophilic or chromophobe adenomas. The commonest hormone-secreting tumour is a lactotroph adenoma, which produces prolactin. Post-mortem studies suggest that 25% of the general population develop an asymptomatic lactotroph microadenoma. Clinical tumours present much less frequently than this but should always be considered as a potential cause of secondary amenorrhoea. Patients may also present with headache, impotence, galactorrhoea or visual field defects. In contrast, thyrotroph adenomas are very rare, accounting for less than 1% of pituitary tumours. Corticotroph adenomas are the cause of Cushing's disease. If bilateral adrenalectomy is performed for this condition, the inhibitory feedback effect of cortisol on the pituitary is lost. A high proportion of these patients then develop Nelson's syndrome with excess adrenocorticotrophic hormone and melanocyte-stimulating hormone causing hyperpigmentation. This condition is serious and requires treatment (eg surgery) as the uninhibited pituitary adenoma grows rapidly and is locally invasive. Somatotroph adenomas produce growth hormone resulting in acromegaly. This may present with enlarging hands and feet, voice changes, skin changes, malocclusion of jaws, headache, diabetes and visual field defects. Glycoprotein-producing adenomas may secrete α-subunit (physiologically inert) or less commonly luteinising hormone or follicle-stimulating hormone. A craniopharyngioma is a tumour arising from epidermal cells from the embryological remnant of Rathke's pouch. Craniopharyngiomas do not secrete hormones but may cause local pressure effects including hypopituitarism and visual field defects.

Q23. GASTROINTESTINAL DISEASE (☆)

1. B   2. E   3. D   4. F   5. C

Coeliac disease is a gluten-sensitive enteropathy, which causes subtotal villous atrophy of the small intestinal mucosa. This is a not uncommon and frequently unrecognised cause of iron-deficiency anaemia. There may also be fatigue, oral ulcers and symptoms suggesting irritable bowel syndrome. Anti endomyseal antibodies are a useful screening test with high sensitivity and specificity. Ulcerative colitis always involves the rectum and spreads continuously to involve a variable amount of the large intestine. Other parts of the gastrointestinal tract are not involved. Patients present with diarrhoea, abdominal pain, rectal bleeding and sometimes weight loss. The onset may be subacute or with acute fulminant colitis. Rectal biopsy histology reveals inflammation confined to the mucosa and the presence of crypt abscesses. Crohn's disease can involve any part of the gastrointestinal tract from the mouth to the anus. As a result, the presenting symptoms can be extremely varied. Many patients present with diarrhoea, malabsorption and anaemia (due to deficiency of iron, folate and/or vitamin B_{12}). Biopsy of affected tissue reveals transmural inflammation and frequently the presence of granulomas. Ischaemic colitis causes abdominal pain, diarrhoea and bleeding per rectum. Barium enema characteristically shows 'thumbprinting' of the bowel wall due to submucosal swelling. Acute ischaemic colitis may lead to bowel infarction indicated by the presence of intramural gas on abdominal imaging. Pseudomembranous colitis commonly occurs in patients who have recently received broad-spectrum antibiotics. The toxin produced by *Clostridium difficile* causes this condition. Hirschprung's disease causes chronic diarrhoea and the development of a grossly distended colon (called megacolon). It is a congenital condition caused by an aganglionic segment of bowel.

Q24. GASTROINTESTINAL DISEASE (☆☆)

1. F   2. A   3. E   4. D   5. B

Achalasia is dilation of the oesophagus due to incomplete relaxation of the gastro-oesophageal sphincter and impaired peristalsis during swallowing. Large amounts of food may collect in the oesophagus leading to regurgitation and risk of tracheal aspiration. The underlying defect is probably most commonly the degeneration of myenteric inhibitory neurones. Barrett's oesophagus is caused by chronic reflux oesophagitis. The oesophageal squamous epithelium undergoes metaplasia to become gastric-type columnar epithelium. This condition is associated with an increased risk of adenocarcinoma of the oesophagus. The sliding type is the commonest form of hiatus hernia accounting for approximately 90% of cases. The gastro-oesophageal junction is displaced upwards and there is a portion of the stomach in the thorax. This predisposes to reflux oesophagitis. In the rolling type of hiatus hernia, a part of the fundus of the stomach herniates into the thorax alongside the undisplaced gastro-oesophageal sphincter. A Schatzki ring causes a luminal stenosis at the gastro-oesophageal junction. The ring consists of mucosa and submucosa. It can be shown by a carefully performed barium swallow but its presence is easily missed. Plummer-Vinson syndrome (also known as Patterson-Brown-Kelly) is the presence of a post-cricoid web in association with iron-deficiency anaemia. Plummer-Vinson syndrome and achalasia are both associated with oesophageal carcinoma.

Q25. HORMONE-SECRETING TUMOURS (☆☆)

1. E   2. A   3. F   4. B   5. D

Pancreatic endocrine tumours are rare, the commonest being gastrinoma and insulinoma. Glucagonoma is a tumour of the pancreatic α cells. This causes a characteristic skin rash known as necrolytic migratory erythema, impaired glucose tolerance, weight loss, venous thrombosis and occasionally paraneoplastic neurological syndromes. Insulinomas arise from the pancreatic β cells. Recurrent attacks of hypoglycaemia occur after fasting, typically on waking in the morning. Hypoglycaemia is not always suspected as the cause of the patient's drowsiness and confusion. Many patients are referred to neurologists or psychiatrists before the diagnosis is established. Gastrinomas cause hypersecretion of gastric acid leading to severe and recurrent peptic ulceration. This condition is known as Zollinger-Ellison syndrome. Diarrhoea also frequently occurs. A VIPoma produces watery diarrhoea of such severity it has been compared to cholera. Patients typically pass more than 3 litres of stool per day resulting in weight loss, hypokalaemia and dehydration. There is also frequently achlorhydria and the condition is sometimes called WDHA syndrome (for **w**atery **d**iarrhoea, **h**ypokalaemia, **a**chlorhydria). A somatostatinoma is a very rare tumour. Approximately 50% arise from the pancreas. The classic triad of symptoms is cholelithiasis, diabetes mellitus and steatorrhoea. Carcinoid tumours (which produce 5-hydroxytryptamine) may occur in many parts of the gastrointestinal tract (or lung) but they usually arise in the appendix or rectum. Systemic symptoms are usually only seen when midgut tumours metastasise to the liver. The classic presentation is with paroxysmal attacks of facial flushing accompanied by tachycardia, wheezing and a feeling of heat. Patients may develop pellagra (nicotinamide deficiency) because the nicotinamide precursor, 5-hydroxytryptophan, is used to produce 5-hydroxytryptamine.

Q26. INVESTIGATION OF GASTROINTESTINAL PROBLEMS (☆☆)

1. B   2. E   3. D   4. C   5. F

The investigation of malabsorption is complex and there are a large number of tests that can be performed. Measurement of faecal fat is used to diagnose malabsorption. However, the quantity of fat in stools can be affected by the quantity ingested and this can vary markedly.

Ideally, faecal fat is measured over five days and expressed as a percentage of the fat ingested. To avoid the unpleasant collection of such large quantities of stool several radioisotope tests of fat absorption are also available. The xylose absorption test is used to investigate suspected carbohydrate malabsorption. A standard dose of xylose is given (usually 5 g) and the amount excreted in the urine is measured over the following five hours. If less than 22% of the dose is excreted this is consistent with carbohydrate malabsorption (also caused by delayed gastric emptying or renal impairment). Small intestinal biopsy allows histological diagnoses to be made and it can be used to assay specific intestinal enzymes such as lactase, enabling the diagnosis of lactase deficiency. The Schilling test involves administration of oral radioactive vitamin B_{12} and intramuscular unlabelled B_{12} and subsequent measurement of urine radioactivity. If urine excretion of radioactivity is reduced, this suggests failure of vitamin B_{12} absorption and the test is repeated after giving intrinsic factor (to exclude intrinsic factor deficiency). If the excretion is decreased on repeat testing this suggests terminal ileal disease (the specific site of vitamin B_{12} absorption). The bile acid breath test is used to demonstrate bacterial overgrowth of the small intestine. ^{14}C labelled conjugated bile acids are given by mouth. If bacteria are present in the small intestine they break down the bile salt and radioactive carbon monoxide is detected in the breath. In normal subjects the unconjugated bile acids are reabsorbed from the terminal ileum and radioactive carbon dioxide is not exhaled. False-positive results occur in terminal ileal disease because the unconjugated bile salts then pass into the colon and are broken down by the bacteria there. Although the glucose tolerance test is abnormal in carbohydrate malabsorption (slower rise in blood glucose than normal), it is not useful in investigating this condition as it is affected by many other factors.

Q27. NYSTAGMUS (☆☆☆)

1. E   2. A   3. F   4. D   5. C

Nystagmus is described as jerky (where beats have a fast and slow component) or pendular (where magnitude and speed of oscillations are equal). Pendular nystagmus occurs in one plane only. It is usually caused by visual impairment in early life. Jerky nystagmus is described as beating in the direction of the fast component. In fact the fast component is really a corrective response for the abnormal slow component. Physiological nystagmus occurs in normal people if they are instructed to gaze to the extreme of one direction. Pathological nystagmus can usually be demonstrated with the patient only gazing around 30° beyond the forward position. Nystagmus caused by problems in the labyrinth or vestibular apparatus is usually only present in one direction. Looking away from the side of the lesion induces the nystagmus. Vestibular nystagmus shows fatigability and is generally associated with vertigo. Nystagmus caused by lesions in the central nervous system may be present in more than one direction. Nystagmus caused by cerebellar lesions usually changes direction with the direction of gaze. It is more marked when looking towards the affected side. Upbeat nystagmus is characteristically caused by lesions of the floor of the fourth ventricle (eg multiple sclerosis, Wernicke's encephalopathy). Downbeat nystagmus is due to lesions around the foramen magnum (eg Arnold-Chiari malformation). A lesion in the medial longitudinal fasciculus produces failure of adduction in the eye on the affected side and simultaneous nystagmus on abduction in the other eye, when looking away from the side of the lesion. This combination of signs is known as an internuclear ophthalmoplegia. Causes include multiple sclerosis, brainstem infarction, pontine glioma, Wernicke's encephalopathy, encephalitis and phenytoin toxicity.

Q28. PATHOLOGY (☆☆☆)

1. A   2. D   3. C   4. F   5. B

The pathological hallmark of Parkinson's disease is Lewy bodies (eosinophilic inclusion bodies) in the pigmented nuclei of the pars compacta of the substantia nigra and the locus coeruleus. There is a marked loss of dopamine from the putamen, caudate nucleus and substantia nigra. Progressive supranuclear palsy (Steele-Richardson-Olszewski syndrome) is the combination of Parkinsonian symptoms plus a disorder of voluntary eye movements. Neurofibrillary tangles are the typical histological feature. There is damage to the basal ganglia nuclei, the periaqueductal grey matter and the red nucleus but the cerebral cortex remains unaffected. Multisystem atrophy includes three entities: (i) cerebellar ataxia, (ii) Parkinsonian symptoms and (iii) autonomic failure (known as Shy-Drager syndrome). The clinical features respectively correlate with the variable pattern of damage to the inferior olives, pontine nuclei and Purkinje cells of the cerebellar cortex (correlate with i); pigmented nuclei of the substantia nigra (ii); and intermediolateral columns in the thoracic spinal cord (iii). Glial cytoplasmic inclusions are characteristically found on histology. In corticobasal degeneration there is atrophy of the frontal and parietal cortex, striatum, globus pallidus, subthalamus and substantia nigra. This leads to an akinetic-rigid syndrome with apraxia, myoclonic jerks, motor and sensory deficits and the alien limb syndrome. Carbon monoxide poisoning and other causes of severe cerebral anoxia (eg cardiac arrest) may cause bilateral necrosis of the striatum or globus pallidus. Signs of damage develop over several days after the anoxic episode and lead to a progressive akinetic-rigid syndrome with dystonias, athetosis, dysarthria and dysphasia. Huntington's disease results in extensive neuronal loss in the caudate nucleus, putamen, thalamus, hypothalamus and deep cerebellar nuclei. There is a marked reduction in aminobutyric acid in the zona reticulata of the substantia nigra. The pigmented zona compacta is usually undamaged.

Q29. CRANIAL NERVE LESIONS (☆☆)

1. B   2. E   3. A   4. F   5. C

A lone CN III palsy can occur due to pressure from a lesion in the location of the cavernous sinus (eg posterior communicating artery aneurysm) or as a false localising sign when there is generalised raised intracranial pressure. In these cases the parasympathetic fibres which accompany CN III are also affected and there is pupillary dilatation. Vascular conditions which produce mononeuritis multiplex (eg diabetes mellitus, rheumatoid arthritis and the connective tissue diseases) are also a common cause of a CN III palsy. In these conditions the pupil is not involved (described as sparing of the pupil). Cavernous sinus thrombosis affects CN III, IV and VI. There is usually also swelling of the eyelid, conjunctival suffusion and proptosis. Other causes of combined CN III, IV and VI palsies include midbrain damage due to stroke, tumour or Wernicke's encephalopathy. The combination of ipsilateral CN V, VII and VIII palsies suggests a cerebellopontine angle tumour (eg acoustic neuroma). The combination of ipsilateral CN V and VI palsies is called Gradenigo's syndrome. This is usually caused by damage to the apex of the petrous part of the temporal bone. Infection spreading from chronic suppurative otitis media is the classical cause. Unilateral anosmia occurs when a frontal tumour produces damage to the optic bulb (CN I). The combination of ipsilateral CN IX, X and XI palsies suggests a lesion in the region of the jugular foramen (eg malignant neck tumour). Lesions in the medulla can produce the same effects.

Q30. GAIT ABNORMALITY (☆)

1. E   2. B   3. C   4. A   5. F

Upper motor neurone damage causes limb spasticity. In the upper limbs this produces a flexion deformity of the hand and wrist and in the lower limbs it produces extension at the hip and knee and plantarflexion of the ankle. A patient with a hemiplegia walks with a circumductive gait, swinging the rigid extended leg around in a wide arc. A patient with a bilateral upper motor neurone lesion walks with a scissoring gate, the toes scraping the floor at each step and swinging in front of the foot that is planted on the ground. Proximal myopathy produces weakness of the limb girdle muscles especially iliopsoas. In order to walk, the patient must swing their entire trunk forwards and the elevated limb then follows through. This is described as a waddling gait. Patients with early proximal myopathy will complain of difficulty climbing stairs and in standing up from a chair. A peripheral motor neuropathy produces a foot drop due to weakness of ankle dorsiflexion. To prevent the toes from scraping the ground when walking, the patient lifts the leg high with the knee bent. This is called a high-stepping gait. When the foot lands on the floor it comes down with a slapping sound. Patients can be examined for early peripheral muscle weakness by testing their ability to walk on tiptoe. Patients with a cerebellar problem walk with a broad-based gait and have a tendency to fall to the side of the cerebellar lesion. These patients cannot walk heel-toe without falling. A patient with an extrapyramidal syndrome (eg Parkinson's disease) walks with a flexed posture and short, shuffling steps. There is postural instability and difficulty in starting and stopping when directed to. Patients with a peripheral sensory neuropathy stamp the foot on the ground to ensure that it is firmly on the floor (stamping gait). Features of a sensory and motor peripheral neuropathy are often combined.

Q31. HISTOLOGY OF RESTRICTIVE LUNG DISEASE (☆☆☆)

1. E   2. A   3. C   4. B   5. F

The cause of diffuse restrictive lung disease is usually established by histology. In bronchiolitis obliterans with organising pneumonia there is oedematous granulation tissue and fibrin within the alveoli and bronchi. In contrast, in cryptogenic fibrosing alveolitis the inflammatory infiltrate, oedema and fibrosis predominantly affect the alveolar walls. Intra-alveolar macrophages are present. In advanced disease alveolar destruction and fibrosis lead to cyst formation producing a 'honeycomb' appearance. In extrinsic allergic alveolitis there are small non-necrotising granulomas around the bronchioles and a lymphocytic infiltrate in the alveolar walls. Mucosal ulceration is generally present and this aids distinction from the other non-necrotising, granulomatous lung disease, sarcoidosis. In histiocytosis X there are eosinohilic granulomas and Langerhan's cells in the interstitial tissues. Langerhan's cells can be seen on electron microscopy or detected by staining for S100 protein. Ferruginous bodies are large asbestos fibres coated with a protein-ferritin complex. Small uncoated fibres are also detected but are best seen by electron microscopy. Asbestos-induced pleural plaques appear as a densely woven pattern of collagen fibres. Lymphangioleiomyomatosis is a rare disease causing recurrent pneumothoraces and chylothorax. On histology proliferation of smooth muscle cells is seen in the walls of the bronchioles.

Q32. INVESTIGATIONS (☆☆)

1. E   2. A   3. D   4. C   5. F

High-resolution computed tomography (HRCT) is the optimal method for imaging interstitial lung disease (eg pulmonary fibrosis). HRCT has also largely replaced bronchography for diagnosing and quantifying the extent of bronchiectasis. Magnetic resonance imaging (MRI) is inferior to HRCT for imaging the lungs but is very useful for mediastinal structures. MRI is useful in the diagnosis of thoracic aortic dissection and is used sequentially in monitoring the rate of progression of thoracic aortic aneurysms. Transoesophageal echocardiography is also widely used for diagnosis of thoracic aortic dissection. Ventilation-perfusion (V/Q) scanning is a useful non-invasive technique for confirming a clinically suspected diagnosis of pulmonary embolism. This technique uses technetium-99m to study perfusion and xenon-133, krypton-81m or technetium-99m aerosol to

study ventilation. However, this technique often gives intermediate results and the gold standard method of pulmonary arteriography may be required to establish the diagnosis. Spiral CT is also increasingly being used to diagnose pulmonary embolism. Transthoracic ultrasound provides good images of pleural effusions. It is particularly useful for diagnosing small effusions not clearly seen on plain chest X-ray and for determining if an effusion is loculated (where simple aspiration is unlikely to be successful).

Q33. ASTHMA (☆☆)

1. F   2. A   3. B   4. C   5. E

The pattern of asthma symptoms can provide useful clues in identifying the underlying cause. Irritant-induced asthma is usually accompanied by symptoms affecting the eye, nose, throat and bronchi. Causes include ammonia, chlorine, phosgene and toluene and measures should be taken to protect workers from these agents. Hypersensitivity-induced asthma can occur to a wide range of allergens particularly proteins (eg animal excreta, grains, flour and moulds) and low molecular weight chemicals (eg acid anhydrides, isocyanates, platinum salts and antibiotics). The diagnosis should be suspected when symptoms get better after a period of absence from work and recur upon repeated exposure. Early responders develop symptoms within minutes of exposure and these then persist for one to two hours. Late responders do not develop symptoms until at least an hour after exposure and these persist for up to 36 hours. The diagnosis is more likely to be missed in late responders. Seasonal atopic asthma develops during one particular time of year. If the allergy is to pollen from flowering plants this is usually in early summer. Continuous atopic asthma may have many different causes. Faeces from the house dust mite, *Dermatophagoides pteronyssinus*, are one of the commonest allergens and symptoms are often worse at night. However, asthma of any cause may be worse at night and this pattern is not diagnostic of dust mite allergy. Byssinosis is acute airway narrowing on exposure to cotton dust. This form of occupational asthma typically develops in cotton mill workers after 20 or more years of exposure. Churg-Strauss is a syndrome of pANCA-positive (pANCA stands for perinuclear antineutrophil cytoplasmic antibodies), autoimmune vasculitis, asthma and eosinophilia and is not known to be linked to an external precipitant.

Q34. INHALED DRUGS (☆)

1. F   2. A   3. B   4. D   5. E

Drugs used in the treatment of asthma are preferably given by the inhaled route to minimise systemic side-effects. Salbutamol and terbutaline are short-acting β_2-agonists taken on an as needed basis. They can be used prophylactically just before an activity known to produce an attack. The dose of salbutamol is 200 μg by inhaler or 2.5–5 mg by nebuliser for severe breathlessness. Patients should not use short-acting β_2-agonists when they are asymptomatic as there is some evidence that regular use may cause worsening of disease and an increase in mortality. Salmeterol and eformoterol are long-acting β_2-agonists used in the prevention of asthmatic attacks. They are often taken before bedtime to reduce nocturnal symptoms. They can be added to high-dose inhaled steroids to improve asthmatic control or can be used with standard dose inhaled steroids as a potential steroid-sparing agent. However, they should not be used in place of inhaled steroids, which are the mainstay of prevention of asthma attacks. Beclomethasone, fluticasone and budesonide are inhaled corticosteroids. They should be commenced in all asthmatic patients who need to use a short-acting β_2-agonist more than once daily. Standard dose is up to 400 μg twice daily. If a higher dosage is used the steroid should be delivered via a spacer device to maximise delivery to the airways and minimise deposition in the oropharynx (which leads to *Candida infection* and a hoarse voice). Ipratropium and oxitropium are anticholinergic agents, which decrease bronchial smooth muscle spasm. They are most useful in older patients with chronic obstructive airways disease. The dose via inhaler is 18 to 36 μg taken as required. Nebulisers can be used to deliver 250 to 500 μg. Sodium cromoglicate is an inhaled mast cell stabiliser most commonly prescribed for children. It is used as an alternative to inhaled corticosteroids but if good asthma control is not achieved, a corticosteroid inhaler should be commenced. Zafirlukast and montelukast are leukotriene receptor antagonists, which are being introduced for improvement of asthma control. The exact place of these oral agents in asthma therapy is not yet clear. They should be used as an adjunct to inhaled steroids not a replacement.

Q35. RHEUMATOLOGICAL DISEASE RISK FACTORS (☆☆)

1. B   2. E   3. A   4. F   5. C

Gout is associated with conditions resulting in increased uric acid production (eg glucose-6-phosphatase deficiency, Lesch-Nyhan syndrome, lymphomas) and those resulting in decreased uric acid excretion (eg idiopathic, sickle cell disease, Down's syndrome, renal impairment). Glucose-6-phosphatase deficiency is also known as von Gierke's disease or glycogen storage disease type I. Pyrophosphate arthropathy is associated with haemochromatosis, hyperparathyroidism, hypophosphatasia and hypomagnesaemia. A systemic lupus erythematosus-like syndrome can be caused by several drugs including gold, hydralazine, isoniazid and penicillamine, but procainamide is the drug most commonly implicated. Drug-induced lupus predominantly affects the lungs. The kidneys are rarely affected. Adult-onset dermatomyositis is frequently associated with bronchial carcinoma or other malignancies. Dermatomyositis can also be associated with other connective tissue diseases or immune-deficiency states and can be drug induced. Reiter's syndrome is the triad of reactive arthritis, conjunctivitis and urethritis. Other features that may be found include acute iritis, circinate balanitis and keratoderma blennorrhagia. This syndrome is associated with genital chlamydia infection or gastrointestinal infection with *Campylobacter jejuni*, non-typhoid *Salmonella* species, *Shigella flexneri* and *Yersinia* species. Fibromyalgia is a condition characterised by generalised body aches, trigger points that elicit pain when pressed and sleep disruption (particularly loss of rapid eye movement sleep). It has substantial overlap with the chronic fatigue syndrome.

Q36. LESIONS AND NODES (☆)

1. F   2. E   3. A   4. D   5. B

Osler's nodes are small, well-circumscribed tender, erythematous nodules that occur in endocarditis and vasculitis (eg severe Raynaud's disease). They most commonly occur on the pulps of the fingers and toes. Heberden's and Bouchard's nodes are bony swellings which occur in osteoarthritis. Heberden's nodes affect the distal interphalangeal joints and Bouchard's nodes affect the proximal interphalangeal joints. Gouty tophi occur in chronic tophaceus gout. Tophi are irregular, firm nodules caused by deposition of uric acid crystals. They occur around the extensor surfaces of the fingers and hands, on the ulnar surface of the forearm, over the olecranon bursae, over the Achilles tendons and on the cartilaginous helix of the ear. The Aschoff nodule is a perivascular lesion with a central core of necrotic material surrounded by an inner layer of polymorphonuclear cells and an outer layer of lymphocytes. The Aschoff nodule is the hallmark of rheumatic fever and is found in joints, tendons, blood vessels and the heart. Rheumatoid nodules are subcutaneous and intracutaneous, non-tender swellings predominantly occurring over the extensor surfaces in rheumatoid arthritis.

Q37. FACIAL ERUPTIONS (☆)

1. C   2. A   3. F   4. E   5. D

Rosacea is a common condition commencing in middle age. This chronic condition often resembles acne rosacea. Erythematous papules and pustules with soreness and itching occur on the greasy areas of the face. Treatment is with antibiotics or isotretinoin. Angular cheilitis is maceration of the skin at the edge of the mouth. It usually occurs in the elderly because sagging facial muscles and poorly fitting dentures allow saliva to produce permanently moist areas, which then become infected with candida. Seborrhoeic dermatitis is caused by the yeast *Pityrosporum ovale*. There is redness and scaling of the eyelids, eyebrows, nasolabial folds and ears. There is usually little pruritus in this condition in contrast to contact dermatitis where there is intense pruritus. Contact dermatitis commonly involves the areas where make-up is applied, eg the cheeks, neck and eyelids. The presence of eyelid oedema is highly suggestive of this condition. In lupus erythematosus there is a 'butterfly rash' which has a similar distribution to that of seborrhoeic dermatitis. Sunlight is a precipitating factor and sufferers should wear a high protection factor sunscreen. Erysipelas is superficial cellulitis usually caused by a Lancefield group A β-haemolytic *Streptococcus*.

Q38. CUTANEOUS DRUG ERUPTIONS (☆☆)

1. D   2. A   3. B   4. E   5. F

Toxic erythema is the most common form of drug eruption accounting for approximately 45% of total cases. It is frequently caused by penicillins, sulphonamides and non-steroidal anti-inflammatory drugs. It is a widespread erythematous, maculopapular, morbilliform eruption, most marked on the trunk. It usually lasts around five to ten days but in severe cases erythroderma and severe exfoliative dermatitis may occur. Urticaria accounts for around 25% of drug eruptions and is often caused by penicillins, sulphonamides and opioids. It is usually due to an immunoglobulin-E-mediated, immediate type I hypersensitivity reaction. However, in some cases urticaria can be caused by serum sickness, which is a type III reaction that takes several days to develop. Erythema multiforme is responsible for around 7% of drug eruptions and can be caused by sulphonamides, barbiturates and carbamazepine. The target lesion is the classical one but macules, papules and blisters also occur. The extremities are affected more than the trunk and lesions also occur on the palms and soles. Severe cases that involve the mucosa are known as Stevens-Johnson syndrome. This may result in epidermal necrolysis and can be fatal. Eczematous eruptions account for around 5% of drug eruptions and are often due to sulphonamides or β-blockers. These eruptions are type IV hypersensitivity reactions and often follow sensitisation to topically administered agents. Patch testing to identify the cause of a rash is most useful in this form of eruption. Fixed drug eruptions are relatively uncommon. These reactions occur at the same anatomical site each time the offending drug is administered and there are usually very few lesions present. The lesions are usually erythematous plaques but bullae may also occur. Psoriasiform reactions and photosensitivity reactions can also be caused by drugs.

Q39. CLOTTING (☆☆☆)

1. D   2. A   3. F   4. E   5. C

The prothrombin time (known as international normalised ratio or INR when compared to the control value) is a measure of the function of the extrinsic clotting pathway. APTT is a measure of the intrinsic pathway and thrombin time a measure of the final stages of the common pathway. Bleeding time is a clinical test where the time taken to stop bleeding after a standard forearm incision is measured. Heparin affects the intrinsic and common pathways and produces a prolonged APTT and thrombin time. Prolonged use may also lead to thrombocytopenia. Warfarin administration and vitamin K deficiency predominantly affect the extrinsic pathway and prolong the PT. In disseminated intravascular coagulation, many of the clotting factors become depleted and thrombocytopenia develops. All of the clotting tests are prolonged and the blood levels of

D-dimers and fibrin degradation products are elevated. In idiopathic thrombocytopenic purpura, the platelet deficiency leads to a prolonged bleeding time but the laboratory tests of coagulation are normal. Haemophilia A (deficiency of factor VIII, a component of the intrinsic pathway) produces a markedly prolonged APTT. In von Willebrand's disease (deficiency of a component of factor VIII) the APTT and the bleeding time are both prolonged.

Q40. WHITE BLOOD CELL ABNORMALITIES (☆☆☆)

1. B   2. F   3. E   4. A   5. C

Normal neutrophils have nuclei with three to five lobes. Pelger-Huët cells are neutrophils with bilobed or monolobed nuclei. These cells are seen in myeloproliferative disease. There is also a hereditary form of this phenomenon. When neutrophils contain nuclei with seven to eight lobes they are described as hypersegmented. This finding is associated with megaloblastic anaemia due to vitamin B$_{12}$ or folic acid deficiency. Chediak-Higashi syndrome is an autosomal recessive lysosomal disorder affecting granulocytes, epithelial cells, melanocytes and nerve cells. Patients' neutrophils have giant lysosomes containing hydrolases and other enzymes. Clinical features include anaemia, thrombocytopenia, leucopenia, decreased skin, iris and hair pigmentation and increased susceptibility to infections. Dohle bodies are large, round, pale blue masses in the periphery of the neutrophil cytoplasm thought to be due to aggregated rough endoplasmic reticulum. They are present when there is severe metabolic derangement because of severe infection, burns, malignancy and other causes of the systemic inflammatory response syndrome. Dohle bodies are often associated with toxic granulation, which is the presence of coarsely staining cytoplasmic granules. Atypical lymphocytes are activated T cells. They are seen in acute infections caused by Epstein-Barr virus (known as infectious mononucleosis or glandular fever), cytomegalovirus and other viruses. A drumstick appendage to the nucleus is occasionally seen in normal females and represents the inactivated X chromosome (Barr body).

Q41. HAEMOLYSIS (☆☆)

1. C   2. E   3. A   4. B   5. F

Haemolysis can occur within the circulation (intravascular) or in the reticuloendothelial system (extravascular). Causes of haemolysis where damage is predominantly intravascular include: transfusion reactions, microangiopathy, glucose-6-phosphate dehydrogenase deficiency, malaria, paroxysmal nocturnal haemoglobinuria and paroxysmal cold haemoglobinuria. Causes of extravascular haemolysis include: autoimmune haemolysis ('warm' or 'cold' agglutinins), hereditary spherocytosis, sickle cell disease and haemolytic disease of the newborn. In intravascular haemolysis, haemoglobin is released into the serum and this becomes bound to haptoglobin and albumin resulting in decreased serum haptoglobin and the formation of methaemalbumin (the basis of Schumm's test). Free haemoglobin can also be detected in the urine. Examination of the peripheral blood film allows calculation of the reticulocyte count, which indicates the degree of bone marrow activity in replacing lost red blood cells. The peripheral blood film may also reveal helmet cells and fragmented cells, which occur when fibrin strands damage red blood cells in microangiopathy. Conditions causing microangiopathic haemolysis include disseminated intravascular coagulation, thrombotic thrombocytopenic purpura and haemolytic uraemic syndrome. The direct Coombs' antiglobulin test detects antibodies that are coated on red blood cells. These antibodies can cause haemolysis by opsonisation, complement fixation or agglutination. The indirect antiglobulin test uses the patient's serum and antigen-coated red blood cells to detect serum antibodies capable of causing haemolysis. This test is the basis of crossmatching blood to ensure the patient will not react to the donor red blood cells.

Q42. DIAGNOSIS OF INFECTION (☆☆)

1. F   2. B   3. D   4. C   5. A

Falciparum malaria is usually diagnosed by examination of thick and thin blood films. However, antigen detection kits are now available which have high sensitivity and specificity. These are particularly useful complementary tests when expertise in blood film examination is not readily available, eg outside routine laboratory working hours. Onchocerciasis affects the skin and eye and is a common cause of blindness. These filarial worms are not seen in blood films and demonstration of the worm on skin biopsy is the usual diagnostic method. Syphilis is diagnosed by specific (TPHA) and non-specific (RPR or VDRL) serological tests. If the patient has neurological symptoms or signs or is HIV positive, CSF examination is also required to detect neurosyphilis. Neonatal HIV infection cannot be detected by serology as maternal antibody can produce false-positive results. Viral RNA detection by nucleic acid sequence binding assay or the polymerase chain reaction is diagnostic. Negative tests make infection unlikely but do not exclude it, as the viral load could be low. Disseminated *Mycobacterium avium* can be diagnosed by culture of many different tissues including blood, lymph node or bone marrow aspirate. Hookworm infection is diagnosed by examination of the stool for eggs.

Q43. INFECTIOUS ORGANISM TRANSMISSION (☆☆)

1. E   2. B   3. F   4. D   5. C

Haemophilus ducreyi causes chancroid, a sexually transmitted disease characterised by painful necrotising genital ulcers and suppurative regional lymphadenopathy. *Dracunculus medinensis*, the guinea worm, is acquired by drinking water containing infected copepods (cyclops). Guinea worms mature over about one year and the large female worm (up to 70 cm) then emerges to release larvae into water. The site of emergence of the worm can become secondarily infected by bacteria and lead to significant tissue destruction and disability. *Schistosoma haematobium* affects the urinary tract and eggs are passed in urine. After the eggs hatch, the larvae multiply in *Bulinus* snails to produce free-swimming cercariae. Human infection occurs when the cercariae penetrate human skin during bathing or standing in shallow water. *Neisseria meningitidis* requires close contact for transmission of respiratory droplets. In true airborne spread, as occurs with *Mycobacterium tuberculosis* and measles virus, infectious particles can remain suspended in the air for some time. These infections can occur without direct face-to-face contact.

Q44. ANTIBIOTICS (☆☆☆)

1. C   2. E   3. D   4. B   5. A

Antibiotic resistance among many species of bacteria is becoming an increasing problem worldwide. *Burkholderia pseudomallei* is a Gram-negative bacterium that causes melioidosis in South East Asia. Skin and soft tissue infections are a common presentation especially among those who work in rice fields. Pneumonia and septicaemia have high mortality even with optimal treatment and supportive care. Treatment of serious infection is with high-dose intravenous ceftazidime for one month followed by six months of oral antibiotics to reduce the risk of relapse. Co-trimoxazole can be used as an adjunct to ceftazidime even if in vitro tests suggest co-trimoxazole resistance is present. *Stenotrophomonas maltophilia* is an increasing cause of hospital-acquired infections particularly in patients treated with multiple broad-spectrum antibiotics in intensive care units. Co-trimoxazole is the recommended treatment. Extended spectrum β-lactamase production among *Klebsiella pneumoniae* and other coliforms is a major problem in treating hospital-acquired infections. These organisms are resistant to penicillins and cephalosporins and are often resistant to quinolones and aminoglycosides. Carbapenems have been

found to be the most effective treatment. Imipenem is the most widely used carbapenem but increases the risk of seizures. Meropenem is therefore preferred in meningitis. Vancomycin-resistant *Enterococcus faecalis* is often also resistant to penicillins and aminoglycosides. The combination streptogramin antibiotic dalfopristin/quinupristin is not effective against *E. faecalis* but may be used for *E. faecium*. If resistance is caused by the Van B phenotype rather than Van A then teicoplanin may be used. Linezolid belongs to a new class of antibiotics known as oxazolidinones. At present it appears highly effective against enterococci but there have already been reports of resistant organisms being identified. Treatment of *Escherichia coli* O157:H7 is controversial, as antibiotics have been reported to increase the risk of haemolytic uraemic syndrome.

Q45. MALIGNANCY ASSOCIATED WITH MICROORGANISMS (☆☆)

1. E   2. A   3. F   4. B   5. D

Epstein-Barr virus is associated with nasopharyngeal carcinoma in China and Burkitt's lymphoma in Africa. In HIV patients, it also appears to be associated with non-Hodgkin's lymphoma. HTLV1 (human T cell leukaemia/lymphoma virus) is an RNA retrovirus associated with adult T cell leukaemia and lymphoma and with tropical spastic paraparesis. Human papilloma virus, the cause of warts, is associated with carcinoma of the cervix in women and of the anal canal in homosexual men. Human herpes virus 8 is associated with all four variants of Kaposi's sarcoma: that which occurs in elderly men of Mediterranean or Jewish origin; the African endemic form; the HIV-associated disease; and the type which occurs in organ transplant recipients. Lymphomas of mucosa-associated lymphoid tissue are the commonest form of gastrointestinal lymphoma and they most frequently arise in the stomach. They are frequently associated with *Helicobacter pylori* and eradication of this bacterium can lead to tumour regression. Hepatocellular carcinoma is associated with hepatitis B virus.

Q46. GENITOURINARY CONDITIONS (☆)

1. E   2. B   3. C   4. D   5. F

A copious foamy discharge suggests infection with the free-swimming flagellate *Trichomonas vaginalis*. This organism can be readily demonstrated by microscopy of a wet preparation. A malodorous odour and the presence of 'clue cells' is suggestive of bacterial vaginosis. This condition is often polymicrobial including *Bacteroides*, *Mobiluncus*, *Peptostreptococci* and *Mycoplasma hominis* in addition to *Gardnerella vaginalis*. Metronidazole is the standard treatment for both of these causes of vaginitis. A single dry penile ulcer is suggestive of primary syphilis. Treatment is with 2.4 mega units of intramuscular penicillin G. Quantitative VDRL is performed at 3, 6, 12 and 24 months to ensure treatment has been successful. If the titre increases fourfold or if it remains high at 12 months, re-treatment is indicated. The causes of prostatitis are similar to those of epididymo-orchitis. Under 35 years, *Neisseria gonorrhoea* and *Chlamydia trachomatis* are likely, over 35 years and in those performing insertive anal intercourse coliforms should be suspected. A group of multiple painful ulcers suggest infection with herpes simplex I or II. Aciclovir therapy for a first attack increases the rate of healing but does not prevent recurrences. *Treponema pertenue* is the cause of yaws, a tropical spirochaetal infection spread by non-sexual, direct contact. Multiple cutaneous frambesial (raspberry-like) lesions develop and periostitis of the long bones may occur.

Q47. PRESCRIBING FOR INFECTIOUS DISEASES (☆☆)

1. B   2. C   3. E   4. F   5. A

Established hepatitis B infection can be treated with the nucleoside analogue lamivudine (3TC). If the patient is also infected with HIV this drug should not be used alone as it will encourage the development of HIV virions with lamivudine resistance. Hepatitis B virus may also develop resistance to this drug. Zidovudine is also a nucleoside analogue but its use is restricted to the treatment of HIV. The National Institute for Clinical Excellence (NICE) has issued guidelines on treatment of hepatitis C. Those with moderate to severe disease on liver biopsy should be treated with the combination of interferon α and ribavirin. Foscarnet can be used to treat cytomegalovirus pneumonia if the patient fails to tolerate or respond to ganciclovir. Ganciclovir causes neutropenia in 25% of patients and foscarnet causes renal impairment in more than 30%. Cidofovir is another available treatment but it causes both nephrotoxicity and neutropenia. NICE has also issued guidelines on the treatment of influenza with the neuraminidase inhibitor zanamivir. It can be prescribed for patients with influenza A or B infection who are at increased risk of severe disease and complications, eg diabetics, renal failure patients and those over 65 years. Palivizumab is a monoclonal antibody against respiratory syncytial virus (RSV) that is licensed for the prevention of infection during the RSV season in pre-term infants (<35 weeks gestation) aged less than six months.

Q48. PHARMACOKINETIC INTERACTIONS (☆☆☆)

1. B   2. C   3. F   4. D   5. A

Rifampicin increases the metabolism of oestrogens causing increased risk of pregnancy in those taking oral contraceptives. Erythromycin decreases metabolism of theophylline, which can lead to increased toxicity producing nausea, tachycardia, cardiac arrhythmias and convulsions. Amiodarone decreases renal tubular secretion of digoxin resulting in decreased excretion. If these drugs need to be used in combination, the dose of digoxin should be reduced. Thiazide diuretics increase renal tubular reabsorption of lithium (as do other causes of hyponatraemia as lithium is reabsorbed from the renal tubule like a sodium ion) causing raised lithium levels and increased risk of adverse effects including nausea, tremor, blurred vision and ataxia. Colestyramine binds bile salts in the gastrointestinal tract and also binds vitamin K and drugs such as warfarin. It can therefore increase or decrease the effects of warfarin. To reduce the potential for interaction these drugs should be given several hours apart. Fibrates and HMGCoA reductase inhibitors (commonly known as 'statins') both cause serious myositis and the risk is greatest when used in combination.

Q49. CONDITIONS AND DRUGS TO BE AVOIDED (☆☆☆)

1. E   2. A   3. C   4. D   5. F

Drugs that have a definite risk of haemolysis in G6PD-deficient subjects include: primaquine, nitrofurantoin, dapsone and other sulphones, sulphonamides and quinolones (including ofloxacin). There is a very long list of drugs that should be avoided in porphyria. Modest changes in chemical structure may lead to changes in porphyrinogenicity; therefore, a drug may be unsafe even though closely related drugs can be given. Examples of common drugs that are unsafe are tricyclic antidepressants, the oral contraceptive, hormone replacement therapy, cephalosporins, sulphonamides, sulphonylureas and loop and thiazide diuretics. Whenever prescribing for a patient with acute porphyria it is essential to check up on the safety of the selected drug. Tetracycline is anti-anabolic and in renal failure it causes further deterioration in renal function. If tetracyclines must be used in renal failure either minocycline or doxycycline should be chosen. Itraconazole is a potent cause of liver toxicity and should not be used in liver disease. The list of drugs that should be avoided or used at reduced dose in liver or renal failure is extensive. Appendices 2 and 3 respectively, in the *British National Formulary*, are useful for reference. Intravenous quinine is the treatment of choice for severe malaria and can be used in all of the above situations. Quinine may cause haemolysis in some G6PD-deficient subjects, but the benefits in severe malaria outweigh the risks. All of the drugs listed can be prescribed for patients with diabetes.

Q50. ADVERSE DRUG REACTIONS (☆☆)

1. C   2. D   3. F   4. A   5. B

Systemic lupus erythematosus, usually without renal involvement, can occur as a consequence of therapy with phenytoin, procainamide, hydralazine or ethosuximide. Long-term use of amiodarone can cause a large number of adverse effects due to the accumulation of lipofuscin. These include pulmonary alveolitis, corneal microdeposits, slate grey discoloration of skin, hyper- and hypothyroidism and hepatitis. Ethambutol may cause colour-blindness, decreased visual acuity and narrowing of the peripheral visual fields. Subjective symptoms develop before abnormalities can be demonstrated on examination and are reversible if the drug is stopped early. All patients should therefore be warned to report any visual symptoms immediately. Fever with eosinophilia is the first stage of the dapsone syndrome. Treatment must be discontinued promptly as there is a risk of exfoliative dermatitis, hepatitis, psychosis and even death. Myositis and rhabdomyolysis may occur with treatment with any fibrate or statin (3-hydroxy 3-methylglutaryl coenzyme A reductase inhibitor). However, the overall risk has been estimated to be only 1 in 100,000 person years of treatment by the Committee on Safety of Medicines. Patients should be warned to report any muscle pain. Worsening of psoriasis can be caused by lithium and β-blockers.

Q51. CYTOTOXIC DRUGS AND THEIR ADVERSE EFFECTS (☆☆)

1. C   2. B   3. D   4. F   5. A

Side-effects common to many cytotoxic drugs include tissue necrosis after extravasation, hyperuricaemia and resulting renal dysfunction, nausea and vomiting, bone marrow suppression, decreased immune responsiveness, alopecia, teratogenicity and impaired fertility. Haemorrhagic cystitis occurs with high doses of intravenous cyclophosphamide or the related drug ifosfamide. This is due to a metabolite called acrolein and can be prevented by co-administration of mesna. Cyclophosphamide is widely used for the treatment of chronic lymphatic leukaemia, lymphomas and solid tumours as well as for autoimmune diseases. Progressive pulmonary fibrosis occurs with busulfan, a drug used in chronic myeloid leukaemia. Busulfan and cyclophosphamide are alkylating agents. Cardiomyopathy may occur in those taking doxorubicin, particularly when a high cumulative dose is administered. Doxorubicin is a cytotoxic antibiotic used very widely to treat acute leukaemias, lymphomas and solid tumours. The vinca alkaloid, vincristine, is a potent cause of peripheral and autonomic neuropathy causing peripheral paraesthesiae, abdominal bloating and constipation. The related drug vinblastine causes less neuropathy but greater myelosuppression than vincristine. Following cessation of the drug, recovery is usually slow but complete. Paclitaxel is a taxane used in the treatment of ovarian and metastatic breast cancer. Hypersensitivity reactions are common and to prevent these premedication with a corticosteroid and antihistamines (both H_1 and H_2 receptor antagonists) is given.

Q52. CORTICOSTEROID POTENCY (☆)

1. F   2. C   3. B   4. A   5. E

Topical corticosteroids are widely used in the treatment of inflammatory skin conditions including eczematous conditions, discoid lupus erythematosus, lichen simplex, lichen planus and palmoplantar pustulosis. Potent and very potent corticosteroids may exert systemic effects resulting in Cushing's syndrome and adrenal suppression. Side-effects are related to the quantity of the preparation applied. Greater absorption will occur through damaged skin and absorption is also increased by occlusive dressings. It is important to recognise the relative potency of commonly used preparations to ensure that excessive steroid doses are not administered inadvertently. Steroids should be avoided or used only under specialised supervision in psoriasis as although

short-term benefits occur, withdrawal can result in vigorous flares of disease. Calcipotriol is a vitamin D derivative that is suitable for mild to moderate psoriasis. Fludrocortisone is a mineralocorticoid used in combination with a glucocorticoid in replacement therapy for adrenal insufficiency.

Q53. ECG (☆☆)

1. E   2. A   3. F   4. B   5. C

Analysis of electrocardiographs (ECG) is complex and requires practice. It is important to adopt a systematic approach, eg:

1. Find QRS complexes
2. Work out rate and rhythm
3. Identify relationship between P wave and QRS complex (any heart block?)
4. Check width of QRS (if >120 ms suspect bundle branch block)
5. Identify frontal axis (normal is usually but not always 0° to 90°)
6. Look for abnormal Q waves (greater than 1 mm tall in leads other than III, aVR, V_1)
7. Check for position of ST segment (if >1 mm elevated in two limb leads or >2 mm in chest leads consider myocardial infarct; if depressed consider ischaemia)
8. Examine T wave morphology (changes are non-specific).

The typical ECG pattern of left ventricular hypertrophy is an R wave in leads V_1 or V_2 greater than 27 mm or an S wave in V_5 or V_6 greater than 30 mm or the combination of the tallest R and deepest S greater than 40 mm. There is often secondary ST depression and T wave inversion in the left precordial leads (V_4 to V_6). In right ventricular hypertrophy there is a dominant R wave in lead V_1 and the frontal QRS axis is greater than 90°. There is often secondary ST depression and T wave inversion in the right precordial leads (V_1 to V_3). The QRS width must be less than 100 ms in both types of ventricular hypertrophy. If the QRS width is greater than 120 ms this suggests bundle branch block. In left bundle branch block there is absence of the R wave in lead V_1 and there may be secondary ST depression and T wave inversion in the left precordial leads. In right bundle branch block there is a dominant R wave in lead V_1 and secondary ST depression and T wave inversion may be seen in the right precordial leads. In acute, transmural myocardial infarction there is initially ST elevation, followed by T wave inversion and the development of Q waves. These changes are seen in leads V_1 to V_{3-4} in an anteroseptal infarct and in leads II, III and aVF in an inferior one.

Q54. HEART MURMURS (☆)

1. C   2. E   3. F   4. B   5. A

Cardiac murmurs can be due to turbulent flow through an abnormal valve or regurgitant flow through a leaking valve. Most cardiac murmurs are produced by blood flow through valves on the left side of the heart as the pressures are much higher than on the right side. However, when there is pulmonary hypertension and right ventricular hypertrophy, loud right-sided cardiac murmurs may also occur. Murmurs arising from the right side of the heart are louder during inspiration and this provides a useful clue to their origin. An ejection systolic murmur (ESM) is a crescendo-decrescendo murmur heard in the middle of systole. The first and second heart sounds are both heard distinct from the murmur. An ESM is usually caused by aortic stenosis or aortic sclerosis. It can also occur in the left ventricular outflow tract obstruction seen in hypertrophic obstructive cardiomyopathy and in pulmonary stenosis. A pansystolic murmur has uniform intensity throughout systole and merges with the second heart sound. The commonest cause is mitral regurgitation but it is also heard in tricuspid regurgitation and ventricular septal defect. A late systolic murmur occurs with a prolapsing mitral valve if it produces mitral regurgitation. The prolapsing valve produces a mid-systolic click that precedes the murmur. Early diastolic murmurs are usually quiet and are easily missed. It is frequently suggested that to hear this decrescendo, high-pitched murmur one must listen for the 'absence of silence'

following the second heart sound. The murmur is usually produced by aortic regurgitation but uncommonly is caused by pulmonary regurgitation due to pulmonary hypertension. If the pulmonary hypertension is caused by mitral stenosis this is called the Graham Steell murmur. A mid-diastolic murmur is a low-pitched, rumbling sound usually caused by mitral stenosis. When the underlying cause is rheumatic fever the murmur is called a Carey-Coombs' murmur. This murmur may also be heard in aortic regurgitation due to vibration of the mitral valve (called an Austin Flint murmur). Patent ductus arteriosus causes a continuous 'machinery shop' murmur.

Q55. BROAD COMPLEX TACHYARRHYTHMIA (☆☆☆)

1. E   2. A   3. B   4. C   5. D

Careful examination of the ECG and of any previous ECGs may assist in discriminating between broad complex tachycardias of ventricular and supraventricular origin. However, if there is any doubt a broad complex tachycardia should be treated as ventricular tachycardia as this is the safest approach. In atrial fibrillation with bundle branch block (BBB) the rhythm is irregular and the QRS morphology is typical of the bundle branch block (eg absent R in V_1, ST depression and T wave inversion in the left precordial leads for left BBB). A previous resting ECG may confirm the BBB was present before the arrhythmia. However, the resting ECG may also be normal as the BBB may be a temporary functional one produced by the rapid depolarisation rate. In atrial fibrillation with an accessory pathway between the atria and ventricles, the rhythm is irregular and there may be episodes of a slower rhythm. In Wolff-Parkinson-White (WPW) syndrome the resting ECG has a short PR interval and delta wave (slurred upstroke to QRS), but in Lown-Ganong-Levine it is normal. Torsade de pointes is a form of polymorphic ventricular tachycardia in which the QRS axis changes continuously. The rate is irregular and P waves are usually not visible. A preceding

ECG may show a long QT syndrome. In ventricular tachycardia the rhythm is usually regular. Most P waves are obscured by the large QRS complexes but occasional P waves may be seen with varying relationship to the QRS because of atrioventricular dissociation. These P waves may occasionally lead to a solitary capture beat (which has the normal QRS morphology) interspersed with the broad QRS complexes of ventricular origin. In ventricular tachycardia the QRS complex is usually very wide (greater than 140 ms) and shows marked axis deviation. In atrioventricular re-entry tachycardia with BBB the rhythm is regular and the QRS complex has a typical BBB morphology. If the BBB is a function of the rapid rhythm the resting ECG will be normal or will show the features of WPW syndrome. In atrioventricular nodal re-entry tachycardia with functional BBB the resting ECG will be normal.

Q56. CARDIAC PROBLEMS ASSOCIATED WITH OTHER CONDITIONS (☆☆)

1. E   2. D   3. F   4. C   5. B

Mitral regurgitation can arise after myocardial infarction because of papillary muscle dysfunction or chordae tendinae rupture. The latter condition may cause severe regurgitation leading to cardiac failure and a need for valve replacement. Mitral regurgitation occurs in any condition producing left ventricular dilatation and may also be caused by rheumatic fever (the most commonly affected valve in this condition), endocarditis and mitral valve prolapse. Aortic coarctation is associated with Turner's syndrome and Noonan's syndrome. Aortic regurgitation may be caused by rheumatic fever, aortic dissection, endocarditis, syphilitic aortitis, Takayasu's arteritis, Ehlers-Danlos syndrome, osteogenesis imperfecta, Marfan syndrome and ventricular septal defect. Endocarditis affecting the right side of the heart is most commonly associated with intravenous drug abuse and may result in tricuspid regurgitation. Other causes of this valve lesion include the carcinoid syndrome and rheumatic fever. In the latter cause, mitral valve disease is almost invariably also seen. Pulmonary stenosis is usually congenital and is a part of Fallot's tetralogy (pulmonary stenosis, ventricular septal defect, overriding aorta and right ventricular hypertrophy).

Q57. CLASSIFICATION (☆☆)

1. C   2. E   3. B   4. D   5. F

Three conditions must be fulfilled for the diagnosis of anorexia nervosa. The patient's weight is greater than 15% less than that expected for height, sex and age; there is amenorrhoea (females account for over 90% of cases); and there is distortion of body image with a morbid fear of fatness. Patients may use dieting, exercise, laxatives, diuretics and self-induced vomiting to achieve weight loss. Bulimia nervosa is a similar condition. However, in bulimia there are episodes of binge eating where there is a feeling of loss of control. These are interspersed with behaviour aimed at losing weight, such as self-induced vomiting. Patients may be of normal weight and have regular menstruation and still suffer from bulimia. The diagnosis of anorexia has primacy over bulimia so if a patient fulfils the criteria for anorexia and also has binge eating they are only defined as having anorexia nervosa. In contrast to bulimia, vomiting which is psychogenic in origin is involuntary. Psychogenic vomiting tends to occur in middle age and there are no abnormal ideas about weight or body image. Pica is the eating of things that are not generally regarded as food. Common examples include soil, paper and other household objects. This phenomenon may occur in developmentally normal children, but is occasionally indicative of emotional distress or mental retardation. Alcohol dependence syndrome is characterised by the following:

- narrowing of drinking repertoire
- priority given to alcohol over other activities
- increased tolerance
- withdrawal symptoms
- drinking to avoid withdrawal
- awareness of compulsion to drink

Hallucinations are a common feature of alcohol-related brain damage and usually take the form of threatening auditory hallucinations. The hallucinations that characterise abuse of lysergic acid diethylamide (LSD) include synaesthesia, the bizarre perception of a stimulus being recognised by another sensory modality (eg sound may be perceived as a visual impulse). Flashbacks occurring after the drug has been taken are also a typical feature of LSD abuse.

Q58. PSYCHIATRIC SYMPTOMS (☆☆)

1. D   2. A   3. F   4. B   5. C

Elementary hallucinations are simple stimuli such as flashes of light, bangs, claps or crashes. There are many underlying causes of these symptoms. Complex hallucinations are those which consist of speech, formed visual images or other complex sensations. Third person auditory hallucinations address the patient as 'he' or 'she'. They may take the form of two voices discussing the patient or of a voice giving a running commentary on the patient's actions. Autoscopic hallucination is the experience of seeing one's own body projected into space. This rare symptom is sometimes seen in temporal lobe epilepsy. Second person hallucinations address the patient directly. They may criticise the patient or give him or her an order to do something. Delusions are incorrect beliefs that are held with unshakeable conviction even if conclusive evidence is produced to disprove them. They are not explicable by the patient's religion, political views or culture. Delusional perception occurs when a normal sensory stimulus (eg a traffic light changing colour) is interpreted as having abnormal significance (eg a message from God to perform a mission). The perception itself is not abnormal, only its interpretation. These delusions are also called primary or autochthonous as they are not explained by some prior mood or thought process. In delusional mood the delusion occurs secondary to the patient's affect. A manic patient may believe he is the son of God and a depressed patient may believe he is dying. Delusional

mood and second person auditory hallucinations occur in affective disorders. Second and third person auditory hallucinations and delusional perception occur in schizophrenia.

Q59. SCHIZOPHRENIA (☆☆)

1. D   2. C   3. E   4. F   5. B

Stereotypies are repeated, regular movements that do not have obvious significance. Examples include rocking and head-nodding movements. Mannerisms are repeated movements that do have significance. The patient may salute, wave or clap hands together repeatedly. Echolalia is the persistent uttering of the same sounds or words as another person. Echopraxia is persistent imitation of another's actions. Echolalia and echopraxia occur without the patient being asked to imitate and do not stop when the patient is requested to do so. Posturing is the adoption of an unusual position such as standing on one leg, raising one arm above the head or standing with both arms outstretched. Tics are a common problem which do not suggest schizophrenia. They are irregular, involuntary, jerky movements which it is difficult for the sufferer to control. Common examples are blepharospasm due to contraction of orbicularis oculi and raising of the eyebrows due to contraction of frontalis.

Q60. IMPAIRED DECISION-MAKING CAPACITY (☆☆)

1. C   2. A   3. F   4. E   5. B

When a patient has impaired decision-making abilities and cannot give his/her own consent for treatment it may be difficult to decide what is in the patient's best interests. This problem is particularly acute when it regards life-sustaining treatment in a terminal illness, advanced dementia, vegetative state or in a patient with a very poor quality of life. A caregiver (which can be a relative, friend or health professional) is usually in a good position to provide information on the patient's quality of life before the acute episode. However, the caregiver is not always an adequate surrogate decision-maker. An objective surrogate decision-maker informally represents the patient's premorbid wishes. However, he/she may not always be aware of these or may be influenced by his/her own values and wishes rather than those of the patient. Caregivers may also disagree with each other regarding what the patient would have wanted. A legal guardian is a person who has been formally appointed by the courts to make decisions on behalf of the patient. This helps to overcome arguments about who is the patient's best surrogate representative but does not guarantee that a patient's premorbid wishes will be followed. A patient who fears he may become incompetent may make a living will to direct future treatment. This is a formal written statement specifying particular situations and the limits of treatment the patient would wish to receive. It is essential that this statement be made with the help of an expert medical advisor to ensure that the patient fully understands the implications of the statement. Doctors should follow the instructions made by a patient in a living will unless they believe that the patient did not fully understand the consequences. Problems may arise with living wills because the instructions do not adequately cover the medical situation which occurs at a later date. An advance directive is a more informal verbal or written statement made by the patient when mentally competent. These statements are often not sufficiently clear to be able to guide therapy adequately. 'Durable power of attorney for healthcare' is a concept from the USA where a competent patient nominates another person to make medical decisions on his or her behalf if he or she later becomes incompetent. In the UK nomination of such a person in a living will makes him/her the preferred surrogate representative. However, in the absence of a legal guardian the doctor in charge of the patient's care retains the legal responsibility for deciding what is in the patient's best interests. The doctor should consider the views of surrogates and caregivers and any advance directives by the patient but he/she is not legally bound to follow them if this is felt not to be in the patient's interests.

PAPER 3 QUESTIONS

-CELLULAR AND MOLECULAR BIOLOGY

1. THEME: CARBOHYDRATE METABOLISM

A   Glucose-6-phosphate dehydrogenase
B   Glucose-6-phosphatase
C   Hexokinase
D   Glucocerebrosidase
E   Pyruvate kinase
F   Diphosphoglycerate mutase

For each of the following descriptions select the appropriate enzyme of carbohydrate metabolism from the above list. The items may be used once or not at all.

☐ 1. Has an important role in conversion of glycogen to glucose
☐ 2. Connects Embden-Meyerhof pathway to hexose monophosphate shunt
☐ 3. Involved in Rapaport-Luebering shunt
☐ 4. Essential for lactate production in red blood cells
☐ 5. Initiates glucose breakdown by converting glucose to glucose-6-phosphate

2. THEME: APOPTOSIS

A   Interleukin 2
B   Fas-ligand
C   p53
D   Interleukin 1β converting enzyme
E   CD95
F   bcl-2

For each of the following descriptions select the appropriate term related to apoptosis from the above list. The items may be used once or not at all.

☐ 1. Member of the caspases that drives changes in the nucleus accompanying apoptosis
☐ 2. Inhibitor of caspases that blocks apoptosis
☐ 3. Transmembrane receptor that activates intracellular caspases
☐ 4. Expressed on membrane of some tumour cells to activate apoptosis in cytotoxic T lymphocytes
☐ 5. Regulator of cell cycle essential for apoptosis in cells with damaged DNA

STATISTICS AND EPIDEMIOLOGY

3. THEME: STUDY DESIGNS

A   Cohort study
B   Cross-sectional survey
C   Cross-over study
D   Case–control study
E   Randomised controlled trial
F   Ecological study

For each of the following descriptions select the appropriate study design from the above list. The items may be used once or not at all.

☐ 1. Frequency of the exposure is compared between those who do and those who do not have a particular disease
☐ 2. Frequency of the outcome is compared between those who have and those who have not had a particular exposure
☐ 3. Frequency of the outcome is compared between those who have received a particular intervention and those who have not. All subjects have the same probability of being allocated to the treatment group
☐ 4. Frequency of outcome and exposure are compared in different groups without information on individuals within the groups being available
☐ 5. Outcome and exposure for each individual in a population are identified simultaneously

IMMUNOLOGY

4. THEME: HYPERSENSITIVITY REACTION

A   Extrinsic allergic alveolitis
B   Goodpasture's syndrome
C   Mycosis fungoides
D   Asthma
E   Grave's disease
F   Contact hypersensitivity

For each of the following type of hypersensitivity reaction select the appropriate disease from the above list. The items may be used once or not at all.

☐ 1. Type I
☐ 2. Type II
☐ 3. Type III
☐ 4. Type IV
☐ 5. Type V

5. THEME: IMMUNODEFICIENCY SYNDROMES

A   Normal lymphocyte count but failure of lymphocyte proliferation with antigen stimulation
B   Bruton's agammaglobulinaemia
C   Common variable immunodeficiency
D   DiGeorge syndrome
E   Severe combined immunodeficiency
F   X-linked immunodeficiency with hyper IgM

For each of the following underlying abnormalities select the associated immunodeficiency syndrome from the above list. The items may be used once or not at all.

☐ 1. B-cell-specific tyrosine kinase deficiency
☐ 2. CD40 ligand deficiency
☐ 3. Microdeletion on chromosome 22
☐ 4. Adenosine deaminase deficiency
☐ 5. MHC class II deficiency

CLINICAL GENETICS

6. THEME: SYNDROMES AND ASSOCIATED ABNORMALITIES

A   Klinefelter's syndrome
B   Down's syndrome
C   Turner's syndrome
D   Homocystinuria
E   Kallman's syndrome
F   Prader-Willi syndrome

For each of the following abnormalities select the associated syndrome from the above list. The items may be used once or not at all.

1. Horseshoe kidney
2. Acute lymphoblastic leukaemia
3. Anosmia
4. Lens dislocation
5. Morbid obesity

7. THEME: FEATURES OF AMINO-ACIDURIA

A Premature intervertebral disc collapse
B Thromboembolism
C Pellagra
D Radiolucent renal stones
E Copper deposition at the corneal limbus
F Pigment deficiency in iris and hair

For each of the following types of amino-aciduria select the condition from the above list that is a characteristic feature. The items may be used once or not at all.

1. Hartnup disease
2. Alkaptonuria
3. Phenylketonuria
4. Homocystinuria
5. Cystinuria

NEUROANATOMY

8. THEME: DERMATOMES AND NERVE ROOT SUPPLY

A L3
B L5
C S1
D S2
E S5
F L2

For each of the following dermatomes select the nerve root supply from the above list. The items may be used once or not at all.

1. The area surrounding the anus
2. The anterior aspect of the thigh and knee
3. The sole and lateral aspect of the foot
4. The medial aspect and dorsum of the foot including the great toe
5. The posterior aspect of the calf and foot

9. THEME: SPINAL CORD TRACTS

A Lateral spinothalamic tract
B Lissauer's tract
C Medial longitudinal fasciculus
D Lateral corticospinal tract
E Fasciculus gracilis
F Fasciculus cuneatus

For each of the following functions select the appropriate spinal cord pathway from the above list. The items may be used once or not at all.

1. Vibration sense for the lower limb
2. Vibration sense for the upper limb
3. Pain and temperature sensation from the contralateral limb
4. Motor supply to limb muscles
5. Pain and temperature sensation from the ipsilateral limb carried up one or two spinal cord segments before decussation

PHYSIOLOGY, BIOCHEMISTRY AND METABOLISM

10. THEME: PLEURAL EFFUSION

A Empyema
B Cirrhosis
C Meigs' syndrome
D Tuberculosis
E Rheumatoid disease
F Uncomplicated parapneumonic effusion

For each of the following characteristic findings of pleural effusion select the appropriate condition from the above list. The items may be used once or not at all.

☐ 1. Straw coloured, 200 WBC/μl mostly mononuclear cells, pleural fluid:serum protein ratio <0.5, pleural fluid:serum glucose ratio =1.0, pH>7.4 *[handwritten: protein exudate]* *[handwritten circled: transudate]*

☐ 2. Turbid, 15,000 WBC/μl mostly polymorphonuclear cells, pleural fluid:serum protein ratio >0.5, pleural fluid:serum glucose ratio =1.0, pH>7.3

☐ 3. Purulent, 80,000 WBC/μl mostly polymorphonuclear cells, pleural fluid:serum protein ratio >0.5, pleural fluid:serum glucose ratio <0.5, pH<7.3

☐ 4. Straw coloured, 8000 WBC/μl mostly mononuclear cells, pleural fluid:serum protein ratio >0.5, pleural fluid:serum glucose ratio 1.0, pH>7.3 *[handwritten: transudate]*

☐ 5. Turbid/yellow, 2000 WBC/μl, pleural fluid:serum protein ratio >0.5, pleural fluid:serum glucose ratio <0.5, pH<7.3 *[handwritten: transudate]*

11. THEME: SIGNAL PATHWAYS

A Insulin
B Atrial natriuretic peptide
C Growth hormone
D Follicle-stimulating hormone
E β-adrenoceptor agonists
F α-adrenoceptor agonists

For each of the following signalling pathways select the appropriate compound from the above list. The items may be used once or not at all.

☐ 1. Activation of cAMP
☐ 2. Inhibition of cAMP
☐ 3. Activation of MAP kinases
☐ 4. Activation of calcium-dependent kinases
☐ 5. Activation of cGMP

12. THEME: ABNORMALITIES OF PORPHYRIN METABOLISM

A Acute intermittent porphyria
B Chronic alcoholism
C Variegate porphyria
D Lead poisoning
E Porphyria cutanea tarda
F Uroporphyria

For each of the following descriptions select the appropriate abnormality of porphyrin metabolism from the above list. The items may be used once or not at all.

☐ 1. A disease with neurological degeneration but no cutaneous features
☐ 2. A commonly acquired skin condition exacerbated by sunlight
☐ 3. An acquired condition with raised urine δ-amino-laevulinic acid and porphobilinogen levels
☐ 4. A hereditary condition with cutaneous and neurological features
☐ 5. A congenital condition with severe skin lesions which usually causes early death

13. THEME: ACID-BASE BALANCE DISORDERS

A Acute paracetamol poisoning
B Acute opioid poisoning
C Pancreatic fistula
D Subarachnoid haemorrhage
E Diabetic ketoacidosis
F Severe burns

For each of the following disorders of acid-base balance select the appropriate causative condition from the above list. The items may be used once or not at all.

☐ 1. Metabolic acidosis with a normal anion gap
☐ 2. Metabolic acidosis with a raised anion gap
☐ 3. Metabolic alkalosis
☐ 4. Respiratory acidosis
☐ 5. Respiratory alkalosis

14. THEME: CLOTTING

A   Acute hepatitis
B   Biliary tract obstruction
C   Cirrhosis
D   Haemolysis
E   Chronic hepatitis
F   Cholestasis

For each of the following results select the appropriate causative condition from the above list. The items may be used once or not at all.

(PT = prothrombin time, ALP = serum alkaline phosphatase, ALT = serum alanine aminotransferase)

☐ 1. Slightly raised bilirubin, normal albumin, normal PT, normal ALP, normal ALT
☐ 2. Moderately raised bilirubin, normal albumin, prolonged PT, slightly elevated ALP, markedly elevated ALT
☐ 3. Slightly raised bilirubin, low albumin, prolonged PT, slightly elevated ALP, slightly elevated ALT
☐ 4. Raised bilirubin, very low albumin, prolonged PT, normal alkaline phosphatase, slightly elevated ALT
☐ 5. Markedly raised bilirubin, normal albumin, prolonged PT, markedly elevated ALP, slightly elevated ALT, markedly decreased urine urobilinogen

RENAL MEDICINE

15. THEME: INHERITED KIDNEY DISEASE

A   Autosomal recessive polycystic kidney disease
B   von Hippel-Lindau syndrome
C   Hyperoxaluria
D   Autosomal dominant polycystic kidney disease
E   Alport's syndrome
F   Juvenile nephronophthisis

For each of the following statements select the appropriate inherited kidney disease from the above list. The items may be used once or not at all.

☐ 1. Commonest inherited renal disease
☐ 2. Renal disease occurs in conjunction with congenital hepatic fibrosis
☐ 3. Chronic tubulointerstitial nephritis causing salt-wasting renal failure
☐ 4. Progressive haematuria, nephritis and bilateral sensorineural deafness
☐ 5. Multiple renal calculi presenting during childhood

16. THEME: RISK FACTORS IN KIDNEY DISEASE

A   Haemolytic uraemic syndrome
B   Papillary necrosis
C   Balkan nephropathy
D   Acute urate nephropathy
E   Rapidly progressive glomerulonephritis
F   Hypercalcaemic nephropathy

For each of the following risk factors select the associated kidney disease from the above list. The items may be used once or not at all.

☐ 1. Analgesic abuse
☐ 2. Glucose-6-phosphatase deficiency
☐ 3. Primary hyperparathyroidism
☐ 4. *Escherichia coli* O157:H7 diarrhoea
☐ 5. Wegener's granulomatosis

17. THEME: INTRAVENOUS UROGRAPHY

A Ureteric stricture at vesicoureteric junction
B Vesicoureteric reflux
C Pelviureteric neuromuscular dysfunction
D Ureteric calculus
E Sloughed renal papilla
F Retroperitoneal fibrosis

For each of the following findings of intravenous urography for suspected urinary tract obstruction select the appropriate condition from the above list. The items may be used once or not at all.

- [ ] 1. Medial deviation of the ureters
- [ ] 2. Bilateral dilated ureters and failure to empty the bladder after micturition
- [ ] 3. Unilateral dilated ureter and no visible stone in a patient with sickle cell anaemia
- [ ] 4. Unilateral dilated ureter in a patient being treated for genitourinary tuberculosis
- [ ] 5. Delayed filling of a dilated renal pelvis and no contrast in the ureter

18. THEME: RENAL IMPAIRMENT

A Gastrointestinal haemorrhage
B Rhabdomyolysis
C Congestive cardiac failure
D Rapidly progressive glomerulonephritis
E Chronic renal failure on very low protein diet
F Chronic renal failure on normal diet

For each of the following plasma urea and creatinine findings in a patient with renal impairment select the appropriate condition from the above list. The items may be used once or not at all.

- [A] 1. Acute elevation of urea disproportionately greater than creatinine
- [F] 2. Chronic elevation of urea disproportionately greater than creatinine
- [ ] 3. Acute elevation of creatinine disproportionately greater than urea

- [ ] 4. Chronic elevation of creatinine disproportionately greater than urea
- [ ] 5. Acute elevation of creatinine and urea in proportion to each other

ENDOCRINOLOGY AND DIABETES

19. THEME: DIAGNOSIS AND TEST RESULTS

A Hypodipsia due to hypothalamic damage
B Normal response
C Primary polydipsia
D Syndrome of inappropriate antidiuretic hormone
E Craniogenic diabetes insipidus
F Nephrogenic diabetes insipidus

For each of the following results select the appropriate causative condition from the above list. The items may be used once or not at all.

- [ ] 1. Increased vasopressin in response to infusion of hypertonic saline; increasing vasopressin and urine osmolality on water deprivation test
- [ ] 2. Increased vasopressin in response to infusion of hypertonic saline; increasing vasopressin but little increase in urine osmolality on water deprivation test
- [ ] 3. No increase in vasopressin in response to infusion of hypertonic saline; no increase in vasopressin or urine osmolality on water deprivation test
- [ ] 4. Hyponatraemia with urine osmolality less than plasma osmolality
- [ ] 5. Hyponatraemia with urine osmolality greater than plasma osmolality

20. THEME: ANTIDIABETIC AGENTS

A Metformin
B Rosiglitazone
C Glibenclamide
D Tolbutamide
E Repaglinide
F Acarbose

For each of the following descriptions select the appropriate antidiabetic agent from the above list. The items may be used once or not at all.

☐ 1. α-glucosidase inhibitor which delays carbohydrate absorption
☐ 2. Biguanide which decreases gluconeogenesis and increases peripheral glucose utilisation
☐ 3. Short-acting sulphonylurea which augments insulin secretion
☐ 4. Long-acting sulphonylurea which augments insulin secretion
☐ 5. Thiazolidinedione which decreases peripheral insulin resistance

21. THEME: DIABETIC NEUROPATHY

A Sensory polyneuropathy affecting large fibres
B Sensory polyneuropathy affecting small fibres
C Mononeuritis
D Radiculopathy
E Autonomic neuropathy
F Amyotrophy

For each of the following presentations select the appropriate type of diabetic neuropathy from the above list. The items may be used once or not at all.

☐ 1. Third cranial nerve palsy
☐ 2. Loss of pain and temperature sensation in the feet
☐ 3. Loss of ankle deep tendon reflexes
☐ 4. Weakness of quadriceps
☐ 5. Urinary retention

22. THEME: DISORDERS OF CALCIUM AND BONE METABOLISM

A Paget's disease
B Vitamin D deficiency
C Vitamin D intoxication
D Primary hyperparathyroidism
E Secondary hyperparathyroidism
F Primary hypoparathyroidism

For each of the following blood test results select the appropriate disorder of calcium and bone metabolism from the above list. The items may be used once or not at all.

☐ 1. Raised calcium, parathyroid hormone and alkaline phosphatase and low phosphate
☐ 2. Normal calcium, parathyroid hormone and phosphate and raised alkaline phosphatase
☐ 3. Raised calcium and phosphate, normal alkaline phosphatase and low parathyroid hormone
☐ 4. Raised phosphate, normal alkaline phosphatase and low calcium and parathyroid hormone
☐ 5. Raised alkaline phosphatase and parathyroid hormone and low calcium and phosphate

GASTROENTEROLOGY

23. THEME: GASTROINTESTINAL ABSORPTION AND EXCRETION

A Bile acids
B Amylase
C Chloride exchanger
D Gastric intrinsic factor
E Trypsin
F Lipase

For the absorption or excretion of each of the following select the appropriate factor from the above list. The items may be used once or not at all.

☐ 1. Vitamin B_{12}
☐ 2. Vitamin A
☐ 3. Carbohydrate
☐ 4. Protein
☐ 5. Water

24. THEME: GASTROINTESTINAL CANCER

A Gastric adenocarcinoma
B Oesophageal adenocarcinoma
C Oesophageal squamous cell carcinoma
D Cholangiocarcinoma
E Enteropathy-associated T cell lymphoma
F Colonic adenocarcinoma

For each of the following predisposing conditions select the associated gastrointestinal cancer from the above list. The items may be used once or not at all.

☐ 1. Barrett's oesophagus
☐ 2. Coeliac disease
☐ 3. Familial adenomatous polyposis
☐ 4. Pernicious anaemia
☐ 5. *Clonorchis sinensis* infection

25. THEME: BOWEL DISEASE

A Cutaneous fistulae
B Primary sclerosing cholangitis
C Sacroiliitis
D Dermatitis herpetiformis
E Virchow's node
F Erythema nodosum

For each of the following statements select the appropriate condition from the above list. The items may be used once or not at all.

☐ 1. Associated with Crohn's disease and ulcerative colitis, but not disease-activity related
☐ 2. Associated with Crohn's disease and ulcerative colitis, occurring during a flare-up of disease
☐ 3. Feature of ulcerative colitis rarely seen in Crohn's disease
☐ 4. Feature of Crohn's disease not generally seen in ulcerative colitis
☐ 5. Associated with gluten-sensitive enteropathy not inflammatory bowel disease

26. THEME: GUT MOTILITY

A Circular muscle layer
B Longitudinal muscle layer
C Auerbach's plexus
D Meissner's plexus
E Coeliac plexus
F Vagus nerve

For each of the following descriptions related to gut motility regulation select the appropriate term from the above list. The items may be used once or not at all.

☐ 1. Part of the sympathetic nerve supply
☐ 2. Part of the parasympathetic nerve supply
☐ 3. The part of the intrinsic nerve supply located between the smooth muscle layers of the gut wall
☐ 4. The part of the intrinsic nerve supply located between the mucosa and smooth muscle
☐ 5. Muscle fibres which constrict the bowel lumen

NEUROLOGY

27. THEME: DYSKINESIA

A Tardive dyskinesia
B Dystonia
C Myoclonus
D Chorea
E Hemiballismus
F Tremor

For each of the following descriptions select the appropriate form of dyskinesia from the above list. The items may be used once or not at all.

☐ 1. Rhythmic sinusoidal motion due to regular muscle contractions
☐ 2. Continuous and explosive, non-rhythmic, purposeless movements flitting from one part of the body to another
☐ 3. Large amplitude, sudden, flinging movements of the limbs
☐ 4. Shock-like involuntary muscle jerks

☐ 5. Prolonged muscle spasms producing abnormal postures

28. THEME: SPEECH DISORDERS

A Extrapyramidal dysarthria
B Cerebellar dysarthria
C Bulbar palsy
D Pseudobulbar palsy
E Wernicke's dysphasia
F Broca's dysphasia

For each of the following descriptions select the appropriate speech disorder from the above list. The items may be used once or not at all.

☐ 1. Slurring of speech which is inappropriately irregular in volume and rhythm
☐ 2. Explosive speech which requires great effort
☐ 3. Indistinct speech with monotonous tone, volume and rhythm
☐ 4. Non-fluent speech with failure to name objects and repeat words but comprehension remains intact
☐ 5. Fluent speech with failure to name objects, repeat words and comprehend others

29. THEME: HEADACHE

A Acute glaucoma
B Raised intracranial pressure
C Giant cell arteritis
D Migrainous neuralgia
E Trigeminal neuralgia
F Migraine

For each of the headaches with the following characteristics select the appropriate diagnosis from the above list. The items may be used once or not at all.

☐ 1. Brief stabbing unilateral facial pain induced by eating and shaving
☐ 2. Severe facial pain around one eye lasting less than one hour but causing lacrimation, flushing and rhinorrhoea and occurring every day for several weeks

☐ 3. Severe headache with jaw pain on eating
☐ 4. Severe pain around one eye with decreased vision and conjunctival redness and a cloudy cornea
☐ 5. Progressive headache exacerbated by lying down and by coughing

30. THEME: CAUSES OF OPTIC DISC SWELLING

A Optic disc drusen
B Papilloedema
C Congenital pseudopapilloedema
D Ischaemic optic neuropathy
E Open-angle glaucoma
F Papillitis due to demyelination

For each of the following findings select the appropriate cause of optic disc swelling from the above list. The items may be used once or not at all.

☐ 1. Bilateral optic disc swelling with abnormal vessels, normal visual acuity and visual fields
☐ 2. Bilateral optic disc swelling, normal visual acuity, increased size of blind spot
☐ 3. Unilateral optic disc swelling, painful rapid loss of visual acuity and development of a central scotoma
☐ 4. Unilateral optic disc swelling, painless rapid loss of visual acuity and partial visual field loss
☐ 5. Unilateral optic disc swelling, progressive visual field loss, pearly white excrescences on disc

RESPIRATORY MEDICINE

31. THEME: RISK FACTORS FOR RESPIRATORY DISEASE

A Pulmonary eosinophilia
B Pulmonary hypertension
C Bronchiectasis
D Mesothelioma
E Chronic obstructive lung disease
F Progressive massive fibrosis

For each of the following risk factors select the associated condition from the above list. The items may be used once or not at all.

☐ 1. Selective immunoglobulin A deficiency
☐ 2. α_1-antitrypsin deficiency
☐ 3. Asbestos exposure
☐ 4. Silica exposure
☐ 5. Sulphonamide therapy

32. THEME: SIGNS OF RESPIRATORY DISEASE

A Right-sided tension pneumothorax
B Right-sided pleural effusion
C Right-sided fibrosis
D Right-sided consolidation
E Right-sided pulmonary embolism
F Right-sided pneumonectomy

For each of the following signs elicited by examination of the chest select the appropriate condition from the above list. The items may be used once or not at all.

☐ 1. Trachea deviated to left, decreased breath sounds and dull percussion on right
☐ 2. Trachea central, bronchial breathing, a pleural rub and dull percussion on right
☐ 3. Trachea deviated to right, decreased breath sounds and dull percussion on right
☐ 4. Trachea deviated to left, decreased breath sounds and resonant percussion on right
☐ 5. Trachea deviated to right, harsh breath sounds, crackles and squawks and dull percussion on right

33. THEME: AETIOLOGY OF PNEUMONIA

A *Pneumocystis carinii*
B *Klebsiella pneumoniae*
C *Staphylococcus aureus*
D *Streptococcus pneumoniae*
E *Pseudomonas aeruginosa*
F *Streptococcus pyogenes*

For each of the following presentations of pneumonia select the appropriate causative organism from the above list. The items may be used once or not at all.

☐ 1. Previously healthy adult with lobar pneumonia
☐ 2. Intravenous drug user with cavitating pneumonia
☐ 3. Diabetic with hospital-acquired, cavitating pneumonia and Gram-negative bacilli seen in the sputum
☐ 4. HIV patient with a six-week history of fever and progressive breathlessness
☐ 5. Cystic fibrosis patient with recurrent bronchiectasis and Gram-negative bacilli in the sputum

34. THEME: RESPIRATORY SUPPORT

A Simultaneous intermittent mandatory ventilation (SIMV)
B High-frequency jet ventilation
C Continuous positive airway pressure (CPAP)
D Pressure-support ventilation
E Assist control ventilation
F Biphasic positive airway pressure (BIPAP)

For each of the following descriptions select the appropriate form of respiratory support from the above list. The items may be used once or not at all.

☐ 1. Non-invasive method where constant airway pressure is maintained throughout the respiratory cycle
☐ 2. Non-invasive method where pressure during inspiration exceeds pressure during expiration

☐ 3. Gaseous exchange is achieved in an intubated patient without chest inflation and deflation

☐ 4. Volume-targeted method where an intubated patient can take additional breaths at own tidal volume

☐ 5. Volume-targeted method where an intubated patient can take additional breaths but machine setting determines the tidal volume

RHEUMATOLOGY

35. THEME: AUTOANTIBODIES

A Microscopic polyangiitis
B Rheumatoid arthritis
C Still's disease
D Wegener's granulomatosis
E Systemic lupus erythematosus
F Antiphospholipid syndrome

For each of the following autoantibodies select the disease from the above list in which it is commonly detected. The items may be used once or not at all.

☐ 1. Cytoplasmic antineutrophil cytoplasmic antibody

☐ 2. Perinuclear antineutrophil cytoplasmic antibody

☐ 3. Antinuclear antibody

☐ 4. Rheumatoid factor

☐ 5. Anticardiolipin antibody

36. THEME: CLINICAL PRESENTATION

A Sarcoidosis
B Polymyalgia rheumatica
C Wegener's granulomatosis
D Behçet's disease
E Systemic sclerosis
F Familial Mediterranean fever

For each of the following clinical presentations select the appropriate disease from the above list. The items may be used once or not at all.

☐ 1. Foul-smelling, bloody nasal discharge, haemoptysis, pleuritic chest pain and proptosis in a middle-aged man

☐ 2. Recurrent peritonitis and recurrent aseptic arthritis in a teenager

☐ 3. Recurrent oral and genital ulcers, a painful red eye and recurrent arthritis in a young man

☐ 4. Acute onset of erythema nodosum, hilar lymphadenopathy and a migratory polyarthritis in a young woman

☐ 5. Chronic Raynaud's phenomenon accompanied by recent onset of swallowing difficulties in a 60-year-old woman

DERMATOLOGY

37. THEME: CUTANEOUS LESIONS

A Dermatitis herpetiformis
B Dermatomyositis
C Acanthosis nigricans
D Erythema nodosum
E Pyoderma gangrenosum
F Ichthyosis

For each of the following descriptions select the appropriate cutaneous lesion from the above list. The items may be used once or not at all.

☐ 1. Painful ulcerating nodules usually occurring on the shins or abdomen

☐ 2. Velvety, thickened lesions in the axillae

☐ 3. Heliotrope oedema of the eyelids with scaly papules on the knuckles

☐ 4. Dry, fish-like scaling particularly affecting the extremities

☐ 5. Panniculitis particularly affecting the shins

38. THEME: PREGNANCY-ASSOCIATED DERMATOSES

A   Chloasma
B   Pruritic urticarial papules and plaques of pregnancy
C   Pruritic folliculitis of pregnancy
D   Telogen effluvium
E   Impetigo herpetiformis
F   Pemphigoid gestationis

For each of the following descriptions select the appropriate pregnancy-associated dermatosis from the above list. The items may be used once or not at all.

☐ 1. Postpartum hair loss
☐ 2. Facial hyperpigmentation
☐ 3. Erythematous pustular psoriasis
☐ 4. Polymorphic abdominal lesions sparing the periumbilical area
☐ 5. Acneiform eruption

HAEMATOLOGY

39. THEME: IRON STATUS

A   Serum ferritin
B   Serum transferrin
C   Bone marrow iron staining
D   Serum soluble transferrin receptor
E   Serum iron
F   Serum transferrin saturation

For each of the following statements related to the assessment of iron status select the appropriate test from the above list. The items may be used once or not at all.

☐ 1. Levels are decreased in systemic inflammatory conditions
☐ 2. Levels are increased in pregnancy
☐ 3. Levels are increased in systemic inflammatory conditions
☐ 4. Gold standard test of availability of iron
☐ 5. Levels raised in iron deficiency

40. THEME: LEUKAEMIA

A   Acute promyelocytic leukaemia
B   Acute lymphoblastic leukaemia
C   Acute myeloid leukaemia
D   Hodgkin's disease
E   Chronic lymphatic leukaemia
F   Chronic myeloid leukaemia

For each of the following statements select the appropriate type of leukaemia from the above list. The items may be used once or not at all.

☐ 1. Most indolent form of leukaemia
☐ 2. Associated with high serum B_{12} level
☐ 3. Predominantly affects children
☐ 4. Around 1% carry the Philadelphia chromosome
☐ 5. Treatable with all-*trans*-retinoic acid

41. THEME: HAEMATOLOGICAL ABNORMALITY

A   Chronic alcoholism
B   Dengue fever
C   Glucose-6-phosphate dehydrogenase deficiency
D   Renal failure
E   Chronic hypoxia
F   α-thalassaemia

For each of the following haematological abnormalities select the appropriate causative condition from the above list. The items may be used once or not at all.

☐ 1. Microcytic anaemia
☐ 2. Normocytic anaemia
☐ 3. Macrocytic anaemia
☐ 4. Haemolytic anaemia
☐ 5. Thrombocytopenia

INFECTIOUS DISEASES AND TROPICAL MEDICINE

42. THEME: CLINICAL PRESENTATION

A *Neisseria gonorrhoea*
B *Pasteurella multocida*
C *Bacillus* species
D *Haemophilus influenzae* group B
E *Streptococcus pneumoniae*
F *Enterococcus* species

For each of the following clinical presentations select the appropriate causative organism from the above list. The items may be used once or not at all.

☐ 1. A 23-year-old man who has had recent sinusitis presents with symptoms of acute meningitis
☐ 2. Localised cellulitis following a cat bite
☐ 3. Bacterial endocarditis in an 80-year-old with a recent change in bowel habit
☐ 4. Endophthalmitis following high-velocity penetrating eye trauma with a metal splinter
☐ 5. Purulent conjunctivitis in a neonate 48 hours after delivery

43. THEME: RICKETTSIAE

A *Rickettsia rickettsii*
B *Rickettsia tsutsugamushi*
C *Bartonella henselae*
D *Rickettsia typhi*
E *Rickettsia conori*
F *Rickettsia prowazekii*

For each of the following diseases select the responsible *Rickettsia* species from the above list. The items may be used once or not at all.

☐ 1. Louse-borne typhus
☐ 2. Murine typhus
☐ 3. Rocky mountain spotted fever
☐ 4. Scrub typhus
☐ 5. Mediterranean spotted fever (tick boutonneuse)

44. THEME: ZOONOTIC INFECTION

A Pig
B Fox
C Domestic cat
D Ungulates, eg cattle, bushbuck, ox
E Small rodents, eg rats and gerbils
F Bat

For each of the following zoonotic infections select the animal from the above list that is the usual reservoir host. The items may be used once or not at all.

☐ 1. *Leishmania major*
☐ 2. *Balantidium coli*
☐ 3. *Echinococcus multilocularis*
☐ 4. *Trypanosoma brucei rhodesiense*
☐ 5. *Bartonella henselae*

45. THEME: DRUG REGIMENS

A Liposomal amphotericin B
B Intrathecal and intravenous amphotericin B
C Praziquantel
D Melarsoprol
E Fluconazole
F Albendazole

For each of the following infections select the appropriate drug regimen from the above list. The items may be used once or not at all.

☐ 1. Disseminated *Encephalitozoon hellem*
☐ 2. *Naegleria fowleri* meningoencephalitis
☐ 3. Indian visceral leishmaniasis
☐ 4. Acute *Schistosoma japonicum* infection
☐ 5. *Trypanosoma brucei* infection with abnormal CSF

GENITOURINARY MEDICINE

46. THEME: HIV-ASSOCIATED INFECTIONS

A *Toxoplasma gondii*
B *Leishmania infantum*
C *Cryptosporidium parvum*
D *Pneumocystis carinii*
E *Cryptococcus neoformans*
F *Candida albicans*

For each of the following descriptions select the appropriate HIV-associated infection from the above list. The items may be used once or not at all.

- ☐ 1. A yeast infection which may be diagnosed by a positive serum antigen test
- ☐ 2. A yeast infection which is best diagnosed by bronchoscopic alveolar lavage
- ☐ 3. A yeast infection which may cause endophthalmitis
- ☐ 4. A systemic protozoan infection which is common in HIV-positive drug users
- ☐ 5. A protozoan infection for which co-trimoxazole is effective prophylaxis

CLINICAL PHARMACOLOGY

47. THEME: ADVERSE DRUG EFFECTS

A Minoxidil
B Amiodarone
C Methysergide
D Lithium
E Metoclopramide
F Phenytoin

For each of the following adverse effects select the appropriate drug from the above list. The items may be used once or not at all.

- ☐ 1. Retroperitoneal fibrosis
- ☐ 2. Gingival hypertrophy
- ☐ 3. Exacerbation of psoriasis
- ☐ 4. Oculogyric crisis
- ☐ 5. Hypertrichosis

48. THEME: DRUGS IN PREGNANCY

A Primaquine
B Benzylpenicillin
C Indomethacin
D Tetracycline
E Carbamazepine
F Stilboestrol

For each of the following problems in pregnancy select the drug most likely to be responsible from the above list. The items may be used once or not at all.

- ☐ 1. Premature closure of the ductus arteriosus if used in third trimester
- ☐ 2. Neonatal haemolysis and methaemoglobinaemia if used in third trimester
- ☐ 3. Believed to be safe
- ☐ 4. Increased risk of later development of vaginal cancer if used in first trimester
- ☐ 5. Increased risk of neural tube defects if used in first trimester

49. THEME: PARKINSON'S DISEASE

A Potent dopamine D_1 and D_2 receptor agonist given by subcutaneous injection
B Catechol-*O*-methyltransferase inhibitor
C Monoamine oxidase B inhibitor
D Dopa-decarboxylase inhibitor which does not cross the blood-brain barrier
E Antimuscarinic drug
F Selective D_2 receptor agonist

For each of the following drugs used to treat Parkinson's disease select the appropriate description from the above list. The items may be used once or not at all.

- ☐ 1. Selegiline
- ☐ 2. Benserazide
- ☐ 3. Ropinirole
- ☐ 4. Apomorphine
- ☐ 5. Benzhexol

50. THEME: GENERAL ANAESTHESIA

A   Inhalational anaesthetic
B   Non-depolarising neuromuscular blocking agent
C   Opioid used to depress respiration
D   Depolarising neuromuscular blocking agent
E   Intravenous anaesthetic agent with high incidence of hallucinations
F   Intravenous anaesthetic agent which can cause fat overload

For each of the following drugs used in general anaesthesia select the appropriate description from the above list. The items may be used once or not at all.

☐ 1. Ketamine
☐ 2. Propofol
☐ 3. Suxamethonium
☐ 4. Atracurium
☐ 5. Fentanyl

51. THEME: LAXATIVE DRUGS

A   Osmotic laxative
B   Stimulant laxative which colours urine pink
C   Potent stimulant laxative with carcinogenic potential
D   Bulk-forming laxative
E   Stimulant laxative used before procedures requiring bowel clearance
F   Stimulant laxative belonging to the anthraquinone group

For each of the following laxative drugs select the appropriate description from the above list. The items may be used once or not at all.

☐ 1. Danthron
☐ 2. Senna
☐ 3. Sodium picosulphate
☐ 4. Phenolphthalein
☐ 5. Lactulose

52. THEME: ANTIBIOTICS

A   Fluconazole
B   Vancomycin
C   Ceftriaxone
D   Ampicillin plus gentamicin
E   Imipenem
F   Liposomal amphotericin B

For each of the following infections select the most suitable antibiotic for treatment from the above list. The items may be used once or not at all.

☐ 1. Methicillin-resistant *Staphylococcus aureus* pneumonia
☐ 2. Invasive *Aspergillus fumigatus*
☐ 3. *Listeria monocytogenes* meningitis
☐ 4. *Candida albicans* urinary tract infection
☐ 5. Penicillin-insensitive *Neisseria meningitidis* meningitis

CARDIOVASCULAR MEDICINE

53. THEME: CARDIAC ARRHYTHMIA

A   Amiodarone
B   DC cardioversion
C   Defibrillation
D   Magnesium sulphate
E   Atropine
F   Adenosine

For each of the following types of cardiac arrhythmia select the appropriate treatment from the above list. The items may be used once or not at all.

☐ 1. Bradycardia with a rate less than 40 beats per minute
☐ 2. Atrial fibrillation at a rate of 130 beats per minute, onset within 24 hours
☐ 3. Pulseless supraventricular tachycardia at a rate of 260 beats per minute
☐ 4. Supraventricular tachycardia at a rate of 200 beats per minute
☐ 5. Pulseless ventricular tachycardia at a rate of 200 beats per minute

54. THEME: NARROW COMPLEX TACHYARRHYTHMIA

A   Atrial tachycardia
B   Atrial fibrillation
C   Atrial flutter
D   Atrioventricular nodal re-entry tachycardia
E   Atrioventricular re-entry tachycardia
F   Sinus re-entry tachycardia

For each of the following findings select the appropriate form of narrow complex tachyarrhythmia from the above list. The items may be used once or not at all.

☐ 1. Rate 130 beats per minute, normal P wave morphology, P:QRS ratio 1:1
☐ 2. Rate 160 beats per minute, abnormal P wave morphology, P:QRS ratio 1:1 with first degree block
☐ 3. Rate 150 beats per minute, saw-toothed baseline at twice ventricular rate
☐ 4. Rate 160 beats per minute, no P waves visible, irregular rhythm
☐ 5. Rate 180 beats per minute, inverted P wave in ST segment, previous ECG shows short PR interval

55. THEME: INVESTIGATIONS

A   Cardiac catheterisation
B   Echocardiography
C   Technetium-99m labelled red blood cell scan
D   Thallium-201 scan
E   Technetium-99m stannous pyrophosphate scan
F   Holter monitoring

For each of the following descriptions select the appropriate investigation from the above list. The items may be used once or not at all.

☐ 1. Useful to diagnose pericardial effusion
☐ 2. Radioisotopic method for measuring ejection fraction
☐ 3. Radioisotopic method for measuring cardiac ischaemia
☐ 4. Gold standard for measuring severity of aortic stenosis

☐ 5. Useful for investigating recurrent palpitations

56. THEME: AMERICAN HEART ASSOCIATION CLASSIFICATIONS

A   Level B
B   Class III
C   Class I
D   Class II
E   Level A
F   Level C

For each of the following descriptions related to American Heart Association classification for levels of evidence and recommendations select the appropriate term from the above list. The items may be used once or not at all.

☐ 1. Data derived from one or more randomised clinical trial involving large numbers of individuals
☐ 2. Consensus opinion of experts
☐ 3. General agreement that a procedure or treatment is beneficial, useful and effective
☐ 4. General agreement that a procedure or treatment is not useful or effective and in some cases may be harmful
☐ 5. Data from a limited number of trials including small numbers of patients or from well-conceived analyses of non-randomised studies or observational data registries

PSYCHIATRY

57. THEME: PSYCHOLOGICAL DEFENCE MECHANISMS

A   Displacement
B   Repression
C   Rationalisation
D   Sublimation
E   Projection
F   Regression

For each of the following descriptions select the appropriate psychological defence mechanism from the above list. The items may be used once or not at all.

☐ 1. Exclusion of memories, emotions or ideas which may cause distress
☐ 2. Attribution of one's own feelings to someone else
☐ 3. Adoption of behaviour characteristic of an earlier stage of development
☐ 4. Transferring emotions into a more socially acceptable outlet
☐ 5. Explaining events in a way which protects one's emotions

58. THEME: PSYCHIATRIC DIAGNOSIS

A Dementia
B Schizophrenia
C Wernicke-Korsakoff syndrome
D Mania
E Depression
F Dysthymia

For each of the following presentations select the appropriate psychiatric diagnosis from the above list. The items may be used once or not at all.

☐ 1. A patient with a two-month history of loss of appetite, weight loss and poor sleep due to early morning wakening
☐ 2. A patient who believes that others can insert thoughts into his mind and control the movements of his limbs
☐ 3. A patient with a two-year history of forgetfulness, change in personality and disorientation occurring at night
☐ 4. A patient who believes he/she has extraordinary powers, dresses flamboyantly and speaks quickly with rapid changes between topics
☐ 5. A patient who has poor short-term memory and ophthalmoplegia

59. THEME: ANTIPSYCHOTIC DRUGS

A Thioridazine
B Clozapine
C Haloperidol
D Sulpiride
E Chlorpromazine
F Fluphenazine

For each of the following statements select the appropriate antipsychotic drug from the above list. The items may be used once or not at all.

☐ 1. A member of the group 1 phenothiazines, which have pronounced sedative effects
☐ 2. A member of the group 2 phenothiazines, which have marked antimuscarinic effects but fewer extrapyramidal effects than groups 1 or 3
☐ 3. A member of the group 3 phenothiazines, which have marked extrapyramidal effects
☐ 4. An atypical antipsychotic with a high risk of agranulocytosis
☐ 5. A substituted benzamide which has an alerting effect in chronic schizophrenia

MISCELLANEOUS

60. THEME: ORAL CONDITIONS

A   Papillary hyperplasia
B   Erythroplakia
C   Parakeratotic leukoplakia
D   Dental caries
E   Acute pseudomembranous candidiasis
F   Periodontal disease

For each of the following descriptions select the appropriate oral condition from the above list. The items may be used once or not at all.

☐ 1. A condition related to poorly fitting dentures which is not of infectious aetiology
☐ 2. Caused by bacterial invasion of the space between the dental root and the gum
☐ 3. Produces soft, white, friable plaques which can be rubbed off the oral mucosa
☐ 4. Diagnosed by the presence of nuclei throughout the keratin layer of the lesion
☐ 5. A generally malignant condition with atrophic epithelium and tissue papillae near the surface

ANSWERS TO PAPER 3

The approximate difficulty rating for the answer to each question is given in brackets.

☆ (the majority of competent final year students will know the answer)

☆☆ (approximately 50% of final year students will be able to answer correctly)

☆☆☆ (only the better students will usually know the answer)

Q1. CARBOHYDRATE METABOLISM (☆☆☆)

1. B   2. A   3. F   4. E   5. C

Carbohydrate is stored as glycogen, which is broken down to glucose-1-phosphate and then to glucose-6-phosphate. This can then be converted to glucose by glucose-6-phosphatase. This enzyme is deficient in type I glycogen storage disease, known eponymously as von Gierke's. Hexokinase converts glucose to glucose-6-phosphate initiating the Embden-Meyerhof pathway of anaerobic carbohydrate metabolism, which leads to the eventual production of lactate. Red blood cells rely on this metabolic pathway as they do not contain the mitochondria necessary for aerobic metabolism. In the final steps of the Embden-Meyerhof pathway, pyruvate kinase converts phosphoenolpyruvate to pyruvate, which is converted to lactate by lactic dehydrogenase. Pyruvate kinase deficiency is a rare, inherited, red cell enzyme deficiency that can lead to haemolytic anaemia. Glucose-6-phosphate dehydrogenase (G6PD) converts glucose-6-phosphate to 6-phosphogluconate, initiating the hexose monophosphate shunt, a process leading to further energy production. G6PD deficiency can lead to haemolysis following ingestion of fava beans or drugs such as dapsone or primaquine. Diphosphoglycerate mutase converts 1,3-diphosphoglycerate to 2,3-diphosphoglycerate (2,3-DPG), part of the Rapaport-Luebering shunt. 2,3-DPG is an important regulator of oxygen-haemoglobin dissociation. Raised levels of 2,3-DPG move the oxyhaemoglobin dissociation curve to the right facilitating oxygen delivery to the tissues. Glucocerebrosidase is a lysosomal enzyme, deficiency of which results in Gaucher's disease, the commonest of the sphingolipidoses.

Q2. APOPTOSIS (☆☆☆)

1. D   2. F   3. E   4. B   5. C

Apoptosis is the term used to describe the morphological changes accompanying programmed cell death. It is an essential part of embryological development and regulation of cellular proliferation. Failure of apoptosis can result in the development of cancer. Caspases, such as interleukin 1β converting enzyme, drive the structural changes in the nucleus that accompany apoptosis. A family of cytoprotective survival signals, including bcl-2, inhibit caspases and prevent apoptosis. Overexpression of bcl-2 correlates with poor survival in cancer. CD95, also known as fas, is a transmembrane receptor that binds fasligands. This leads to activation of intracellular caspases and is a trigger for apoptosis to occur. Expression of fasligands on the cell membrane of tumour cells can activate fas on cytotoxic T lymphocytes (CTL). This stimulates CTL death and facilitates immune evasion by the tumour cells. p53 is an important regulator of the cell cycle which activates apoptosis of cells with damaged DNA. In Li Fraumeni syndrome, inherited mutations of p53 result in failure of apoptosis to occur in cells with damaged DNA and this leads to increased risk of several malignancies. Interleukin 2 is a cytokine that stimulates lymphocyte proliferation and is not involved in apoptosis.

Q3. STUDY DESIGNS (☆☆)

1. D   2. A   3. E   4. F   5. B

In a case–control study, a group of people who have experienced the same outcome (usually a disease) are identified and a group of healthy people from the same population are selected as controls. The controls may be matched to the cases by age, sex, residence, ethnic group, etc. The frequency of the exposure of interest is then compared between the two groups. For example, cases may be lung cancer patients and the exposure may be cigarette smoking. If the frequency of cigarette smoking among the cases is found to be different from that among the controls then smoking and lung cancer are said to be associated. Case–control studies are most useful when the disease outcome is rare, as prospective studies on risk factors for rare diseases often do not contain enough outcome events. The disadvantages of case–control studies are that as they are retrospective they cannot establish the time course of events (ie that the exposure preceded the outcome) and they are susceptible to the effects of bias and confounding. In a cohort study, people who have experienced an exposure are identified and the frequency with which a particular outcome occurs is compared to that in those who were not exposed. For example, a group of smokers and non-smokers can be followed over several years to determine how many will develop lung cancer. Cohort studies can be prospective and can therefore be used to identify the temporal relationship between the exposure and the outcome. They are useful for rare exposures but not for rare outcomes. However, cohort studies are expensive and time-consuming. In a randomised trial, all subjects have the same probability of being assigned to each treatment group. This minimises the risk of confounding factors affecting the frequency with which the outcome occurs in each group. Randomised trials are the best method for establishing causal relationships but in some cases may be unethical. Clearly one cannot randomly allocate people to smoke cigarettes for 20 years, but

there is also much controversy over allocating people to placebo treatments or potentially suboptimal therapies. A cross-over study is a form of intervention trial where each patient receives both treatment arms, one followed by the other. It is suitable for outcomes where the intervention only has an effect during the treatment period. For example, analgesics could be compared for chronic pain management and the patient could state which treatment gave the most benefit. In a cross-sectional survey, individuals are surveyed for the presence of an exposure and an outcome at the same time. In an ecological study the frequencies of outcome and exposure in different populations are compared to determine if there is any relationship between them. The difference between cross-sectional surveys and ecological studies is that in the latter it is not known whether the outcome and exposure occur together in the same individuals. An ecological study looks at risks at the population level but does not distinguish risk between individuals within a population. For example, iodine deficiency is a risk factor for goitre at the population level. Between individuals within a population where iodine intake is constant (or adequate) autoimmune disease is the major risk factor for goitre.

Q4. HYPERSENSITIVITY REACTION (☆)

1. D   2. B   3. A   4. F   5. E

Type I hypersensitivity reactions are mediated by immunoglobulin E (IgE). Crosslinking of IgE molecules on mast cells leads to release of histamine and leukotrienes. T helper (Th$_2$) type lymphocytes have the primary role in this reaction by producing interleukin 4, which leads to B cell stimulation and IgE production. Examples of diseases caused by type I hypersensitivity reactions are anaphylaxis, asthma and atopic disorders. Type II reactions are due to IgG-mediated cellular cytoxicity. Antibody binds to cells and leads to destruction of those cells by phagocytes. Type II reactions can be classified into five groups according to the antigen bound to the immunoglobulin molecule: cell surface receptor, eg acetylcholine receptor; adhesion molecules/extracellular matrix, eg type IV collagen in Goodpasture's syndrome; circulating serum proteins, eg antiphospholipid syndrome; cytoplasmic antigens, eg mitochondrial antigens in primary biliary cirrhosis; nuclear antigens, eg in systemic lupus erythematosus and Sjögren's syndrome. Type III reactions are caused by immune-complex-mediated damage. In serum sickness and in the glomerulonephritides the antigen-antibody complexes are formed in the blood and are then deposited at the renal glomerulus where the damage occurs. In contrast, in extrinsic allergic alveolitis the antigen-antibody complexes are formed at the site of the tissue damage. Type IV hypersensitivity is a cell-mediated reaction involving T cells and macrophages. The tuberculin reaction and contact hypersensitivity are caused by this mechanism. Type V reactions are due to stimulation of a receptor by an autoantibody. In Grave's disease the anti-TSH (TSH is thyroid-stimulating hormone) receptor antibody results in overproduction of thyroid hormone. Type V reactions are now generally classified with type II. Mycosis fungoides is a form of cutaneous T cell lymphoma.

Q5. IMMUNODEFICIENCY SYNDROMES (☆☆☆)

1. B   2. F   3. D   4. E   5. A

Bruton's agammaglobulinaemia is an X-linked recessive condition with normal T cells and cellular immunity but very few circulating B cells. It is caused by deficiency of B-cell-specific tyrosine kinase. In X-linked immunodeficiency with hyper IgM there are low circulating levels of IgG, IgA and IgE and markedly raised IgM and sometimes IgD. The gene for CD40 ligand is defective which prevents T cells switching B cells from IgM to IgG production, as this is dependent on CD40 ligand–CD40 interaction. Patients also suffer from T cell lymphopenia and neutropenia. DiGeorge syndrome is due to failure of development of the third and fourth branchial arches due to a microdeletion on chromosome 22. Affected children suffer from thymic aplasia, dysmorphic facies, cardiac malformations and absent parathyroids. They have a severely reduced number of circulating T cells (<10% normal) resulting in defective cell-mediated immunity. Severe combined immunodeficiency indicates a failure of antibody and cell-mediated immunity and can be caused by mutations in several different genes. Adenosine deaminase deficiency is an autosomal recessive condition presenting in early childhood with severe infections. Children may present when given BCG as they are liable to develop disseminated infection. This condition can be treated by red cell transfusions, adenosine deaminase purified from calf thymus or bone marrow transplantation. It was also the first condition to be treated by gene therapy. In X-linked MHC class II deficiency, the circulating lymphocyte count is normal but proliferation does not occur in response to antigens. Affected patients have a severe immunodeficiency of antibody production and cell-mediated immunity. Common variable immunodeficiency is a heterogeneous group of disorders with a multifactorial aetiology.

Q6. SYNDROMES AND ASSOCIATED ABNORMALITIES (☆☆)

1. C   2. B   3. E   4. D   5. F

Features of Turner's syndrome include short stature, shield-shaped chest, webbed neck, gonadal dysgenesis, poorly developed secondary sexual characteristics, amenorrhoea, aortic coarctation and horseshoe kidney. Down's syndrome is due to trisomy of chromosome 21. Mental retardation, characteristic facies, short stature, atrio ventricular septal defects and hypothyroidism are common features. Life expectancy is reduced and many adult patients develop acute lymphoblastic leukaemia or premature Alzheimer's disease. Kallman's syndrome is the association of hypogonadotrophic hypogonadism and anosmia. Patients with homocystinuria morphologically resemble those with the Marfan syndrome. However, lens dislocation is usually downwards in homocystinuria and upwards in Marfan patients. Prader-Willi syndrome is due to paternal inheritance of an abnormal gene at the imprinted locus on chromosome 15q12. Characteristic features include mental retardation and morbid obesity. Patients with Klinefelter's syndrome have the karyotype XXY. They are phenotypically male but have underdeveloped secondary sexual characteristics.

Q7. FEATURES OF AMINO-ACIDURIA (☆☆)

1. C   2. A   3. F   4. B   5. D

These inborn errors of metabolism are all inherited as autosomal recessive conditions. Hartnup disease is malabsorption and excessive renal loss of tryptophan and other neutral amino acids. Tryptophan is a precursor for the B complex vitamin nicotinamide. Deficiency may result in pellagra, the classical triad of sunlight-induced dermatitis, diarrhoea and dementia. Treatment is with oral nicotinamide. Tryptophan is also a precursor of 5-hydroxytryptamine (5HT) and therefore carcinoid syndrome (where excessive quantities of 5HT are produced exhausting tryptophan) may also cause pellagra. In alkaptonuria, deficiency of the enzyme homogentisate oxidase results in accumulation of homogentisic acid. Oxidation of this substance in urine makes it dark and pigment also accumulates in cartilage, eg the external auricle. The commonest presentation is with premature intervertebral disc collapse and calcification. Eventually a rigid spine develops and patients may also suffer attacks of ochronotic arthritis. Phenylketonuria is due to deficiency of phenylalanine hydroxylase or its cofactors. Patients do not produce melanin and if untreated develop severe mental retardation. The condition is detected in neonates by the Guthrie test and treatment is with a phenylalanine-free diet until age 16 years. This diet is also required for pregnant women preferably commenced before attempting to conceive. Whether it is really safe for adults to

discontinue the dietary restriction is uncertain. Cystathionine synthase deficiency leads to homocystinuria. Patients have a Marfanoid body habitus and frequently suffer thromboembolic, ocular, skeletal and central nervous system complications. A proportion of cases respond to vitamin B$_6$ (pyridoxine). Cystinuria is believed to be due to an amino acid renal transport defect. Radiolucent cystine and occasionally calcium stones form in the kidneys. Stone analysis may establish the diagnosis but if calcium stones form in a teenager or young adult, urinary amino acid chromatography should also be performed. Stone formation is prevented by drinking 3 litres of water per day or by penicillamine, which binds to cystine in urine and increases its solubility. Lithotripsy is often ineffective but high-dose penicillamine may eventually dissolve stones. Cystinuria should not be confused with cystinosis, a rare inborn error of metabolism frequently causing premature death. Copper deposition at the margin of the cornea is known as a Kayser-Fleischer ring and is pathognomonic of hepatolenticular degeneration (Wilson's disease). This inherited deficiency of caeruloplasmin results in cirrhosis and basal ganglia degeneration. Copper deposition in the kidney can cause a secondary amino-aciduria.

Q8. DERMATOMES AND NERVE ROOT SUPPLY (☆)

1. E   2. A   3. C   4. B   5. D

There are 8 cervical nerve roots, 12 thoracic, 5 lumbar and 5 sacral. It is important to know the dermatomes that they supply to localise the nerve root that is affected when cutaneous sensory loss is identified. This is useful for identifying a sensory level in spinal cord damage or to identify the nerve root being compressed by a herniating inter vertebral disc or other pathology. The back of the head and neck is supplied by C1-4, C the upper limb by C5 to T1/2, the trunk by T2 to T12/L1, the lower limb by L1/2 to S3 with S4/5 surrounding the anus. There is overlap between dermatomes and a solitary root lesion may not produce a detectable area of anaesthesia. It is also important to know the individual nerves supplying each cutaneous area as peripheral nerve damage or compression may also cause sensory loss, eg compression of the common peroneal nerve against the fibula may cause sensory loss on the dorsum of the foot. L2 supplies the superior part of the thigh.

Q9. SPINAL CORD TRACTS (☆☆)

1. E   2. F   3. A   4. D   5. B

Vibration sense, proprioception and two-point discrimination are carried in the posterior columns. The nerve supply is from the ipsilateral limb and crossing over occurs in the medulla. The fasciculus gracilis is located medially and carries afferent fibres from the lower limb. The adjacent fasciculus cuneatus carries fibres from the upper limb. Fibres carrying pain and temperature sensation pass from the posterior root ganglia up one or two segments of spinal cord in Lissauer's tract before crossing over to the contralateral side of the cord and ascending in the lateral spinothalamic tract. The lateral corticospinal tract carries ipsilateral motor fibres. Spinal cord hemisection (Brown-Séquard syndrome) therefore causes loss of ipsilateral motor function, proprioception, vibration sense and two-point discrimination and contralateral loss of pain and temperature sensation below the level of the lesion. The medial longitudinal fasciculus connects the contralateral CN III and CN VI nuclei. Damage to this tract produces an internuclear ophthalmoplegia, failure of adduction of the ipsilateral eye on contralateral gaze (ie if the lesion is on the left, the left eye will fail to adduct when looking to the right).

Q10. PLEURAL EFFUSION (☆☆)

1. B   2. F   3. A   4. D   5. E

Pleural effusions can be divided into transudates and exudates. Transudates have low white blood cell (WBC) and red blood cell (RBC) counts, low protein content, a glucose content which equals that in plasma and

pH > 7.40. Common causes of a transudate include left ventricular failure, cirrhosis, nephrotic syndrome and other causes of hypoalbuminaemia. Exudates contain high protein (exceeding 50% of the level found in serum) and frequently contain high WBC and RBC counts. Empyema can be distinguished from an uncomplicated parapneumonic effusion by its frequently purulent appearance, higher WBC count (usually 25,000 to 100,000 WBC/μl compared to 5000 to 25,000 WBC/μl respectively), low glucose content and low pH. A pulmonary infarct may produce an effusion where the contents resemble a parapneumonic effusion but there will frequently be a higher RBC content (up to 100,000 RBC/μl). In tuberculous pleural effusion there are predominantly mononuclear cells present (5000 to 10,000 WBC/μl), protein content is high, pleural fluid:serum glucose ratio is between 0.5 and 1 and pH may be < 7.30 or > 7.30. In pleural effusion secondary to rheumatoid disease the appearance is turbid to green/yellow, there are usually fewer than 2000 WBC/μl (either mononuclear or polymorphonuclear), pleural fluid:serum glucose ratio is < 0.5 and pH is < 7.30. In a malignancy-associated effusion the appearance is turbid to bloody, with a high RBC count and high protein. The pleural fluid:serum glucose ratio is between 0.5 and 1 and pH may be < or > 7.30. Meigs' syndrome is the very rare association of a benign ovarian tumour with ascites and a pleural effusion.

Q11. SIGNAL PATHWAYS (☆☆☆)

1. E   2. F   3. A   4. D   5. B

Hormones and neurotransmitters act by binding to specific receptors. The above compounds all exert their effects via membrane-bound receptors causing activation or inhibition of cellular signalling pathways, known as second messengers. Other hormones (eg steroid hormones, vitamin D) act by binding to intracellular receptors. β-adrenoceptor agonists stimulate cyclic adenosine monophosphate (cAMP) and protein kinase A, via activation of adenylate cyclase and the

G protein Gsα. G protein indicates the ability to bind the guanine nucleotides, guanosine diphosphate and guanosine triphosphate. α-adrenoceptor agonists inhibit cAMP via the G protein Giα. Insulin binds to the insulin receptor and stimulates several cell signalling pathways including mitogen activated pathway (MAP) kinases, phosphatidyl inositol-3-kinases and ribosomal S6 kinases. These multiple signalling pathways enable insulin to exert many different effects on cell metabolism. Luteinising hormone, follicle-stimulating hormone and thyroid hormone are all peptides which exert their effects via calcium-dependent kinases and calmodulin. Atrial natriuretic peptide stimulates cyclic guanosine monophosphate (cGMP) and cGMP-dependent protein kinase via guanylate cyclase. Growth hormone stimulates tyrosine kinases.

Q12. ABNORMALITIES OF PORPHYRIN METABOLISM (☆☆)

1. A   2. E   3. D   4. C   5. F

The porphyrias are defects of iron metabolism. Porphyria can be classified into hepatic and erythropoeitic forms. The hepatic forms are acute intermittent porphyria, variegate porphyria, hereditary coproporphyria (all familial) and porphyria cutanea tarda (in which some familial factors are important). The two erythropoeitic porphyrias, uroporphyria and erythropoeitic protoporphyria, are both hereditary and rare. Defects of porphyrin metabolism also occur in lead poisoning and chronic alcoholism. In acute intermittent porphyria (AIP), urine porphobilinogen (PBG) and δ-amino-laevulinic acid (ALA) levels are raised but faecal porphyrins are not elevated. AIP causes acute psychiatric and neurological disturbances often provoked by alcohol or medication. The deficient enzyme is uroporphyrinogen-1-synthetase. Porphyria cutanea tarda (PCT) is the most common form of porphyria. Urine PBG and ALA levels are normal but urine coproporphyrin (CP) and uroporphyrin (UP) are elevated, as are faecal CP and protoporphyrin (PP). PCT is exacerbated by sunlight and alcohol. It exhibits cutaneous features only. Variegate porphyria is a rare condition caused by either protoporphyrinogen oxidase or ferrochelatase deficiency. Episodic attacks cause neurological and cutaneous disease. Urine PBG and ALA and faecal CP and PP are elevated. When abnormal porphyrin metabolism is due to lead poisoning, blood ALA dehydrase levels are low. Urine ALA and CP levels are elevated but faecal porphyrins are normal. In chronic alcoholism the urine contains excess CP but the other urine metabolites are normal. Uroporphyria is a very rare disease causing severe skin lesions, haemolysis and frequently death in early childhood. It is caused by uroporphyrinogen III co-synthetase deficiency. Urine UP and CP and faecal CP are characteristically elevated.

Q13. ACID-BASE BALANCE DISORDERS (☆)

1. C   2. E   3. F   4. B   5. D

The anion gap is the sum of sodium plus potassium ions minus chloride and bicarbonate ions ($Na^+ + K^+ - Cl^- - HCO_3^-$). An increase in the anion gap indicates the presence of other anions such as ketones. A pancreatic fistula causes metabolic acidosis due to loss of bicarbonate ions. Other causes of a metabolic acidosis with a normal anion gap include renal tubular acidosis, diarrhoea, acetazolamide, Addison's disease and ammonium chloride ingestion. Causes of metabolic acidosis with an increased anion gap include diabetic ketoacidosis, lactic acidosis (eg in septic shock), salicylate, methanol and ethylene glycol poisoning and the presence of inorganic acids in renal failure. Metabolic alkalosis occurs when excessive quantities of hydrogen ions are lost. This occurs in severe vomiting, burns, diuretic-induced hypokalaemia and following ingestion of base. Respiratory acidosis occurs in type II respiratory failure when there is accumulation of excess carbon dioxide. This is likely to be uncompensated when it occurs acutely, eg with suppression of respiration following acute opioid poisoning. Respiratory alkalosis occurs when a patient breathes in excess of requirements resulting in a low blood carbon dioxide concentration. This occurs in anxiety-induced hyperventilation and following sub arachnoid haemorrhage, stroke and meningitis. Acute paracetamol poisoning does not usually cause acid-base abnormalities. The presence of acidosis would suggest that the patient may have taken other medicines in addition.

Q14. CLOTTING (☆☆)

1. D   2. A   3. E   4. C   5. B

The pattern of liver function test abnormalities provides valuable clues in the investigation of jaundice. In haemolysis (pre-hepatic jaundice), bilirubin and urinary urobilinogen are elevated, but the albumin, PT and ALT are normal. Acute hepatitis has many causes including viruses (eg hepatitis viruses A to E, cytomegalovirus and yellow fever virus) and drug reactions. The characteristic picture is that of extremely high serum transaminases (ALT may be several thousand international units per litre) and only slightly elevated ALP. The PT is usually prolonged and this is not reversed by administration of vitamin K. Chronic hepatitis may follow infection with hepatitis B or C or be caused by alcohol or autoimmune disease. It is often idiopathic. The bilirubin is usually less raised than occurs in acute hepatitis and it may be normal. Albumin is usually low and ALP and ALT slightly elevated. The PT is prolonged and not reversible by vitamin K. The distinguishing feature of cirrhosis is that the serum albumin is usually very low. The bilirubin is usually only slightly elevated, the ALP is usually normal and the ALT may be normal or slightly prolonged. The PT is usually slightly prolonged (irreversible with vitamin K) but may be normal. In biliary tract obstruction the bilirubin (and its conjugated subfraction) are usually markedly elevated and the urine and faecal urobilinogen are markedly decreased. Although the PT is prolonged, this can be corrected by giving 10 mg IV vitamin K on three consecutive days. ALP is usually markedly elevated and ALT is only

slightly elevated. In cholestasis the pattern of abnormalities is very similar to that in biliary tract obstruction except that the urine urobilinogen is normal or elevated.

Q15. INHERITED KIDNEY DISEASE (☆☆)

1. D   2. A   3. F   4. E   5. C

Autosomal dominant polycystic kidney disease affects around one in 1000 of the general population and is the commonest inherited kidney disease. Multiple cysts occur in the kidneys and in 70% of affected persons there are also cysts in the liver. Patients may present with renal pain (eg due to haemorrhage into a cyst, stones or blood clots), haematuria, recurrent urinary tract infections, hypertension, renal failure or on ultrasound screening. In some families patients develop intracranial aneurysms which cause strokes. Autosomal recessive polycystic kidney disease is a rare condition that occurs in conjunction with congenital hepatic fibrosis. Patients may present with gastrointestinal haemorrhage secondary to portal hypertension-induced varices or with recurrent urinary tract infections. Juvenile nephronophthisis is an autosomal recessive, chronic tubulointerstitial disorder that results in the development of cysts in the renal medulla or at the corticomedullary junction. There is also tubular atrophy, interstitial fibrosis and thickening of the tubular basement membrane. Patients usually present around age four years with polyuria, polydipsia, salt-wasting renal failure and metabolic acidosis. Alport's syndrome is usually inherited as an X-linked condition and therefore predominantly affects male children. It produces chronic progressive haematuria, proteinuria and the nephrotic syndrome, in association with bilateral sensorineural deafness. Electron microscopy shows thickening of the basement membrane and splitting of the lamina densa. Hyperoxaluria is caused by a group of autosomal recessive inborn errors of metabolism where there is deficiency of a hepatic peroxisomal enzyme. Hyperoxaluria results in the development of multiple calcium oxalate renal stones during childhood and subsequent development of hydronephrosis and renal fibrosis. The von Hippel-Lindau syndrome is a hereditary condition leading to the development of cerebellar haemangiomas, renal cell carcinomas, retinal angiomas and endocrine tumours.

Q16. RISK FACTORS IN KIDNEY DISEASE (☆☆)

1. B   2. D   3. F   4. A   5. E

Excessive consumption of analgesics can cause severe renal damage, particularly if preparations containing a combination of non-steroidal anti-inflammatory agents, codeine and caffeine are consumed. Damage can be caused by acute or chronic interstitial nephritis and papillary necrosis may occur. Phenacetin was previously a major cause of this condition and has now been removed from the market. Papillary necrosis can be caused by a direct toxic effect or by ischaemic injury. It is a feature of diabetes mellitus, pyelonephritis, urinary tract obstruction, shock and sickle cell disease as well as analgesic abuse. Acute urate nephropathy is usually due to a combination of excessive dietary purine intake and a familial predisposition caused by undersecretion of uric acid by the renal tubule. It is also a feature of several uncommon conditions such as glucose-6-phosphatase deficiency (glycogen storage disease type I), hypoxanthine guanine phosphoribosyltransferase deficiency (Lesch-Nyhan syndrome), phosphoribosyl pyrophosphate synthetase deficiency, familial juvenile gout and hereditary xanthinuria. Hypercalcaemic nephropathy is seen in malignancy with bone metastases, cancers producing parathyroid-like hormone, primary hyperparathyroidism, multiple myeloma, sarcoidosis and hypervitaminosis D toxicity. Haemolytic uraemic syndrome is the association of renal failure and intravascular autoimmune haemolysis without clotting abnormalities. It is associated with haemorrhagic colitis caused by *Escherichia coli* O157:H7, *Shigella* infections and ciclosporin

use. Rapidly progressive glomerulonephritis with crescent formation needs urgent diagnosis and treatment. The two commonest causes of the most fulminant presentation are antiglomerular basement membrane antibody disease and Wegener's granulomatosis. Both conditions may also cause pulmonary haemorrhage. Balkan nephropathy is a disease that occurs along the tributaries of the River Danube. The cause is uncertain but it is likely that it is related to chronic toxicity produced by a fungal toxin (probably ochratoxin A).

Q17. INTRAVENOUS UROGRAPHY (☆)

1. F   2. B   3. E   4. A   5. C

Retroperitoneal fibrosis occurs when there is periaortic inflammation. It is associated with the use of certain drugs (eg methysergide, methyldopa and β-adrenoceptor blockers). Intravenous urography typically shows medial deviation of the ureters. In vesicoureteric reflux the ureters become dilated by contrast on micturition. Following this the ureters empty back into the bladder which will therefore not be empty. Dilated ureters and a bladder that does not empty after micturition are also seen in lower urinary tract obstruction. Acute ureteric obstruction may be caused by passage of a renal calculus, a blood clot or a sloughed papilla. Ureteric calculi are the commonest cause and they are usually radio-opaque and visible in the lower third of the ureter on plain films. However, a renal calculus may be missed if it is overlying a bony prominence. Papillary necrosis is a classic complication of sickle cell anaemia and may be a recurrent problem in some patients. Ureteric stricture is a frequent complication of genitourinary tuberculosis and most frequently occurs at the vesicoureteric junction. Steroids are often given with anti-tuberculous therapy to prevent this complication but their efficacy remains unproven. Pelviureteric neuromuscular dysfunction is a common cause of ureteric obstruction. The intravenous urogram shows a dilated renal pelvis which fills with contrast on delayed films. The ureter may show no filling with contrast.

Q18. RENAL IMPAIRMENT (☆☆)

1. A   2. C   3. B   4. E   5. D

Plasma urea is dependent on its rate of production by protein breakdown as well as its rate of excretion. In contrast plasma creatinine is dependent on muscle mass. Clearance of urea decreases at low glomerular filtration rates whereas creatinine clearance increases at low flow rates due to a relatively greater effect of tubular secretion. Causes of elevated plasma urea disproportionate to plasma creatinine therefore include dehydration, cardiac failure, high dietary protein intake, increased catabolism (eg due to corticosteroids, trauma, burns or pyrexia), severe muscle wasting and bilateral above-knee amputations. Causes of elevated plasma creatinine disproportionate to urea include rhabdomyolysis, muscular physique, chronic renal failure with a low protein diet, protein malabsorption and decreased protein synthesis in cirrhosis. Acute and chronic renal failure without the above factors cause a proportionate rise in urea and creatinine.

Q19. DIAGNOSIS AND TEST RESULTS (☆☆)

1. B   2. F   3. E   4. C   5. D

Hypertonic saline infusion and/or the water deprivation test can be used in the investigation of suspected diabetes insipidus (DI). The normal response to an infusion of hypertonic saline is for the serum vasopressin concentration to rise as serum osmolality increases. In nephrogenic DI the response to hypertonic saline infusion is normal whereas in craniogenic DI increasing serum osmolality does not stimulate an increase in vasopressin. The normal response to the water deprivation test is for an increase in vasopressin to occur and stimulate an increase in urine osmolality. In nephrogenic DI, serum vasopressin increases but the increase in urine osmolality is subnormal. In craniogenic DI, the water deprivation test does not produce a rise in serum vasopressin and there is no increase in urine osmolality. Syndrome of inappropriate antidiuretic hormone (SIADH) causes hyponatraemia and low serum osmolality. The urine osmolality is greater than the plasma osmolality and there is persistent renal sodium excretion. In primary polydipsia there may also be hyponatraemia and low serum osmolality. However, the urine osmolality will be less than the serum osmolality. Hypodipsia due to damage to the anterior hypothalamus is a rare but potentially life-threatening condition causing hypernatraemia and high serum osmolality. Serum vasopressin concentration and urine osmolality will be high unless there is accompanying craniogenic DI.

Q20. ANTIDIABETIC AGENTS (☆)

1. F   2. A   3. D   4. C   5. B

Acarbose is an inhibitor of α-glucosidase. It acts by delaying digestion and absorption of carbohydrates and therefore helps to reduce post prandial hyperglycaemia. It can be used alone (though it is relatively ineffective) or in conjunction with other oral hypoglycaemic agents or insulin. Metformin is a biguanide that decreases gluconeogenesis and increases the peripheral utilisation of glucose. It is effective only in the presence of some natural insulin secretion. It promotes weight loss and is therefore widely used for obese type II diabetics. Sulphonylureas increase insulin secretion in those with some residual islet cell function. They tend to promote weight gain and therefore require careful dietary control. Tolbutamide and gliclazide are short-acting sulphonylureas. These agents must be taken before each meal but are less likely to cause hypoglycaemia. They are generally regarded as the safest sulphonylureas for use in the elderly. Glibenclamide and chlorpropamide are long-acting sulphonylureas that have a higher risk of hyperglycaemic attacks particularly during the morning. Symptomatic hypoglycaemia secondary to the use of these agents should usually be treated in hospital. Rosiglitazone and pioglitazone are thiazolidinediones that act by decreasing peripheral insulin resistance. The

National Institute for Clinical Excellence has advised that they should only be used for those with inadequate diabetic control with metformin and/or sulphonylureas or those intolerant of these agents. As they promote weight gain it is better to combine thiazolidinediones with metformin than with a sulphonylurea, particularly for obese diabetics. Repaglinide stimulates insulin release by the pancreas. It has a short duration of action and is taken before each meal. It can be used alone or as part of combination therapy.

Q21. DIABETIC NEUROPATHY (☆)

1. C   2. B   3. A   4. F   5. E

Mononeuritis is caused by microvascular damage to the vasa nervorum. If more than one nerve is involved this is called mononeuritis multiplex. It may affect the third, sixth or fourth cranial nerves or peripheral nerves. Mononeuritis multiplex also occurs in connective tissue diseases (eg systemic lupus erythematosus) and the systemic vasculitides (eg microscopic polyangiitis). Sensory polyneuropathy affecting small nerve fibres results in loss of pain and temperature sensation of the feet. This can lead to the development of painless ulcers and it is one of the major contributing factors in the infected diabetic foot. Peripheral neuropathy affecting large fibres results in loss of ankle deep tendon reflexes. There is also often loss of proprioception and uncommonly this may lead to the development of Charcot's joints. Diabetic amyotrophy affects motor supply to the proximal limb muscles. This may affect quadriceps, the gluteal muscles and the hamstrings. Characteristically the onset is rapid and the affected muscles may be painful. The affected patient has difficulty in rising from a chair and in climbing stairs. Autonomic neuropathy is caused by damage to the sympathetic ganglia. The resulting problems include postural hypotension, urinary retention due to an atonic bladder, diarrhoea, erectile dysfunction and gustatory sweating. Radiculopathy involves one or more nerve roots causing paraesthesia, which is often painful, in a dermatomal distribution.

Q22. DISORDERS OF CALCIUM AND BONE METABOLISM (☆☆)

1. D   2. A   3. C   4. F   5. B

Paget's disease causes high bone turnover resulting in markedly raised alkaline phosphatase. However, serum calcium, phosphate and parathyroid hormone (PTH) levels should be normal. Vitamin D increases both serum calcium and phosphate but does not directly affect alkaline phosphatase levels. In vitamin D deficiency, low calcium causes a compensatory increase in PTH resulting in increased alkaline phosphatase. Calcium levels may also be normal in vitamin D deficiency due to the compensatory effect of hyperparathyroidism. PTH increases calcium and decreases phosphate. Therefore, in primary hypoparathyroidism, calcium and parathyroid hormone levels are low and phosphate levels are high. Other diseases affecting bone and calcium metabolism include renal disease, hypercalcaemia of malignancy, sarcoidosis and pseudohypoparathyroidism. In secondary hyperparathyroidism due to renal disease calcium levels are normal and PTH levels are generally raised. In hypercalcaemia of malignancy, calcium is raised and phosphate and alkaline phosphatase may be raised or normal. If the hypercalcaemia is due to ectopic PTH production, PTH will be raised but it is usually low in hypercalcaemia of malignancy. In sarcoidosis calcium is raised, PTH is low, alkaline phosphatase is normal and phosphate can be normal or low. In pseudohypoparathyroidism calcium is low, PTH and phosphate are elevated and alkaline phosphatase is normal. All four tests should be normal in osteoporosis.

Q23. GASTROINTESTINAL ABSORPTION AND EXCRETION (☆☆)

1. D   2. A   3. B   4. E   5. C

Gastric intrinsic factor is essential for the absorption of vitamin B_{12}. Malabsorption of this vitamin occurs in pernicious anaemia because of autoantibodies produced against parietal cells. Bile acids are important in the absorption of dietary fat and of the fat-soluble vitamins A, D, E and K. Bile acid deficiency may result in vitamin deficiency states. Amylase is secreted in the saliva and in pancreatic fluid. Amylase breaks down starch, which then undergoes further digestion by disaccharidases in the small intestinal brush border. Specific epithelial transporters and disaccharidases enable the absorption of individual sugars and inherited deficiencies (eg alactasia) can result in osmotic diarrhoea. Proteases such as trypsin, pepsin, chymotrypsin and elastase enable intraluminal protein digestion. Amino acids are then absorbed at the brush border using sodium-coupled and sodium-independent transporters for basic, neutral, acidic, imino and hydrophobic amino acids. Water and electrolytes are transported across the enterocyte membrane by the sodium-hydrogen exchanger, sodium channel, potassium-hydrogen ATPase and the chloride exchanger. This latter molecule is involved in diarrhoea due to cholera or enterotoxigenic *Escherichia coli* where large volumes of water are excreted. Pancreatic lipase and phospholipase are involved in the breakdown of dietary fats.

Q24. GASTROINTESTINAL CANCER (☆☆)

1. B   2. E   3. F   4. A   5. D

Squamous cell carcinoma is the commonest form of oesophageal cancer. This cancer shows extremely marked global variation in incidence. Risk factors include spicy foods, pickled vegetables (in the Chinese) and alcohol. Squamous cell carcinoma is also associated with achalasia, Plummer-Vinson syndrome, coeliac disease (weakly) and the rare hereditary condition of tylosis. Adenocarcinomas arise in the lowest one-third of the oesophagus. Barrett's oesophagus (metaplasia resulting in columnar epithelium) carries a 30 to 40-fold increased risk of this cancer. Gastric carcinoma is associated with *Helicobacter pylori* infection, achlorhydria and pernicious anaemia. Dietary factors such as alcohol and nitrate intake may also be involved. Enteropathy-associated T cell lymphoma is associated with coeliac disease and dermatitis

herpetiformis. It is uncertain whether those suffering from coeliac disease have a further increase in risk if they do not strictly avoid gluten-containing foods. Less commonly, patients with coeliac disease develop adenocarcinoma of the small bowel. *Helicobacter pylori* infection is a risk factor for lymphomas arising in mucosa-associated lymphoid tissue in the small intestine. Small intestinal lymphoma is also common in patients with AIDS. Cholangiocarcinoma is most frequently found in Asia. This is because of the association with the bile duct flatworms, *Clonorchis sinensis* (correct name really *Opisthorchis sinensis*) and *O. viverrini*. Cholangiocarcinoma is also associated with ulcerative colitis, congenital hepatic fibrosis and polycystic liver disease. It is uncertain whether gallstones are an independent risk factor for cholangiocarcinoma. Colonic adenocarcinoma is associated with ulcerative colitis, Crohn's disease and the autosomal dominant conditions, hereditary non-polyposis colon cancer and familial adenomatous polyposis (FAP). In FAP, hundreds of polyps occur throughout the large and small intestines.

Q25. BOWEL DISEASE (☆☆)

1. C   2. F   3. B   4. A   5. D

There are many extraintestinal manifestations of ulcerative colitis and Crohn's disease. Those related to disease activity include oral aphthous ulcers, erythema nodosum, pyoderma gangrenosum, peripheral arthropathy, conjunctivitis, episcleritis and anterior uveitis. Features unrelated to disease activity include sacroiliitis, ankylosing spondylitis and liver disease. Primary sclerosing cholangitis occurs in many patients with chronic severe ulcerative colitis but is rare in patients with Crohn's disease. Perianal and abdominal cutaneous fistulae commonly occur in Crohn's disease but are not a feature of ulcerative colitis. Dermatitis herpetiformis is associated with gluten-sensitive enteropathy. The lesions typically appear on the extensor skin surfaces (eg the elbows) and are extremely itchy. They usually resolve if a gluten-free diet is adhered to. Virchow's node is the presence of a palpable lymph node in the supraclavicular fossa in a patient with a gastric carcinoma.

Q26. GUT MOTILITY (☆☆☆)

1. E   2. F   3. C   4. D   5. A

The extrinsic nerve supply to the gut comes from the autonomic nervous system. Sympathetic innervation of the proximal part of the gut is via the coeliac plexus and parasympathetic innervation is via the vagus nerve. It was traditionally believed that the autonomic nervous system was the principal regulator of gut motility. However, it is now realised that gut motility is regulated locally by the enteric nervous system. This intrinsic system includes afferent and efferent neurones, interneurones and a large number of neurotransmitter substances. In many ways it is similar to the central nervous system in that it has all of the components needed for complex regulation of function. Auerbach's (myenteric) plexus is located between the smooth muscle layers of the gut. Meissner's (submucosal) plexus is located between the mucosa and the innermost smooth muscle layer. There are three layers of muscle surrounding the gut. The innermost layer is called the muscularis mucosae. This very thin muscle is of uncertain function. The middle layer consists of circular muscle fibres that contract to constrict the bowel lumen. The outermost layer is made up of longitudinal fibres that shorten the bowel. In the colon the longitudinal layer is not continuous and is present only as bands called the taenia coli. Co-ordinated contractions of circular and smooth muscle produce gut peristalsis.

Q27. DYSKINESIA (☆☆)

1. F   2. D   3. E   4. C   5. B

Tremor is a rhythmic sinusoidal motion caused by regular muscle contractions. Resting tremor is a coarse tremor (approximately 4–6 Hz), which occurs in Parkinson's disease and other extrapyramidal disorders. Intention tremor

occurs on movement in patients with cerebellar disorders (tremor of intermediate frequency) and those with excess sympathetic stimulation due to thyrotoxicosis, anxiety, salbutamol therapy or other causes (fine tremor). Chorea is continuous, non-rhythmic, jerky purposeless movement, which flits from one part of the body to another. Chorea is probably caused by an excess of L-DOPA in the basal ganglia. Classic causes include Huntington's disease, Sydenham's chorea (a rare feature of acute rheumatic fever and pregnancy) and drugs (eg oral contraceptive pill or anticonvulsants). Hemiballismus is a large-amplitude, flinging movement of a limb due to a lesion in the contralateral subthalamic nucleus. Myoclonus is the occurrence of rapid shock-like, involuntary movements that affect part or all of the body. Myoclonus occurs in neurodegenerative diseases (eg Creutzfeldt-Jakob disease or lysosomal storage disorders), metabolic derangements (eg uraemia or hyponatraemia) and myoclonic epilepsy. Dystonia is a prolonged muscle spasm which produces an abnormal posture or repetitive movements. Examples include blepharospasm, writer's cramp, oculogyric crisis and torsion dystonia. It can be generalised in systemic conditions such as Wilson's disease and the organic acidurias. Tardive dyskinesia is a complication of treatment with neuroleptic drugs. Involuntary chewing, grinning and lip-smacking movements occur.

Q28. SPEECH DISORDERS (☆)

1. B   2. D   3. A   4. F   5. E

Cerebellar dysarthria is slurring of speech which is inappropriately irregular in volume and rhythm. Speech in pseudobulbar palsy (upper motor neurone lesion) is slow and indistinct. It takes great effort to produce and the result is explosive speech that has been cruelly compared to the voice of Donald Duck. Extrapyramidal dysarthria produces soft, indistinct speech that is monotonous in tone, volume and rhythm. Bulbar palsy is caused by a lower motor neurone lesion affecting one or more of the seventh, ninth, tenth and twelfth cranial nerves. The patient has difficulty pronouncing letters and words clearly. The speech resembles that of a patient who is not wearing their false teeth. Broca's dysphasia is non-fluent speech with a failure to name objects correctly and to repeat words. Words may be malformed but closely resemble the sound of the word intended (eg pan for pen). This is called phonemic paraphasia. The lesion is in the motor cortex of the dominant frontal hemisphere and comprehension is not impaired. The patient is aware that he/she is making mistakes and will often become frustrated. In Wernicke's dysphasia the lesion is in the dominant temporoparietal region. Comprehension is impaired and the patient seems oblivious of the errors he/she is making. There is fluent speech with failure to name objects and to repeat words. The patient may substitute words with similar meaning (eg wrist-clock rather than watch). This is called semantic paraphasia.

Q29. HEADACHE (☆)

1. E   2. D   3. C   4. A   5. B

The commonest cause of headache is tension. This must be distinguished from headaches of a more sinister nature and from those with specific treatments. Trigeminal neuralgia is a stabbing unilateral pain that lasts seconds at a time but which is so severe that it frequently causes facial spasms (tic douloureux). Individual attacks may be induced by eating, shaving and talking. It is usually the maxillary and mandibular divisions of the trigeminal nerve which are involved. Migrainous neuralgia causes a rapid onset of pain which lasts up to one hour and occurs once or twice per day for one to three months. The patient may be pain-free for one to two years before the cycle of attacks recurs. The periodicity of the attacks has given rise to the name 'cluster headache'. Each attack begins around one eye, which becomes erythematous and is accompanied by eyelid swelling, lacrimation, facial flushing and rhinorrhoea. Giant cell arteritis is a serious

disease occurring predominantly in those over 55 years. The patient complains of a throbbing headache and jaw claudication when eating. There may be tender, pulseless, thickened temporal arteries and a high erythrocyte sedimentation rate (often >100 mm/h). Rapid treatment is essential to prevent retinal artery infarction. Acute glaucoma generally occurs in elderly people with a narrow anterior chamber. Severe pain develops around the eye and radiates to the forehead. The patient has a red eye with a cloudy cornea, dilated pupil and decreased visual acuity. The eyeball feels stony-hard if palpated through the lid. Headache due to raised intracranial pressure is exacerbated by lying down and is therefore worse after waking than later in the day. The pain is also increased by coughing and exertion. In migraine the patient usually has an aura preceding the headache by around 15 minutes. Attacks are accompanied by visual symptoms such as distortion and zigzag fortification spectra.

Q30. CAUSES OF OPTIC DISC SWELLING (☆☆☆)

1. C   2. B   3. F   4. D   5. A

Papilloedema may be difficult to distinguish from other causes of optic disc swelling particularly congenital pseudopapilloedema. In the latter condition the appearance of one or both discs may be abnormal. The disc vessels are often abnormal in size and shape and there may be choroidal pigment. Corrected visual acuity (they are often long-sighted), colour vision, visual fields and pupillary reflexes are usually normal. Papilloedema usually affects both eyes. The optic disc swelling is produced by raised intracranial pressure and the fundus appears normal. There is usually normal visual acuity, colour vision and pupil reflexes until the disease is far advanced. The size of the blind spot is generally increased. Papillitis usually affects only one eye at a time. The other optic disc may be normal or show optic atrophy from a previous episode of demyelination (particularly in multiple sclerosis). The eye is painful particularly on eye movements. There is rapid loss of colour vision and acuity and there is a relative afferent pupil defect. Visual field testing typically demonstrates a central scotoma. Ischaemic optic neuropathy produces unilateral, painless, rapid loss of colour vision and acuity. There is a relative afferent pupil defect and a partial, altitudinal visual field loss. Causes include diabetes, hypertension and temporal arteritis. Drusen at the disc may be present in one or both eyes. These pearly white excrescences are shown as calcific deposits on computed tomography. Drusen may cause progressive visual field loss. Chronic open-angle glaucoma causes optic disc cupping (and eventually optic atrophy) not optic disc swelling.

Q31. RISK FACTORS FOR RESPIRATORY DISEASE (✩✩)

1. C   2. E   3. D   4. F   5. A

Bronchiectasis can occur because of selective immunoglobulin A deficiency, tuberculosis, whooping cough, measles, a foreign body, a tumour obstructing a bronchial lumen or cystic fibrosis. Chronic obstructive lung disease (COLD) is most commonly caused by tobacco smoking. α_1-antitrypsin deficiency is an uncommon cause of emphysematous lung disease, which should be suspected in young patients and in non-smokers. Certain occupational groups were previously at increased risk of developing COLD particularly cadmium workers, gold miners and cotton and grain workers. Mesothelioma is associated with a history of exposure to asbestos. Ship-builders who worked during the 1940s and 1950s were the worst affected. The most damaging fibres are those 1.5–8 μm in length as they are small enough to enter the respiratory bronchi and large enough to be deposited there. The disease frequently takes 20 to 40 years to develop following exposure. Progressive massive fibrosis (PMF) can be caused by exposure to coal dust, talc, kaolin, Fuller's earth and crystalline silica dioxide (quartz). In a minority of cases rheumatoid arthritis plays a role in the development of PMF (Caplan's syndrome). PMF

is defined as a pneumoconiosis where at least one nodule is more than 1 cm in diameter. Silica exposure occurs in masons and workers in slate quarries. Silica is a macrophage poison and silicosis predisposes to infection with *Mycobacterium tuberculosis*, *M. avium* and *M. kansasii*. The causes of pulmonary eosinophilia include infection by the larval stage of helminth infections and drugs such as *para*-amino salicylic acid (PAS), aspirin and sulphonamides. Pulmonary eosinophilia with bronchial involvement is caused by *Aspergillus* and the agents of lymphatic filariasis, *Wuchereria bancrofti* and *Brugia malayi*. Pulmonary hypertension may be secondary to left heart failure, mitral valve disease or pulmonary thromboembolism. It is also associated with the autoimmune vasculitides and with HIV infection.

Q32. SIGNS OF RESPIRATORY DISEASE (✩)

1. B   2. D   3. F   4. A   5. C

With a large pleural effusion there is typically decreased chest expansion and stony dull percussion on the affected side, with the trachea and apex beat shifted away from the effusion. Breath sounds and vocal resonance are decreased over the effusion. There may be a small area of collapse/consolidation detectable above the effusion. The typical signs in consolidation are a centrally placed trachea and decreased expansion and a dull percussion note on the affected side. Bronchial breathing, increased vocal resonance, whispering pectoriloquy, crackles and sometimes a pleural rub may be heard. In pneumonectomy there is a large scar, the trachea and apex beat are deviated to the affected side and there is decreased expansion and dull percussion on that side. Breath sounds are diminished and there are no added sounds (crackles or wheeze). A tension pneumothorax causes deviation of the trachea and apex beat away from the affected side. The percussion note is classically described as hyper-resonant and breath sounds are decreased in volume. In marked unilateral fibrosis (eg post-tuberculosis) the trachea and the apex beat are often deviated to the affected side. There is decreased expansion and a dull percussion note over the fibrotic lung. Loud crackles and squawks may be heard and if the fibrosis extends to the pleura there may be harsh breath sounds and even bronchial breathing. In pulmonary embolism the only abnormal sign on examination of the chest is usually a pleural rub over the affected lung.

Q33. AETIOLOGY OF PNEUMONIA (☆☆)

1. D   2. C   3. B   4. A   5. E

The commonest cause of community-acquired pneumonia in a previously healthy adult is *Streptococcus pneumoniae*. In most case series of lobar pneumonia this organism accounts for around 80% of cases where the cause is identified. *Mycoplasma pneumoniae* is also an important cause of community-acquired pneumonia with epidemics occurring approximately every four years. Other causes include *Chlamydia pneumoniae*, *Haemophilus influenzae* and the influenza virus. *Staphylococcus aureus* is a common cause of pneumonia in intravenous drug abusers. Endocarditis affecting the right side of the heart may cause showers of bacterial emboli producing multiple lung abscesses. In addition, *Staphylococcus aureus* may cause secondary bacterial pneumonia following viral pneumonia (eg post-influenza). *Klebsiella pneumoniae* also has the potential to cause a cavitating pneumonia. This Gram-negative bacillus is a common nosocomial pathogen and diabetics are particularly susceptible. An HIV patient with a subacute history of progressive breathlessness is likely to be suffering from *Pneumocystis carinii* pneumonia. This fungal infection causes systemic disease with patients also suffering from malaise, night sweats and gastrointestinal symptoms. The important differential diagnosis is tuberculosis. Cystic fibrosis patients initially develop infections with *Streptococcus pneumoniae* and *Staphylococcus aureus*. As the disease progresses infection with

the Gram-negative bacilli *Pseudomonas aeruginosa* and *Burkholderia cepacia* frequently occurs. Infection with these organisms carries a poor prognosis in cystic fibrosis patients. *Streptococcus pyogenes* rarely causes pneumonia and is much more frequently a cause of cellulitis.

Q34. RESPIRATORY SUPPORT (☆☆☆)

1. C   2. F   3. B   4. A   5. E

CPAP (continuous positive airway pressure) and BIPAP (biphasic positive airway pressure) are useful in the non-intubated patient. They are delivered via a tightly fitting face mask. CPAP delivers high-flow oxygen at a constant pressure throughout the respiratory cycle. This helps to re-expand collapsed alveoli and improves arterial oxygen concentration. However, CPAP also increases the work of breathing and can lead to a rise in arterial carbon dioxide concentration. It is therefore generally not suitable for type II respiratory failure. In BIPAP, the airway pressure maintained during inspiration exceeds that during expiration. This helps to reduce the effort of breathing and to expel excess carbon dioxide. BIPAP can increase oxygen delivery and reduce carbon dioxide concentration and is thus used in type II respiratory failure. The machine is triggered by patient inspiration. Ventilation via an endotracheal tube has the advantages of protecting the airway from vomit and of delivering more effective gas exchange in the critically ill or unconscious patient. Both the SIMV (simultaneous intermittent mandatory ventilation) and assist control modes of ventilation deliver a fixed rate of breaths of a machine-specified tidal volume. These ventilator modes are therefore described as 'volume-targeted'. In SIMV if the patient takes additional breaths these are allowed to occur at the patient's own (usually lower) tidal volume. The patient therefore has some control over ventilation. In assist control mode the ventilator ensures that the full machine-set tidal volume is also delivered for patient-initiated breaths. This may achieve better gas exchange but can produce hyperventilation. Alternative forms of ventilation include high-frequency jet ventilation (HFJV) and pressure support ventilation (PSV). In PSV the machine is used to specify inflation pressure and the resultant tidal volume depends on the thoracic compliance. In HFJV oxygen is pumped into the lungs extremely rapidly without causing inflation and deflation. This method reduces the pressure required to ventilate patients with very stiff lungs.

Q35. AUTOANTIBODIES (☆☆)

1. D 2. A 3. E 4. B 5. F

Antineutrophil cytoplasmic antibodies (ANCA) are a marker of the autoimmune small vessel vasculitic syndromes. These systemic diseases may affect any organ but predominantly affect the lungs and kidneys. Wegener's disease is a variant of autoimmune small vessel vasculitis in which granulomas are found. More than 90% of patients with this disease have cytoplasmic-staining cANCA, the target of which is proteinase 3. In microscopic polyangiitis without granulomas, perinuclear pANCA is formed against myeloperoxidase. Antinuclear antibodies are present in around 99% of patients with systemic lupus erythematosus (SLE). They are also found in a smaller percentage of patients with rheumatoid arthritis, Sjögren's disease (sicca syndrome), systemic sclerosis and chronic active hepatitis and in up to 2% of the healthy general population. Antiphospholipid syndrome is a variant of SLE in which recurrent spontaneous abortions and venous thromboses occur. Anticardiolipin (a phospholipid) antibodies are the hallmark of this disease. Rheumatoid factor is found in 70–80% of patients with rheumatoid arthritis and in almost all patients with Sjögren's disease and Felty's syndrome (where rheumatoid arthritis is accompanied by hypersplenism and haemolytic anaemia). Rheumatoid factor is also found in a smaller proportion of patients with systemic sclerosis, systemic lupus erythematosus and infective endocarditis. It is also found in close relatives

of patients with rheumatoid arthritis and in 5–10% of the healthy general population. There is frequently an extremely high serum ferritin in adult Still's disease but autoantibodies are rarely found.

Q36. CLINICAL PRESENTATION (☆☆)

1. C 2. F 3. D 4. A 5. E

Wegener's granulomatosis causes a bloody foul-smelling nasal discharge, paranasal sinus pain, nasal ulceration, septal perforation, saddle nose deformity and a chronic cough with pleuritic chest pain and haemoptysis. It also frequently affects the kidneys causing focal proliferative glomerulonephritis and eye problems including conjunctivitis, iritis and a retro-orbital pseudotumour. The latter is a serious problem, which can cause proptosis and optic nerve ischaemia. Familial Mediterranean fever causes recurrent peritonitis and recurrent synovitis of the knees, hips and ankles. There is usually severe arthritis but full recovery of joint function between attacks. Presentation is usually during adolescence and attacks are prevented with colchicine. Behçet's disease is characterised by recurrent oral and genital ulceration, anterior or posterior uveitis, retinal vasculitis, rashes (including erythema nodosum, acneiform, pseudofollicular and papulopustular types). Polyarthritis affecting large joints, central nervous system problems, venous thrombosis and recurrent abdominal pain may also occur. Acute sarcoidosis is characterised by erythema nodosum, bilateral hilar lymphadenopathy and a symmetrical, migratory polyarthropathy. Knees, ankles, the proximal interphalangeal joints, wrists and elbows are most frequently affected. A full recovery usually occurs after a few weeks or months. Systemic sclerosis is often preceded by a long history of Raynaud's phenomenon. The hands eventually become affected by finger swelling, tight skin, painful joints and eventual atrophy of the finger pulps. Patients have tight facial skin with puckering around the mouth, a beaked nose, ectropion and telangiectasia. Involvement of the gut leads to swallowing difficulties and malabsorption. Polymyalgia rheumatica presents with a short history of pain and stiffness of the shoulders and pelvic girdle. Patients are usually over 60 years old. Malaise, fatigue, anorexia, depression, night sweats and fever are common and the erythrocyte sedimentation rate is high.

Q37. CUTANEOUS LESIONS (☆☆)

1. E   2. C   3. B   4. F   5. D

These cutaneous lesions are all associated with systemic diseases. Pyoderma gangrenosum is the occurrence of painful, red, ulcerating nodules with violaceous borders which become inflamed and indurated and characteristically have an undermined edge. They occur on the shins and abdomen and are frequently associated with inflammatory bowel disease, rheumatoid arthritis or leukaemia. Acanthosis nigricans is the presence of velvety thickened skin in the flexural areas of the axillae and neck. This condition is associated with obesity, insulin resistance, polycystic ovary syndrome and adenocarcinoma of the stomach. Dermatomyositis is a form of connective tissue disease sometimes associated with occult malignancy. Patients develop myositis, violaceous (heliotrope) oedema of the eyelids, scaling papules on the knuckles (Gottron's papules) and erythema, telangiectasia and atrophy of sun-exposed skin. Ichthyosis can be hereditary or acquired. The acquired form is associated with Hodgkin's disease, sarcoidosis and internal malignancy. Dry, fish-like scaling of the skin occurs particularly affecting the limbs. Erythema nodosum is a panniculitis or inflammation of the subcutaneous fat. Tender, red nodules develop on the anterior shins and then turn purple and involute. Erythema nodosum is associated with sarcoidosis, inflammatory bowel disease, rheumatic diseases, pregnancy and infections (eg tuberculosis and streptococcal infections). Dermatitis herpetiformis is a pruritic, vesicular rash on the extensor surfaces that is associated with gluten-sensitive enteropathy.

Q38. PREGNANCY-ASSOCIATED DERMATOSES (☆☆☆)

1. D   2. A   3. E   4. B   5. C

Telogen effluvium is the simultaneous movement of large numbers of hair follicles into the telogen stage of the hair growth cycle. This sometimes results in substantial hair loss but as the hair follicles recover the hair regrows several months later. Telogen effluvium can occur postpartum and also following severe illness. Chloasma is facial pigmentation in a butterfly distribution, which occurs during pregnancy. It usually disappears postpartum, but in some cases this may take many months or even years. Impetigo herpetiformis is a form of pustular psoriasis that usually begins in the third trimester. This rare condition may progress from erythematous plaques on the flexural areas to widespread disease with systemic symptoms of fever, diarrhoea, vomiting and delirium. It is known to recur in later pregnancies. Pruritic urticarial papules and plaques of pregnancy are relatively common affecting around one in 200 pregnancies. This condition has acquired several different names including polymorphic eruption of pregnancy and toxic erythema of pregnancy. Macules, papules, target lesions, vesicles and blisters may all occur. They most frequently develop in the final month before delivery or in the early puerperium. The lesions mostly arise on the abdomen, along the lines of cutaneous striae, and there is typically periumbilical sparing. Pruritic folliculitis of pregnancy is an itchy, acneiform eruption associated with infection by the yeast *Pityrosporum ovale*. Pemphigoid gestationis is a severe bullous/urticarial eruption that typically commences around the periumbilical region. The rash begins in the last two trimesters and over a few weeks may become widespread. It typically resolves after delivery and is believed to be caused by an autoimmune reaction to trophoblastic antigens.

Q39. IRON STATUS (☆☆)

1. E   2. B   3. A   4. C   5. D

Serum iron levels are an unreliable marker of body iron stores. Serum iron is decreased in iron deficiency but is also decreased in systemic inflammation. Recent treatment with iron may produce elevated serum iron levels. Transferrin (also known as total iron binding capacity) is increased in iron deficiency, in pregnancy and in those taking oestrogens. Transferrin saturation is the serum iron divided by transferrin and this is a better marker of iron stores than either of the individual measurements alone. Ferritin is a major transport and storage form of iron. Levels correlate with total body iron stores but ferritin is also an acute phase protein. Ferritin levels therefore rise in acute inflammation. It is reasonable to assume that when C-reactive protein levels are elevated serum ferritin is an unreliable guide to iron status. Serum soluble transferrin receptor levels are high in iron deficiency and low in iron overload. This marker is increasingly being used as the most practical measure of iron status. The gold standard test of iron availability is specific staining of bone marrow but this invasive investigation is rarely performed solely to evaluate iron status.

Q40. LEUKAEMIA (☆☆)

1. E   2. F   3. B   4. C   5. A

Chronic lymphatic leukaemia (CLL) is the most indolent form of leukaemia. It is often diagnosed incidentally when a high lymphocytosis is detected on a peripheral blood count. CLL is associated with lymphadenopathy, hepatosplenomegaly, thrombocytopenic purpura, glomerulonephritis and warm autoimmune haemolytic anaemia. Chronic myeloid leukaemia often presents with fatigue, weight loss and anaemia. Many patients have massive splenomegaly. The white cells produce a B_{12} binding protein leading to raised serum B_{12}. The Philadelphia chromosome (a 9;22 translocation producing the *bcr-abl*

fusion gene) is found in most cases. In cases where it is not seen on karyotyping there is usually a translocation at the molecular level. The Philadelphia chromosome is also found commonly in acute lymphoblastic leukaemia (ALL) and is seen occasionally (1%) in acute myeloid leukaemia (AML). ALL most commonly affects children and has the best prognosis of all leukaemias with over 60% being cured. The prognosis is worse for those with the Philadelphia chromosome. AML generally affects adults and the prognosis is around 30%. The most favourable prognosis in AML is for the subtype called acute promyelocytic leukaemia (APML; type M3 on the French-American-British classification). This subtype is characterised by hypergranular promyelocytes and a translocation between chromosomes 15 and 17 involving the retinoic acid receptor α gene. The treatment includes all-*trans*-retinoic acid. Hodgkin's disease is a form of lymphoma not leukaemia.

Q41. HAEMATOLOGICAL ABNORMALITY (☆)

1. F   2. D   3. A   4. C   5. B

The commonest cause of microcytic anaemia (cell volume <80 μl) is iron deficiency which is often due to blood loss from the gastrointestinal tract (eg in peptic ulcer disease, colitis or hookworm infection), inadequate dietary iron intake or heavy periods. α- and β-thalassaemia are common causes of microcytosis among ethnic groups originating from malaria-endemic regions. A useful clue suggesting thalassaemia is that, compared to iron deficiency, the microcytosis is more marked than expected for the degree of anaemia. Congenital sideroblastic anaemia is a rare X-linked disease that also causes a microcytic blood film. Causes of normocytic anaemia include bone marrow failure, renal failure, anaemia of chronic disease, hypothyroidism (can be macrocytic) and pregnancy. Common causes of macrocytic anaemia (>110 μl) include vitamin B_{12} or folate deficiency, chronic alcoholism, myelodysplastic syndrome, drugs (eg azathioprine, zidovudine, hydroxyurea), reticulocytosis and liver disease. Mixed anaemias with combined microcytes and macrocytes may also arise (eg in combined vitamin B_{12} and iron deficiency) giving rise to a normal average red cell volume. However, the Coulter counter measurements will show that the red cell distribution width is increased and the presence of abnormal erythrocytes can then be confirmed by examination of a blood film. Inherited causes of haemolytic anaemia include enzyme deficiencies (eg glucose-6-phosphate dehydrogenase deficiency and pyruvate kinase deficiency), haemoglobin abnormalities (eg sickle cell disease) and membrane abnormalities (eg hereditary spherocytosis and elliptocytosis). Acquired causes include infections, drug-induced haemolysis, cardiac prosthetic valve trauma, microangiopathic haemolytic anaemia and paroxysmal nocturnal haemoglobinuria. Thrombocytopenia is characteristic of dengue and other viral haemorrhagic fevers. It is also seen in marrow failure, connective tissue diseases and as an idiopathic autoimmune disease (idiopathic thrombocytopenic purpura). Chronic hypoxia causes polycythaemia due to increased erythropoietin production.

Q42. CLINICAL PRESENTATION (☆☆)

1. E   2. B   3. F   4. C   5. A

Acute bacterial meningitis in a young adult is usually caused by *Neisseria meningitidis* or *Streptococcus pneumoniae*. A preceding history of pneumonia, sinusitis or otitis media suggests *S. pneumoniae* is the cause. Eighty per cent of cat bites become infected compared to only around 5% of dog bites. Antibiotic prophylaxis with co-amoxiclav is appropriate following cat bites. The commonest infecting organism is *Pasteurella multocida*. Causes of bacterial endocarditis on a native valve include viridans group *Streptococci*, *Enterococci*, *Staphylococcus aureus* and HACEK organisms (*Haemophilus aphrophilus/parainfluenzae*, *Actinobacillus actinomycetemcomitans*, *Cardiobacterium hominis*, *Eikenella corrodens* and *Kingella*

kingae). Enterococcal endocarditis is most common in the elderly and is associated with gastrointestinal disease, particularly colonic cancer. Endophthalmitis has a wide range of causes. Although *Bacillus* species are often regarded as contaminants (eg in blood cultures), they are a common cause of serious endophthalmitis following penetrating eye trauma. Vitrectomy, intravitreal and systemic antibiotics are all required. Common causes of ophthalmia neonatorum are *Neisseria gonorrhoea*, *Chlamydia trachomatis* and herpes simplex. *N. gonorrhoea* usually presents two to four days after birth, whereas the other infections develop more slowly. For confirmed *N. gonorrhoea* and *C. trachomatis* infections, the mother and her sexual partner(s) require treatment in addition to the baby. *Haemophilus influenzae* group B predominantly affects young children and is a cause of upper and lower respiratory tract infections, otitis media, meningitis and epiglottitis.

Q43. RICKETTSIAE (☆☆☆)

1. F   2. D   3. A   4. B   5. E

Rickettsia prowazekii causes epidemic or louse-borne typhus. This infection is spread by human lice and has caused major epidemics among refugees during famine and wars. It can lie dormant in humans for many years and then produce a recurrent infection known as Brill-Zinsser disease. It has a high case-fatality rate if not treated. *Rickettsia prowazekii* is also a zoonosis of flying squirrels which has resulted in occasional transmission to humans. Endemic or murine typhus is a less serious illness caused by *Rickettsia typhi*. This is a zoonosis that is spread to humans living in rat-infested dwellings. When a rat flea feeds it defecates and the rickettsia-containing faeces are rubbed into the bite site by scratching. Rocky Mountain spotted fever is a tick-borne infection caused by *Rickettsia rickettsii*. Infection follows visits to tick-infested areas, but it is not restricted to the Rocky Mountains. Rodents and dogs act as reservoir hosts and treating domestic dogs with anti-flea treatments can reduce the risk of human infection. Scrub typhus is spread by trombiculid mites, which bite humans entering infected scrub land or overgrown terrain. Epidemics have been described among army personnel. The infecting organism, *Rickettsia tsutsugamushi*, produces an eschar at the bite site. Mediterranean spotted fever is caused by *Rickettsia conori* which is spread by tick bites. A necrotic eschar forms at the tick bite site and is known as a tache noire. This infection is widely distributed in Africa, India and the Mediterranean region. Rickettsioses were traditionally diagnosed by the Weil-Felix reaction. This test lacks specificity and it is preferable to use immunofluorescence-based serological tests. The treatment for all rickettsioses is doxycycline. *Bartonella henselae* is a rickettsia-like organism which causes cat-scratch fever.

Q44. ZOONOTIC INFECTION (☆☆☆)

1. E   2. A   3. B   4. D   5. C

Leishmania major causes the Old World form of cutaneous leishmaniasis known as 'wet sore'. The large rodent reservoir has made it difficult to control this disease in rural North Africa. *Leishmania tropica*, the cause of the Old World form of cutaneous leishmaniasis known as 'dry sore', does not have a significant animal reservoir and predominantly occurs in urban areas. *Balantidium coli* is the only ciliate protozoon known to infect humans. Its natural host is the pig and communities that use pig faeces as fertiliser have the highest risk of infection. It is a rare cause of diarrhoea and dysentery in developed countries, occasionally causing outbreaks in mental institutions. *Echinococcus multilocularis*, the fox tapeworm, causes alveolar hydatid disease when eggs are accidentally ingested. This infection is much more serious than *E. granulosus* disease as the larvae grow more quickly and metastasise to other organs. Both surgery and antimicrobial treatment with albendazole are required. Although *E. multilocularis* is not found in Britain, there is a concern that it may be introduced from Europe following the

relaxation of quarantine regulations. *Trypanosoma brucei* is the cause of sleeping sickness. The West African form of the disease *T. brucei gambiense* has no significant animal reservoir but the East African form, *T. brucei rhodesiense*, occurs in many species of domestic and wild ungulates. The Gram-negative bacillus *Bartonella henselae* is the cause of cat-scratch fever and is an occasional cause of culture-negative endocarditis. In HIV patients it also causes peliosis hepatis (venous lakes in the liver) and bacillary angiomatosis (a cutaneous lesion resembling Kaposi's sarcoma). Bats are one of many animals that act as a reservoir host for rabies.

Q45. DRUG REGIMENS (☆☆☆)

1. F   2. B   3. A   4. C   5. D

Encephalitozoon hellem is a microsporidian parasite. It can cause disseminated disease in those who are severely immunocompromised such as patients with advanced AIDS. Albendazole is currently the treatment of choice for intestinal and extraintestinal microsporidia infections. *Naegleria fowleri* is an amoeba that penetrates the CNS through the cribriform plate, when swimming or particularly diving into contaminated water. Mortality is >95% justifying the use of intraventricular as well as intravenous amphotericin B. Pentavalent antimonials such as sodium stibogluconate or meglumine antimonate have traditionally been used to treat visceral leishmaniasis (kala-azar). Resistance to these drugs has now rendered them ineffective in Indian kala-azar and the much more expensive liposomal or lipid complex preparations of amphotericin B are required. Fortunately studies suggest a single infusion may be sufficient treatment in many cases. Acute schistosomiasis, known as Katayama fever, may present with fever, chills, urticaria, cough, haemoptysis and hepatitis. This acute reaction is more severe in *Schistosoma japonicum* infection than with *S. mansoni* or *S. haematobium* and can be fatal. Treatment is with praziquantel for acute or chronic infection with any *Schistosoma* species.

Trypanosoma brucei is the cause of African sleeping sickness. In early infection without CNS involvement suramin can be used but for those with abnormal CSF, the more toxic drug melarsoprol is needed. Ten per cent of patients treated with melarsoprol develop encephalopathy and Jarisch-Herxheimer reactions are not uncommon either. Pre-treatment with steroids is given to reduce these risks. Fluconazole is effective treatment for yeast infections.

Q46. HIV-ASSOCIATED INFECTIONS (☆☆)

1. E   2. D   3. F   4. B   5. A

Cryptococcus neoformans is an encapsulated yeast that causes meningitis in severely immunocompromised patients, particularly those with advanced AIDS. It can be diagnosed by CSF or blood culture or by a positive antigen test in CSF or blood. Treatment is with amphotericin B and flucytosine followed by long-term secondary prevention with fluconazole. *Pneumocystis carinii* is a yeast infection that was previously the commonest cause of death in AIDS patients in the West. Regular prophylaxis with co-trimoxazole (or if allergic with dapsone or nebulised pentamidine) should be given to all HIV patients with a CD4 count below 200/mm³ to prevent *Pneumocystis carinii* pneumonia. Sputum rarely yields a positive diagnosis and bronchoalveolar lavage is generally performed for diagnosis. *Candida albicans* is a common cause of mucosal infections in HIV-infected and other immunosuppressed patients and in those receiving antibiotics. When invasive disease produces fungaemia there is a high risk of endophthalmitis which can rapidly cause blindness and may require surgical intervention. All patients with *Candida* in blood cultures should therefore have a thorough fundoscopic examination. *Leishmania infantum* is traditionally spread by sandflies and predominantly causes visceral leishmaniasis in children. However, it has now become an increasingly important problem in HIV patients in countries surrounding the Mediterranean. It is

increasingly common among injecting drug users with over 10% of HIV-positive drug users in Spain being infected. Treatment in HIV patients is more difficult than in the immunocompetent and may require liposomal amphotericin B. *Toxoplasma gondii* is acquired from cat faeces or eating uncooked meat. It can lie dormant for many years and be reactivated in AIDS patients to cause cerebral toxoplasmosis. Those with positive serology and a CD4 count below 100/mm³ should receive prophylaxis with co-trimoxazole. If allergic to this drug then dapsone should be given together with pyrimethamine and folinic acid. *Cryptosporidium parvum* is a protozoon that commonly causes chronic diarrhoea in AIDS patients. No antibiotic has been shown to eradicate this infection.

Q47. ADVERSE DRUG EFFECTS (☆☆)

1. C   2. F   3. D   4. E   5. A

Methysergide is a drug that is uncommonly used for the prevention of severe recurrent migraine and cluster headache. In addition to retroperitoneal and other fibrotic reactions including the heart valves and pleura it may cause angina, hair loss, mental and behavioural disturbance. It should only be administered under specialist supervision. Phenytoin is used in tonic-clonic and partial seizures. This drug exhibits zero-order kinetics so a small change in dosage or absorption can have large effects on plasma concentration. It has a narrow therapeutic window and monitoring of plasma concentration is therefore required. Side-effects include dizziness, coarse facies, acne, hirsutism and gingival hyperplasia and less commonly leucopenia, thrombocytopenia, megaloblastic or aplastic anaemia, osteomalacia and severe skin reactions including erythema multiforme and toxic epidermal necrolysis. β-blockers and lithium are both implicated as causes of exacerbations of psoriasis. Lithium may also cause ataxia, psychosis, nephrogenic diabetes insipidus and thyroid dysfunction. Measuring of plasma concentrations is required and patients should be given a lithium treatment card listing medicines with potential interactions.

Metoclopramide is an antiemetic with actions on the gut and the chemoreceptor trigger zone. The risk of oculogyric crisis and other dystonic reactions is highest in young persons, and for those under 20 years use should be restricted to severe intractable vomiting and for anaesthetic premedication. Minoxidil is used in the treatment of severe hypertension and has been found to cause hypertrichosis. This discovery led to the incorporation of minoxidil into a topical preparation to be used in the treatment of male pattern baldness.

Q48. DRUGS IN PREGNANCY (☆☆)

1. C   2. A   3. B   4. F   5. E

Drugs should be used in pregnancy only if the expected benefit to the mother outweighs the risk to the fetus. No drug is safe beyond all doubt in the first trimester and all drugs should therefore be avoided unless they are really necessary. Indomethacin and other non-steroidal anti-inflammatory drugs may cause premature closure of the ductus arteriosus and this may lead to neonatal pulmonary hypertension. They may also delay the onset and increase the duration of labour. The antimalarial primaquine may cause neonatal haemolysis and methaemoglobinaemia, as may sulphonamides and dapsone. Although chloroquine and quinine may also involve some risk in pregnancy, the benefit outweighs the risk in the treatment and prophylaxis of malaria. Penicillins have a long record of safety for use in pregnancy and should generally be preferred to other antibiotics if treatment of infection is required. Stilboestrol is an anti-oestrogen that is still occasionally used in the treatment of breast cancer. Its use during pregnancy has been linked to the later development of vaginal adenocarcinomas in adolescent girls and young women. It should now only be used in postmenopausal women. Carbamazepine and folate antagonists such as trimethoprim cause an increased risk of neural tube defects. If carbamazepine use cannot be avoided folate supplements are recommended. Tetracyclines cause dental discoloration and may affect skeletal development.

Q49. PARKINSON'S DISEASE (☆☆)

1. C   2. D   3. F   4. A   5. E

Treatment of Parkinson's disease is complex and balancing bradykinesia and drug-induced dyskinetic involuntary movements can be difficult. With increasing duration of treatment, 'on-off' symptoms, characterised by marked fluctuation in performance between doses, may become problematic. Selegiline is a monoamine oxidase B inhibitor which helps to reduce this fluctuation. Before starting treatment, patients should be informed of its limitations and the common side-effects. Levodopa is a pro-drug of dopamine and is administered with a decarboxylase inhibitor that does not cross the blood-brain barrier. Dopa decarboxylase inhibitors include benserazide, which is a component of co-beneldopa and carbidopa, which is found in co-careldopa. Peripheral decarboxylase inhibitors allow therapeutic brain concentrations of dopamine with a lower dose of levodopa. After several years of therapy, levodopa frequently becomes less effective. Patients may then respond to dopamine receptor agonists, such as apomorphine, which is given by subcutaneous injection or continuous infusion. Several new selective dopamine receptor stimulants are now available including ropinirole and pramipexole. Ropinirole is a D_2 receptor agonist that is used as an adjunct to levodopa. It is also used as single therapy to try to avoid the dyskinetic side-effects that occur with levodopa. Antimuscarinic drugs are used in conjunction with levodopa particularly to reduce tremor. These drugs include benzhexol, benztropine, orphenadrine and procyclidine. Entacapone is a catechol-*O*-methyltransferase inhibitor used as an adjunct to levodopa/dopa-decarboxylase inhibitor for patients who experience end of dose deterioration.

Q50. GENERAL ANAESTHESIA (☆☆☆)

1. E   2. F   3. D   4. B   5. C

Specialist registrar training in general internal medicine involves management of patients in high-dependency and intensive care units. A knowledge of anaesthetic drugs used to facilitate intubation and ventilation is therefore essential. Ketamine and propofol are intravenous anaesthetic agents that have a rapid onset of action, making them suitable for induction of anaesthesia. Propofol can be used for the sedation of ventilated patients for up to three days. The drug is administered in a fat-rich emulsion and blood lipid concentrations should be monitored to avoid fat overload. Ketamine has good analgesic properties when used at subanaesthetic dose but has a high incidence of hallucinations. It has become an occasional illegal recreational drug. Suxamethonium is a depolarising muscle relaxant with a rapid onset and short duration of action which is widely used to facilitate endotracheal intubation. Repeated use can produce a non-depolarising block with a more prolonged duration of action. People with pseudocholinesterase deficiency may also develop prolonged paralysis. Atracurium is one of several non-depolarising muscle relaxants. Its principal advantage over other drugs in this class is that it is degraded by non-enzymatic Hoffmann elimination, which is independent of liver and kidney function. This makes it particularly useful for patients with multiorgan failure. Fentanyl is an opioid with good analgesic properties and is a potent suppressor of respiration. This is useful in mechanical ventilation to reduce the pressures required to produce chest movement. Inhalational anaesthetics include halothane, enflurane and isoflurane.

Q51. LAXATIVE DRUGS (☆☆)

1. C   2. F   3. E   4. B   5. A

A balanced diet with adequate fluid intake is important in preventing constipation. Many people suffer from constipation because of inadequate dietary fibre. If improved fibre intake is not successful or not achievable then bran and other bulk-forming agents are the most rational choice of laxative. The widespread use of stimulant laxatives is costly

and may lead to hypokalaemia and a poorly functioning colon. Poor mobility promotes constipation, particularly in the elderly and those in hospital. If increasing mobility and providing time and privacy are ineffective then stimulant or osmotic laxatives may occasionally be required. Senna is an anthraquinone that is widely used as a stimulant laxative. It is cheaper, more palatable and usually more effective than lactulose, a frequently used osmotic agent. Phenolphthalein is available in many laxative preparations on direct sale to the public. It is a cause of rashes and can colour urine pink. Danthron is used in two combination preparations called co-danthramer and co-danthrusate. Danthron is carcinogenic in rat studies and its use should be restricted to patients known to have a terminal illness. Sodium picosulphate should only be used as a bowel cleanser, eg prior to colonoscopy, barium enema or bowel surgery. It should not be used as a treatment for constipation. Bulk-forming laxatives include bran, methylcellulose and ispaghula husk.

Q52. ANTIBIOTICS (☆☆)

1. B   2. F   3. D   4. A   5. C

Methicillin-resistant *Staphylococcus aureus* is resistant to multiple antibiotics. Standard treatment is with the glycopeptide antibiotic vancomycin. If vancomycin cannot be used then teicoplanin (a glycopeptide), linezolid (an oxazolidinone) or the streptogramin combination of dalfopristin/quinupristin (Synercid™) are alternatives. *Aspergillus* species are resistant to fluconazole and infections require treatment with systemic amphotericin B. Liposomal formulations are less nephrotoxic enabling higher doses to be used. *Listeria* meningitis usually occurs in the immunocompromised, neonates and the elderly. Treatment is difficult as most antibiotics are only bacteriostatic against this organism, resulting in a high relapse rate. The combination of ampicillin and gentamicin is synergistic and is the standard treatment. *Candida* is frequently isolated from the urine of catheterised patients. Changing the catheter is usually all that is required. The frequent practice of using amphotericin B bladder washouts is of no proven benefit and is not recommended. If there is convincing evidence of *Candida* cystitis then oral fluconazole is a suitable treatment. Penicillin insensitivity in *Neisseria meningitidis* is an increasing problem worldwide. In Spain more than 50% of isolates are penicillin-insensitive. Fortunately this organism remains sensitive to ceftriaxone and other third-generation cephalosporins. Imipenem is useful for treating serious infection caused by highly resistant Gram-negative bacteria.

Q53. CARDIAC ARRHYTHMIA (☆☆)

1. E   2. A   3. B   4. F   5. C

Ventricular arrhythmias compromise cardiac function more markedly than supraventricular arrhythmias of an equivalent rate. Ventricular arrhythmias should therefore be treated with greater urgency to prevent serious adverse consequences such as myocardial ischaemia or systemic shock. Patients with a symptomatic bradycardia of 40 beats per minute or less (or 40 to 60 if severe problems such as a systolic blood pressure less than 90 mmHg or heart failure are present) should initially be treated with atropine (500 µg intravenously, repeated up to a total dose of 3 mg). If atropine fails, the patient requires urgent cardiac pacing. Atrial fibrillation is often markedly undertreated in hospital. Those with a heart rate above 100, where the onset is believed to be within 24 hours, should be anticoagulated and treated with intravenous amiodarone (300 mg) over one hour. If this attempt at medical cardioversion fails then DC cardioversion should be considered. Supraventricular tachycardia is occasionally pulseless, particularly if the rate is above 250 beats per minute. The patient should be DC cardioverted with an initial shock of 100 J, followed by 200 J then 360 J if the arrhythmia persists. Ventricular tachycardia where the rate is above 150 beats per minute should usually be treated in the

same way unless the patient is very stable, when medical cardioversion with amiodarone may be attempted. Pulseless ventricular tachycardia should be treated by defibrillation and not by DC cardioversion. A supraventricular tachycardia with a rate below 250 beats per minute can be treated with bolus doses of adenosine (6 mg then 12 mg repeated up to three times if needed). This has diagnostic and treatment value. It will often revert a junctional tachycardia or circus rhythm involving the sinus node to sinus rhythm. In addition it will slow the ventricular rate in fast atrial fibrillation or atrial flutter revealing the underlying rhythm. Torsade de pointes is a very rapid, polymorphic ventricular tachycardia where the ventricular complexes revolve around a central axis. This arrhythmia is associated with the long QT syndrome and, if the patient is stable, it can be treated with magnesium sulphate (5 ml of 50% over 30 minutes). If this fails overdrive pacing is an alternative.

Q54. NARROW COMPLEX TACHYARRHYTHMIA (☆☆)

1. F   2. A   3. C   4. B   5. E

Careful examination of the ECG can usually reveal the cause of a narrow complex tachycardia. The ECG of sinus re-entry tachycardia resembles that of sinus tachycardia. The rate is typically 100 to 140 beats per minute, the P wave is normal and every P wave is followed by a QRS complex. The history should help to distinguish the two causes as an arrhythmia has a very abrupt onset (and termination) whereas sinus tachycardia usually increases and decreases gradually. Atrial tachycardia occurs when a part of the atrium other than the nodal tissue discharges more rapidly than the sinus node. The features are similar to sinus re-entry except that the P wave morphology is abnormal and the PR interval is usually long. Atrial tachycardia may also produce 2:1 heart block. In atrial flutter the atrial depolarisation rate is 300 per minute. This produces a 'saw-toothed' pattern of flutter waves on the ECG. These flutter waves are usually negative in the inferior leads II, III and aVF. The ratio between P waves and QRS complexes is usually between two and four, producing a regular ventricular response rate of 150, 100 or 75 beats per minute. Occasionally the ventricular response rate may be irregular or there may be 1:1 conduction producing a ventricular rate of 300 beats per minute. In atrial fibrillation the rate of atrial depolarisation is 450 to 600 beats per minute. This may produce an isoelectric baseline or small 'f' waves. The ventricular response is irregularly irregular. The rate varies rapidly between patients depending on the ability of the atrioventricular node to transmit the electrical stimulus. Atrioventricular re-entry tachycardia is a consequence of an additional electrical connection between the atria and ventricles (called the Bundle of Kent). In Wolff-Parkinson-White syndrome this pathway can be identified on the resting ECG because of a short PR interval and slurred upstroke to the QRS complex (delta wave) but in Lown-Ganong-Levine syndrome the resting ECG is normal. During the re-entry tachycardia the ventricular rate is typically 150 to 220 beats per minute and an inverted, retrograde P wave may be seen in the ST segment. In atrioventricular nodal re-entry tachycardia the P wave is synchronous with the QRS complex and is therefore invisible. The resting ECG is normal.

Q55. INVESTIGATIONS (☆☆)

1. B   2. C   3. D   4. A   5. F

Echocardiography is a non-invasive investigation that is useful in the investigation of many cardiac problems. It is widely used to estimate the left ventricular ejection fraction (percentage of ventricular blood expelled with each contraction) in suspected cardiac failure, to estimate the severity of cardiac valve disease and to identify cardiac aneurysms, dyskinesia and pericardial effusions. Echocardiography can also be performed using a transoesophageal probe to obtain better views of the right-sided cardiac chambers (eg to investigate suspected pulmonary hypertension),

to look for vegetations in suspected endocarditis and to diagnose aortic dissection. Radionuclide ventriculography can also be used in the imaging of global and focal dyskinesias. Two methods are available: multigated acquisition and the first pass technique. Technetium-99m labelled red blood cells are used in the multigated acquisition technique where information from multiple cardiac cycles is obtained. In the first pass technique (only one cardiac cycle used) technetium-99m labelled DTPA is used. A thallium-201 scan can be performed with a treadmill exercise-tolerance test to increase its sensitivity. This scan can discriminate infarcts, which appear as fixed perfusion defects, and ischaemia, which appears as initial poor perfusion that improves after rest. Technetium-99m stannous pyrophosphate is taken up by newly infarcted cardiac tissue. This radionuclide scan was formerly performed to diagnose myocardial infarcts but is now seldom used. Cardiac catheterisation is the gold standard method of identifying coronary artery occlusions that have caused previous infarcts (complete occlusions) and are a cause of continuing angina (partial occlusions). Cardiac catheterisation is also used to measure the gradients across valves to determine the severity of valve lesions (eg in aortic stenosis). Twenty-four-hour ECG monitoring (Holter monitoring) is useful in the investigation of palpitations and in syncope to identify whether a cardiac arrhythmia is the cause.

Q56. AMERICAN HEART ASSOCIATION CLASSIFICATIONS (☆☆☆)

1. E   2. F   3. C   4. B   5. A

Different guidelines committees have used different grading systems (ie with different numbers of levels) for ranking levels of evidence and strength of recommendations. It is not necessary to memorise these but it is essential to understand that the alphabetical letters refer to the level of evidence supporting a recommendation and that the Roman numerals refer to the strength of the recommendation itself. It is also important to be able to distinguish what constitutes strong evidence and what should be regarded as weak evidence. Recommendations based on weak evidence may change when more data become available but this is unlikely for recommendations based on strong evidence. In addition it is much more difficult for the individual clinician to ignore recommendations based on strong evidence. Level A evidence is the strongest evidence and it must be based on one or preferably more, well-designed, randomised clinical trials with large enough numbers of individuals to provide adequate power. Level B evidence represents data derived from randomised trials with comparatively small numbers of subjects or data from well-designed analyses of data from non-randomised studies or observational data registries. Level C evidence is the weakest level. This is the consensus view of experts usually based on their own clinical experience and interpretation of theoretical principles. Class I recommendations are those for which there is general agreement that the procedure or treatment is beneficial, useful and effective. Class III recommendations indicate that a procedure or treatment is not beneficial, useful or effective. In some cases the procedure or treatment may even be harmful. Class II recommendations are those for which there is conflicting evidence or opinion regarding the usefulness of a procedure. In class IIa evidence the opinion is slightly in favour of the procedure or treatment and for class IIb the evidence of benefit is less well established. This system has been widely used for guidelines on management of hypertension, ischaemic heart disease, cardiac failure, etc.

Q57. PSYCHOLOGICAL DEFENCE MECHANISMS (☆☆)

1. B   2. E   3. F   4. D   5. C

Defence mechanisms are subconscious methods of coping with stressful stimuli. Initially these are understandable reactions to stress and may be beneficial. Freud believed

that these mechanisms were largely responsible for mental illness. Although this is now generally not believed to be true, they can be damaging when taken to extremes. Repression is the exclusion from consciousness of emotions, memories or ideas which may cause distress. One example is forgetting a stressful event such as witnessing a violent death. Repression is similar to denial, a mechanism where the patient will not believe the facts (eg that he/she has cancer). Projection is the attribution of one's own feelings onto someone else. For example, if I am jealous of someone else I may imagine that he or she is really jealous of me. Regression is the unconscious adoption of behaviour that is characteristic of an earlier stage of development. This may occur when someone wants others to feed, dress or wash him/her even when he/she is still able to perform these tasks him/herself. Displacement is transferring emotions from one person to another. If I am angry with myself for making a mistake, I may blame someone else and be angry with him/her even though he/she has done nothing wrong. Displacement commonly occurs in grief reactions. Rationalisation is producing an incorrect (and often implausible) explanation for something in order to protect one's own emotions. For example if I fail an exam because I have not worked hard enough, I may reason that the exam itself was unfair. Sublimation is channelling one's emotions into a more socially acceptable outlet. Repressed anger may be channelled into a contact sport.

Q58. PSYCHIATRIC DIAGNOSIS (☆)

1. E   2. B   3. A   4. D   5. C

Depression and dementia can be very difficult to distinguish in elderly patients. If there is a long history of gradually increasing forgetfulness, loss of concentration and disorientation at night, this is suggestive of dementia. The patient may also have a flattened affect and lack of spontaneity leading to suspicions that the patient is really depressed. Depression causes low mood, negative thoughts and biological symptoms such as loss of appetite, weight loss, constipation and early morning wakening. The patient may have poor concentration and memory impairment and this may lead to confusion with dementia. In practice many patients with cognitive impairment, where the cause is uncertain, are given a trial of antidepressants. Dysthymia is a persistent state of low mood that overlaps with the diagnosis of depression. However, when biological features (such as early morning wakening) are present the patient should be classified as depressed. Passivity phenomena, such as the belief that others can control one's thoughts and movements or can insert thoughts into one's head, are highly suggestive of schizophrenia. Patients typically lack insight into their illness and may also experience primary delusions and third person auditory hallucinations. Schizophrenic patients with longstanding illness may have negative symptoms such as social withdrawal, abnormal movements and catatonia. The manic patient is usually overactive, dresses flamboyantly and has grandiose ideas which may be held with delusional conviction. Flight of ideas occurs leading to rapid speech with changes in topic that are very difficult for the interviewer to follow. Wernicke-Korsakoff syndrome occurs in chronic alcoholics with thiamine deficiency (vitamin B₁). There is a loss of short-term memory leading to confabulation. The patient is often ataxic and has an external ophthalmoplegia due to damage around the third and fourth ventricles.

Q59. ANTIPSYCHOTIC DRUGS (☆☆)

1. E   2. A   3. F   4. B   5. D

Phenothiazines can be divided into groups 1, 2 and 3. Group 1 agents include chlorpromazine and promazine. These drugs have the most pronounced sedative effects and have moderate antimuscarinic (dry mouth, urine retention, constipation, etc) and moderate extrapyramidal side-effects (akathisia, dystonia, Parkinsonism, tardive dyskinesia). Thioridazine is a group 2 agent. These drugs have moderate sedative effects, marked antimuscarinic effects and

fewer extrapyramidal effects compared to group 1 drugs. The use of thioridazine is now restricted by the committee on Safety of Medicines, because of the risk of cardiotoxicity. Fluphenazine, prochlorperazine and trifluoperazine are group 3 phenothiazines. These have the least sedative and antimuscarinic effects, but they have the most pronounced extrapyramidal side-effects. Other traditional antipsychotic drugs such as haloperidol (a butyrophenone), sulpiride (a substituted benzamide), flupentixol and pimozide have similar side-effect profiles to the group 3 phenothiazines. Low-dose sulpiride has an alerting effect in schizophrenic patients with negative symptoms. Clozapine is an atypical antipsychotic that is highly effective in the treatment of schizophrenia, which is resistant to other drugs. It has a high risk of agranulocytosis and full blood counts must be performed weekly for 18 weeks, then every fortnight for one year and then every four weeks thereafter.

Q60. ORAL CONDITIONS (☆☆)

1. A   2. F   3. E   4. C   5. B

Papillary hyperplasia is swelling of the papillae on the hard palate due to an ill-fitting denture, poor oral hygiene and/or wearing the denture during the night. It is a benign condition. Periodontal disease occurs when plaque leads to bacterial colonisation and subsequent penetration of the space between the dental roots and the gums. This condition may lead to severe gingivitis and to dental root abscesses. Transient bacteraemia can occur particularly following dental procedures and this may be hazardous in those with cardiac valve abnormalities. Dental caries are also caused by plaque. Bacterial invasion of the tooth surface and subsequent acid production results in decalcification of enamel and lysis of protein matrix. This eventually destroys the affected tooth. Acute pseudomembranous candidiasis appears as white friable patches that can be scraped off the oral mucosa. This condition is associated with antibiotic usage, immunosuppression, inadequate saliva production and poor care of dentures. Hyperkeratotic and parakeratotic leukoplakia cannot be scraped off the mucosa. The former condition is a benign thickening of the keratin layer and this can usually simply be observed. Parakeratosis is diagnosed by a biopsy, which shows nuclei and cell membranes throughout all of the keratin layers. These lesions should be excised completely as a small percentage is malignant. Erythroplakia is the presence of red lesions with thinned epithelium and connective tissue papillae near the surface. More than 90% of these lesions are malignant.

PAPER 4 QUESTIONS

CELLULAR AND MOLECULAR BIOLOGY

1. THEME: NITRIC OXIDE

A   Endothelial NO synthase
B   Macrophage NO synthase
C   Guanylate cyclase
D   Endothelin 1
E   L-arginine
F   Sodium nitroprusside

For each of the following descriptions related to nitric oxide (NO) select the appropriate compound from the above list. The items may be used once or not at all.

☐ 1. Source of nitrogen atoms for synthesis of NO
☐ 2. Cell messenger directly activated by NO
☐ 3. Constitutive enzyme produced in response to calcium and calmodulin
☐ 4. Inducible enzyme produced in response to cytokines
☐ 5. Synthetic nitrate activated when converted to NO

2. THEME: TISSUE INFLAMMATION AND REPAIR

A   Free radicals
B   Superoxide dismutase
C   Tumour necrosis factor α
D   Transforming growth factor β
E   Heat shock proteins
F   Interleukin 1

For each of the following descriptions related to tissue inflammation and repair select the appropriate term from the above list. The items may be used once or not at all.

☐ 1. Family of three related polypeptides which potentiate local inflammatory damage
☐ 2. Induce(s) granulocyte-monocyte colony-stimulating factor production
☐ 3. Induce(s) production of extracellular matrix leading to development of fibrosis
☐ 4. Function(s) as molecular chaperone(s) for proteins moving in and out of cells
☐ 5. Molecule(s) containing unpaired electrons

STATISTICS AND EPIDEMIOLOGY

3. THEME: STATISTICAL TERMS

A   Risk ratio
B   Risk difference
C   Risk
D   Incidence
E   Prevalence
F   Rate

For each of the following definitions select the appropriate term from the above list. The items may be used once or not at all.

☐ 1. Frequency of new cases of disease occurring in a specified time interval
☐ 2. Frequency of cases of disease at a specified point in time
☐ 3. Probability of developing a disease during a specified time period
☐ 4. Probability of developing a disease per unit of time
☐ 5. Reciprocal of the number needed to treat

IMMUNOLOGY

4. THEME: COMPLEMENT

A CD59 deficiency
B C6 deficiency
C C3 deficiency
D C1 esterase inhibitor deficiency
E C1q deficiency
F C2 deficiency

For each of the following clinical problems select the complement deficiency responsible from the above list. The items may be used once or not at all.

☐ 1. Hereditary angio-oedema
☐ 2. Systemic lupus erythematosus-like syndrome
☐ 3. Membranoproliferative glomerulonephritis
☐ 4. Recurrent *Neisseria* infections
☐ 5. Severe skin infections

5. THEME: COMPLEMENT RECEPTORS

A CR1
B CR2
C CR3
D CR4
E C5aR
F C4b-binding protein

For each of the following descriptions select the appropriate complement receptor (CR) from the above list. The items may be used once or not at all.

☐ 1. A ligand for C3d which protects renal podocytes from immune complexes
☐ 2. A cofactor for C3b cleavage found on erythrocytes and monocytes
☐ 3. A mast cell receptor which triggers release of inflammatory mediators
☐ 4. A tissue macrophage receptor which is needed for crossing endothelium
☐ 5. A neutrophil and monocyte receptor involved in phagocytosis

CLINICAL GENETICS

6. THEME: GENETIC SYNDROMES

A Optic nerve astrocytoma
B Corneal clouding
C Cherry red spot at macula
D Retinal haemangioblastoma
E Retinal phakoma
F Angiokeratoma corporis diffusum

For each of the following genetic syndromes select the recognised associated feature from the above list. The items may be used once or not at all.

☐ 1. Tuberous sclerosis
☐ 2. von Hippel-Lindau
☐ 3. von Recklinghausen neurofibromatosis
☐ 4. Fabry disease
☐ 5. Hexosaminidase A deficiency (Gm$_2$-gangliosidosis)

7. THEME: FAMILIAL PATTERNS OF INHERITANCE

A Incomplete penetrance
B Germline mosaicism
C Anticipation
D Mitochondrial inheritance
E Balanced translocation
F Autosomal recessive inheritance

For each of the following familial patterns of inheritance select the appropriate mechanism from the above list. The items may be used once or not at all.

☐ 1. Two siblings share a dominant gene mutation not present in either parent
☐ 2. A couple have two children with Down's syndrome
☐ 3. A child and grandparent have the same disease but the parents are unaffected
☐ 4. Symptoms develop at a progressively younger age in successive generations
☐ 5. Females with a disease transmit it to all offspring but affected males never do

PAPER 4 QUESTIONS

NEUROANATOMY

8. THEME: AUTONOMIC NERVE SUPPLY

A   Midbrain
B   T5-T11
C   L3-L4
D   Medulla
E   T1
F   T2-T4

For each of the following autonomic nerve supplies select the appropriate area of origin from the above list. The items may be used once or not at all.

☐ 1. Sympathetic nerve supply to levator palpebrae superioris
☐ 2. Parasympathetic nerve supply to the iris
☐ 3. Sympathetic nerve supply to the lungs
☐ 4. Sympathetic nerve supply to the stomach
☐ 5. Parasympathetic nerve supply to the stomach

9. THEME: NERVE ROOTS

A   C3-C5
B   C8
C   T1
D   L1-L2
E   L2-L3
F   L4-L5

For each of the following muscle groups select the appropriate nerve root from the above list. The items may be used once or not at all.

☐ 1. Hip flexors
☐ 2. Diaphragmatic muscles
☐ 3. Intrinsic muscles of the hand
☐ 4. Knee extensors
☐ 5. Long finger extensors

PHYSIOLOGY, BIOCHEMISTRY AND METABOLISM

10. THEME: HYPONATRAEMIA

A   Cirrhosis
B   Conn's syndrome
C   Diuretic therapy
D   Excessive intravenous fluid therapy
E   Severe vomiting
F   Syndrome of inappropriate antidiuretic hormone

For each of the following findings select the appropriate cause of hyponatraemia from the above list. The items may be used once or not at all.

☐ 1. Dehydration and urine sodium >20 mmol/l
☐ 2. Dehydration and urine sodium <20 mmol/l
☐ 3. Not dehydrated and oedema is present
☐ 4. Not dehydrated and not oedematous and urine osmolality >500 mosmol/kg
☐ 5. Not dehydrated and not oedematous and urine osmolarity <500 mosmol/kg

11. THEME: SERUM ENZYMES

A   Alkaline phosphatase
B   Amylase
C   Troponin T
D   Lactate dehydrogenase
E   Alanine aminotransferase
F   Aldolase

For each of the following conditions select the serum enzyme from the above list that would be most useful in establishing the diagnosis. The items may be used once or not at all.

☐ 1. Myocardial infarction
☐ 2. Acute myositis
☐ 3. Mumps
☐ 4. Paget's disease
☐ 5. Acute hepatitis

12. THEME: ELECTROLYTE ABNORMALITIES

A Hypocalcaemia
B Hypercalcaemia
C Hyponatraemia
D Hypernatraemia
E Hypokalaemia
F Hyperkalaemia

For each of the following conditions/situations select the resulting electrolyte abnormality from the above list. The items may be used once or not at all.

1. Subarachnoid haemorrhage
2. Haemolysis of sample after phlebotomy
3. Diabetes insipidus
4. Insulin infusion
5. Hyperparathyroidism

13. THEME: BILIRUBIN METABOLIC PATHWAY

A Cholic acid
B Bilirubin
C Urobilinogen
D Biliverdin
E Bilirubin diglucuronide
F Haem

For each of the following descriptions related to the bilirubin metabolic pathway select the appropriate compound from the above list. The items may be used once or not at all.

1. Immediate precursor of bilirubin
2. Bilirubin metabolite secreted into the bile ducts
3. Water-soluble form which undergoes extensive enterohepatic recirculation
4. Water-insoluble form carried in plasma bound to albumin
5. Immediate main precursor of biliverdin

14. THEME: SITES OF COMPOUND PRODUCTION

A Kidney
B Thyroid
C Skin
D Liver
E Stomach
F Pancreas

For each of the following compounds select the appropriate organ of production from the above list. The items may be used once or not at all.

1. Thrombopoietin
2. Erythropoietin
3. Cholecalciferol
4. Calcitonin
5. Glucagon

RENAL MEDICINE

15. THEME: METHODS OF GLOMERULAR FILTRATION RATE MEASUREMENT

A Twenty-four-hour urinary creatinine clearance
B Plasma β_2-microglobulin
C Radioactively labelled DTPA clearance
D Inulin clearance
E Plasma creatinine
F Plasma urea

For each of the following limitations of measures of glomerular filtration rate select the appropriate method from the above list. The items may be used once or not at all.

1. Depends on muscle mass
2. Depends on protein synthesis
3. Estimated clearance is overestimated at low glomerular filtration rates due to tubular secretion
4. Measurement requires an expensive immunoassay
5. Estimated clearance is unreliable at low flow rates due to extrarenal clearance

16. THEME: RENAL STONES

A Magnesium ammonium phosphate stone
B Calcium phosphate stone
C Cystine stone
D Xanthine stone

E   Calcium oxalate stone
F   Uric acid stone

For each of the following descriptions select the appropriate type of renal stone from the above list. The items may be used once or not at all.

☐ 1. Commonest renal stone in men in the United Kingdom
☐ 2. Commonest renal stone in women in the United Kingdom
☐ 3. Commonest type of radiolucent stone
☐ 4. Radiolucent stone which forms in patients with the commonest inherited form of amino-aciduria
☐ 5. Radiolucent stone which is a rare complication of treatment with allopurinol

17. THEME: RENAL TOXICITY

A   Acute interstitial nephritis
B   Nephrogenic diabetes insipidus
C   Distal renal tubular acidosis
D   Fanconi syndrome
E   Membranous glomerulopathy
F   Acute tubular necrosis

For each of the following toxic agents select the associated renal condition from the above list. The items may be used once or not at all.

☐ 1. Acute lead poisoning
☐ 2. Amphotericin B
☐ 3. Lithium
☐ 4. Aminoglycoside antibiotics
☐ 5. Penicillin

18. THEME: DRUG CHARACTERISTICS

A   Vancomycin
B   Gentamicin
C   Tetracycline
D   Lithium
E   Quinidine
F   Aspirin

For each of the following statements select the appropriate drug from the above list. The items may be used once or not at all.

☐ 1. An organic acid, the excretion of which is increased in alkaline urine
☐ 2. A nephrotoxic drug which is not excreted by haemodialysis
☐ 3. A drug which shows increased tubular reabsorption in hyponatraemia
☐ 4. An antianabolic drug which may worsen uraemia
☐ 5. A nephrotoxic drug which is excreted by haemodialysis

ENDOCRINOLOGY AND DIABETES

19. THEME: DISORDERS OF THYROID FUNCTION

A   Graves' disease
B   Struma ovarii
C   De Quervain's thyroiditis
D   Riedel's thyroiditis
E   Choriocarcinoma
F   Hashimoto's thyroiditis

For each of the following statements select the appropriate condition from the above list. The items may be used once or not at all.

☐ 1. Causes hypothyroidism and a goitre
☐ 2. Causes hyperthyroidism and a painful thyroid gland
☐ 3. Commonest cause of hyperthyroidism in the United Kingdom
☐ 4. Thyroid-containing teratoma which secretes thyroid hormones
☐ 5. Causes hypothyroidism and a hard fibrotic thyroid gland

20. THEME: THYROID CANCER

A   Medullary carcinoma
B   Hürthle cell carcinoma
C   Follicular carcinoma
D   Papillary carcinoma
E   Thyroid lymphoma
F   Anaplastic carcinoma

For each of the following statements select the appropriate type of thyroid cancer from the above list. The items may be used once or not at all.

☐ 1. Commonest cause of thyroid cancer
☐ 2. Treatment is with total thyroidectomy and radioiodine ablation of residual thyroid tissue
☐ 3. Rapidly growing tumour with a five-year survival of only around 7%
☐ 4. Tumour arising from the parafollicular cells
☐ 5. Uncommon tumour which can usually be treated with external irradiation alone

21. THEME: DISORDERS OF CALCIUM METABOLISM

A   Pseudohypoparathyroidism
B   Pseudohyperparathyroidism
C   Primary hypoparathyroidism
D   Primary hyperparathyroidism
E   Secondary hyperparathyroidism
F   Tertiary hyperparathyroidism

For each of the following descriptions select the appropriate disorder of calcium metabolism from the above list. The items may be used once or not at all.

☐ 1. Excess parathyroid hormone production by an autonomous parathyroid adenoma
☐ 2. Peripheral resistance to parathyroid hormone
☐ 3. Excess parathyroid hormone production in response to low serum calcium
☐ 4. Prolonged low serum calcium results in autonomously functioning parathyroid glands
☐ 5. Autoimmune destruction of the parathyroid glands leads to decreased or absent parathyroid hormone

22. THEME: ENDOCRINE DISORDERS

A   Addison's disease
B   Ectopic adrenocorticotrophic hormone (ACTH) syndrome
C   Hyporeninaemic hypoaldosteronism
D   Conn's syndrome
E   ACTH deficiency
F   Cushing's disease

For each of the following findings select the appropriate condition from the above list. The items may be used once or not at all.

☐ 1. Central obesity, moon face and buffalo hump
☐ 2. Weight loss, hyperpigmentation and hyperkalaemia
☐ 3. Weight loss, amenorrhoea, hypoglycaemia and no hyperpigmentation
☐ 4. Weight loss, hyperpigmentation and hypokalaemic alkalosis
☐ 5. Hypertension, hypokalaemic alkalosis and no hyperpigmentation

GASTROENTEROLOGY

23. THEME: CONGENITAL PROBLEMS

A   Pyloric stenosis
B   Oesophageal atresia
C   Meconium ileus
D   Meckel's diverticulum
E   Exomphalos
F   Gastroschisis

For each of the following presentations select the appropriate congenital condition from the above list. The items may be used once or not at all.

☐ 1. Newborn infant with copious frothy saliva causing choking, dyspnoea and cyanosis
☐ 2. Newborn infant with herniation of the gastrointestinal tract through abdominal wall adjacent to the umbilicus

3. Four-week-old infant with projectile vomiting of feeds
4. Six-month-old infant with passage of bright red blood per rectum
5. One-day-old infant with bile-stained vomiting and abdominal distension

24. THEME: GASTROINTESTINAL DISORDERS

A Laxative abuse
B Irritable bowel syndrome
C Functional constipation
D Diverticular disease
E Angiodysplasia
F Rectal carcinoma

For each of the following presentations select the appropriate condition from the above list. The items may be used once or not at all.

1. Chronic history of abdominal pain relieved by defaecation, abdominal distension and passage of mucus in stools
2. Chronic history of constipation with pigmented rectal mucosa on sigmoidoscopy
3. Chronic history of passing hard stools, infrequent defaecation and a sensation of incomplete evacuation
4. Recent history of constipation and regular passage of blood mixed with stools
5. Regular passage of blood mixed with stools and a normal barium enema

25. THEME: VIRAL HEPATITIS

A Hepatitis A virus
B Hepatitis B virus
C Hepatitis C virus
D Hepatitis D virus
E Hepatitis E virus
F Cytomegalovirus

For each of the following descriptions select the appropriate cause of viral hepatitis from the

above list. The items may be used once or not at all.

1. Parenterally transmitted RNA-containing flavivirus
2. Enterally transmitted RNA-containing picornavirus
3. RNA virus requiring hepatitis B envelope antigen for successful replication
4. Parenterally transmitted DNA-containing hepadnavirus
5. Enterally transmitted calicivirus

26. THEME: INFECTIONS

A *Escherichia coli* O157:H7
B *Clostridium difficile*
C *Clostridium perfringens*
D *Campylobacter jejuni*
E Enterotoxigenic *Escherichia coli*
F *Cryptosporidium parvum*

For each of the following conditions select the appropriate causative microorganism from the above list. The items may be used once or not at all.

1. Travellers' diarrhoea
2. Haemolytic uraemic syndrome
3. Chronic diarrhoea in an immunocompromised patient
4. Antibiotic-associated diarrhoea
5. Guillain-Barré syndrome following gastroenteritis

NEUROLOGY

27. THEME: NEUROLOGICAL FINDINGS

A Extrinsic compressive lesion in cervical spine
B Syringomyelia
C Guillain-Barré syndrome
D Botulism
E Subacute combined degeneration of the cord
F Transverse myelitis

For each of the following clinical findings select the appropriate condition from the above list. The items may be used once or not at all.

☐ 1. Peripheral paraesthesia, loss of proprioception, absent ankle reflexes and an extensor plantar response
☐ 2. Wasting of small muscles of the hands, absent upper limb reflexes, absent pain and temperature sensation but preservation of proprioception
☐ 3. Acute onset of paraplegia and loss of sensation with a definable dermatomal level
☐ 4. Back pain, peripheral paraesthesia and a lower motor neurone facial palsy
☐ 5. Cranial nerve palsies, descending paralysis and no sensory abnormalities

28. THEME: NARCOLEPSY

A Cataplexy
B Hypnopompic hallucinations
C Hypnagogic hallucinations
D Sleep paralysis
E Automatic behaviours
F Sleep attacks

For each of the following descriptions select the appropriate feature of narcolepsy from the above list. The items may be used once or not at all.

☐ 1. Sudden loss of consciousness usually lasting less than 30 minutes with no recall of the event
☐ 2. Sudden onset of paralysis usually lasting less than 30 seconds with consciousness and recollection of the event preserved
☐ 3. Total inability to perform voluntary movements despite being alert and aware of surroundings lasting up to ten minutes
☐ 4. Frightening visual phenomena occurring on falling asleep
☐ 5. Fugue-like state reminiscent of sleep-walking with no recall of events

29. THEME: GLASGOW COMA SCALE

A E-1 V-1 M-1
B E-0 V-0 M-0
C E-4 V-3 M-5
D E-2 V-2 M-3
E E-4 V-3 M-4
F E-2 V-2 M-2

For each of the following responses select the appropriate assessment using the Glasgow Coma Scale (E = eye; M = motor; V = verbal) from the above list. The items may be used once or not at all.

☐ 1. Eyes open to pain, makes incomprehensible sounds, has flexion response to pain
☐ 2. Eyes open to pain, makes incomprehensible sounds, has extension response to pain
☐ 3. Eyes open spontaneously, makes inappropriate words, localises to pain
☐ 4. Eyes open spontaneously, makes inappropriate words, withdrawal response to pain
☐ 5. Eyes never open, no verbal response, no motor response

30. THEME: DEMENTIA

A Creutzfeldt-Jakob disease
B Lewy body disease
C Multi-infarct dementia
D Wilson's disease
E Pick's disease
F Alzheimer's disease

For each of the following findings select the appropriate cause of dementia from the above list. The items may be used once or not at all.

☐ 1. Stepwise deterioration and focal neurological signs

☐ 2. Inheritance of the apolipoprotein E_4 allele

☐ 3. Focal lobar atrophy demonstrated on brain imaging

☐ 4. Rapidly progressive dementia with myoclonus

☐ 5. Global dementia with marked Parkinsonian symptoms

RESPIRATORY MEDICINE

31. THEME: ATYPICAL PNEUMONIA

A *Mycoplasma pneumoniae*
B *Legionella pneumophila*
C *Coxiella burnetii*
D *Chlamydia pneumoniae*
E *Chlamydia psittaci*
F *Pneumocystis carinii*

For each of the following descriptions select the appropriate cause of atypical pneumonia from the above list. The items may be used once or not at all.

☐ 1. Acquired from parrots and other birds

☐ 2. Periodic epidemics occur approximately every four years

☐ 3. Multiplies in warm still water and may be spread via air-conditioners

☐ 4. Common in patients with HIV infection

☐ 5. Acquired from farm animals, abattoirs and unpasteurised milk

32. THEME: LUNG TUMOURS

A Adenocarcinoma
B Carcinoid tumour
C Large cell carcinoma
D Mesothelioma
E Squamous cell carcinoma
F Small cell carcinoma

For each of the following descriptions select the appropriate lung tumour from the above list. The items may be used once or not at all.

☐ 1. Commonest type of bronchial carcinoma

☐ 2. The bronchial carcinoma which is least smoking related

☐ 3. Highly malignant carcinoma with little or no evidence of differentiation

☐ 4. Rapidly metastasising tumour which secretes clinically significant hormones in 10% of cases

☐ 5. Exerts systemic effects due to serotonin secretion

33. THEME: CHEST X-RAYS

A Anteroposterior film
B Fluoroscopy
C Posteroanterior film
D Apical film
E Lateral film
F Lateral decubitus film

For each of the following descriptions select the appropriate chest X-ray view from the above list. The items may be used once or not at all.

☐ 1. Standard view

☐ 2. Useful for portable radiography to replace the standard view

☐ 3. Useful to detect abnormalities hidden behind the heart on the standard view

☐ 4. Useful to detect small pleural effusions

☐ 5. Useful to study diaphragmatic movement

34. THEME: COLLAGEN VASCULAR DISEASE

A   Systemic lupus erythematosus
B   Systemic sclerosis
C   Sjögren's syndrome
D   Ankylosing spondylitis
E   Rheumatoid arthritis
F   Dermatomyositis

For each of the following respiratory conditions select the associated collagen vascular disease from the above list. The items may be used once or not at all.

☐ 1. Cricoarytenoid arthritis
☐ 2. Alveolar haemorrhage
☐ 3. Recurrent aspiration pneumonia
☐ 4. Bronchial carcinoma
☐ 5. Upper zone fibrosis and cavitation

RHEUMATOLOGY

35. THEME: INFECTIOUS AETIOLOGY OF RHEUMATIC DISEASE

A   Parvovirus B19 infection
B   Atypical mycobacterial arthritis
C   Staphylococcal arthritis
D   Lyme disease
E   Gonococcal arthritis
F   Sporotrichosis

For each of the following presentations related to arthritis of infectious aetiology select the appropriate causative condition from the above list. The items may be used once or not at all.

☐ 1. Acute polyarthritis following a tick bite
☐ 2. Symmetrical polyarthropathy following an acute febrile illness with marked facial flushing
☐ 3. Arthritis affecting large joints after skin penetration by a rose thorn
☐ 4. Insidious onset of pain and swelling in a single joint after intra-articular steroid injection
☐ 5. Acute onset of pain and swelling in a single joint in a patient with rheumatoid arthritis

36. THEME: AUTOANTIBODIES AND CONNECTIVE TISSUE DISEASE/VASCULITIDES

A   Mixed connective tissue disease
B   Dermatomyositis
C   Sjögren's syndrome
D   Churg-Strauss syndrome
E   Scleroderma
F   Systemic lupus erythematosus

For each of the following autoantibodies select the most commonly associated connective tissue disease/vasculitides from the above list. The items may be used once or not at all.

☐ 1. Anti-dsDNA
☐ 2. Anti-Jo1
☐ 3. Anti-Scl-70
☐ 4. Anti-Ro
☐ 5. pANCA

DERMATOLOGY

37. THEME: PHOTODERMATOSES

A   Xeroderma pigmentosum
B   Actinic reticuloid syndrome
C   Actinic prurigo
D   Solar urticaria
E   Polymorphic light eruption
F   Hydroa vaccineforme

For each of the following descriptions select the appropriate photodermatosis from the above list. The items may be used once or not at all.

☐ 1. Commonest photosensitive drug eruption
☐ 2. Persistent pruritic papular eruption usually commencing in childhood
☐ 3. Pseudolymphomatous condition of the elderly
☐ 4. UVA-induced type I hypersensitivity reaction
☐ 5. DNA-repair defect resulting in high risk of skin tumours

38. THEME: SKIN TUMOURS

A Melanoma
B Squamous cell carcinoma
C Basal cell papilloma
D Keratoacanthoma
E Basal cell carcinoma
F Pyogenic granuloma

For each of the following descriptions select the appropriate skin tumour from the above list. The items may be used once or not at all.

☐ 1. Aggressive tumour which metastasises early
☐ 2. Locally destructive slow-growing tumour which never metastasises
☐ 3. Tumour associated with sites of chronic inflammation and immunosuppression
☐ 4. Rapidly growing, benign tumour resembling squamous cell carcinoma
☐ 5. Benign proliferation of blood vessels resembling amelanotic melanoma

HAEMATOLOGY

39. THEME: ANAEMIA

A Folate deficiency
B Haemolysis
C Sideroblastic anaemia
D Iron deficiency
E B_{12} deficiency
F Aplastic anaemia

For each of the following conditions select the resulting type of anaemia from the above list. The items may be used once or not at all.

☐ 1. Coeliac disease
☐ 2. Vegan diet
☐ 3. Lead poisoning
☐ 4. Pyrimethamine
☐ 5. Parvovirus B19

40. THEME: HAEMOGLOBIN

A $\alpha_2\delta_2$
B $\alpha_2\gamma_2$
C β_4
D γ_4
E $\alpha_2\beta_2$-NH-glucose
F $\alpha_2\beta_2$

For each of the following descriptions select the appropriate type of haemoglobin from the above list. The items may be used once or not at all.

☐ 1. Constitutes 92% of haemoglobin in normal adults
☐ 2. Constitutes 5% of haemoglobin in normal adults
☐ 3. Constitutes 2% of haemoglobin in normal adults
☐ 4. Constitutes predominant haemoglobin in the fetus
☐ 5. Non-functional haemoglobin found in adults with α-thalassaemia

41. THEME: CLOTTING FACTORS

A Prothrombin (factor II)
B Factor XIII
C Fibrinogen (factor I)
D Factor IX
E Factor VII
F Factor VIII

For each of the following descriptions select the appropriate clotting factor from the above list. The items may be used once or not at all.

☐ 1. A vitamin-K-dependent factor in the common pathway
☐ 2. A vitamin-K-dependent factor in the extrinsic pathway
☐ 3. A vitamin-K-dependent factor in the intrinsic pathway
☐ 4. A non-vitamin-K-dependent factor produced by megakaryocytes
☐ 5. A common pathway factor which stabilises fibrin

INFECTIOUS DISEASES AND TROPICAL MEDICINE

42. THEME: VIRAL DISEASE

A   Cytomegalovirus
B   Measles virus
C   Herpes simplex virus 1
D   JC polyoma virus
E   Adenovirus
F   Parvovirus B19

For each of the following diseases select the recognised causative virus from the above list. The items may be used once or not at all.

☐ 1. Subacute sclerosing panencephalitis
☐ 2. Progressive multifocal leucoencephalopathy
☐ 3. Guillain-Barré syndrome
☐ 4. Bell's palsy
☐ 5. Erythema infectiosum

43. THEME: STREPTOCOCCI

A   *S. milleri*
B   *S. pneumoniae*
C   *S. mutans*
D   *S. bovis*
E   *S. agalactiae*
F   *S. pyogenes*

For each of the following conditions select the causative species of streptococci from the above list. The items may be used once or not at all.

☐ 1. Neonatal meningitis
☐ 2. Deep soft tissue abscess
☐ 3. Rheumatic fever
☐ 4. Primary peritonitis
☐ 5. Dental caries

44. THEME: RISK FACTORS FOR INFECTION

A   Cirrhosis
B   Diabetes mellitus
C   Splenectomy
D   Cystic fibrosis
E   HIV infection
F   Gastric achlorydria

For infection with each of the following organisms select the appropriate condition from the list above that is an established risk factor. The items may be used once or not at all.

☐ 1. *Cryptococcus neoformans*
☐ 2. *Babesia divergens*
☐ 3. *Burkholderia pseudomallei*
☐ 4. *Burkholderia cepacia*
☐ 5. *Vibrio cholerae*

45. THEME: BACTERIAL TAXONOMY

A   Gram-negative bacillus
B   Gram-negative diplococcus
C   Spirochaete
D   Non-spore-forming Gram-positive bacillus
E   Gram-positive, filamentous branching bacterium
F   Anaerobic Gram-negative bacillus

For each of the following bacteria select the appropriate description from the above list. The items may be used once or not at all.

☐ 1. *Listeria monocytogenes*
☐ 2. *Acinetobacter baumannii*
☐ 3. *Neisseria gonorrhoea*
☐ 4. *Bacteroides fragilis*
☐ 5. *Nocardia asteroides*

GENITOURINARY MEDICINE

46. THEME: ANTIMICROBIAL THERAPY IN AIDS

A   Co-trimoxazole
B   Amphotericin B plus flucytosine
C   Clindamycin plus quinine
D   Pentamidine
E   Albendazole
F   Pyrimethamine plus sulphadiazine

For each of the following opportunistic infections in an AIDS patient select the appropriate standard first-line antimicrobial therapy from the above list. The items may be used once or not at all.

- ☐ 1. Cerebral toxoplasmosis
- ☐ 2. Intestinal cyclosporiasis
- ☐ 3. Cryptococcal meningitis
- ☐ 4. *Babesia microti* parasitaemia
- ☐ 5. Intestinal microsporidiosis

CLINICAL PHARMACOLOGY

47. THEME: ANTIARRYTHMIC DRUGS

A   Amiodarone
B   Lignocaine
C   Atenolol
D   Flecainide
E   Quinidine
F   Verapamil

For each of the following descriptions related to the Vaughan-Williams classification select the appropriate antiarrhythmic drug from the above list. The items may be used once or not at all.

- ☐ 1. Class I agent which increases the duration of the action potential
- ☐ 2. Class I agent with no effect on the duration of the action potential
- ☐ 3. Class I agent which decreases the duration of the action potential
- ☐ 4. An agent with complex class I, II, III and IV actions
- ☐ 5. Class IV agent

48. THEME: ANTIFUNGAL AGENTS

A   An allylamine used systemically for dermatophyte infections
B   A polyene with activity against yeasts and *Aspergillus*
C   A triazole active only against yeasts
D   A polyene which is too toxic for systemic use
E   A triazole active against yeasts and *Aspergillus*
F   An allylamine used as a lacquer in nail infections

For each of the following antifungal agents select the appropriate description from the above list. The items may be used once or not at all.

- ☐ 1. Amorolfine
- ☐ 2. Terbinafine
- ☐ 3. Amphotericin B
- ☐ 4. Itraconazole
- ☐ 5. Fluconazole

49. THEME: ANTIBIOTIC PROPHYLAXIS

A   No antibiotic required
B   Ceftriaxone
C   Benzylpenicillin
D   Amoxicillin
E   Ciprofloxacin
F   Phenoxymethylpenicillin

For each of the following situations select the recommended prophylactic antibiotic from the above list. The items may be used once or not at all.

- ☐ 1. Prevention of meningococcal meningitis in a pregnant household contact of a primary case
- ☐ 2. Prevention of pneumococcal infection in an adult following splenectomy
- ☐ 3. Patient with valvular heart disease undergoing dental scaling
- ☐ 4. Prevention of gas gangrene in a hindquarter amputation
- ☐ 5. Patient with total hip replacement undergoing dental extraction

50. THEME: DRUG SIDE-EFFECTS

A   Ciprofloxacin
B   High strength pancreatin
C   Prazosin
D   Rifampicin
E   Ciclosporin
F   Mesalazine

For each of the following warnings related to side-effects select the associated drug from the above list. The items may be used once or not at all.

☐ 1. Lie down if dizziness, fatigue or sweating develops after the first dose
☐ 2. Avoid grapefruit juice for 1 hour before taking dose
☐ 3. Discontinue drug if tendon pain or inflammation occurs
☐ 4. Report any unexplained bleeding, bruising, fever, malaise or sore throat
☐ 5. Ensure adequate hydration at all times

51. THEME: DRUGS USED TO TREAT MALIGNANCY

A   Melphalan
B   Fludarabine
C   Carboplatin
D   Hydroxyurea
E   Liposomal daunorubicin
F   Ciclosporin

For each of the following types of malignancy select the appropriate drug from the above list. The items may be used once or not at all.

☐ 1. Myeloma
☐ 2. Kaposi's sarcoma
☐ 3. B cell chronic lymphatic leukaemia
☐ 4. Small cell lung cancer
☐ 5. Chronic myeloid leukaemia

52. THEME: INFLAMMATORY BOWEL DISEASE

A   Budesonide
B   Sulfasalazine
C   Mesalazine
D   Infliximab
E   Prednisolone
F   Olsalazine

For each of the following descriptions select the appropriate treatment for inflammatory bowel disease from the above list. The items may be used once or not at all.

☐ 1. Monoclonal antibody to tumour necrosis factor α
☐ 2. Modified release steroid used to treat terminal ileitis
☐ 3. Enteric-coated modified-release preparation of 5-aminosalicylic acid
☐ 4. Dimer of 5-aminosalicylic acid
☐ 5. Steroid used as an enema to treat distal colitis

CARDIOVASCULAR MEDICINE

53. THEME: HYPERTENSION

A   β-blockers
B   Angiotensin-converting enzyme inhibitors
C   Thiazide diuretics
D   Angiotensin II receptor antagonists
E   Calcium channel blockers
F   α-blockers

For each of the following descriptions select the appropriate treatment for hypertension from the above list. The items may be used once or not at all.

☐ 1. Highly suitable for those with coexistent heart failure, not suitable for those with gout
☐ 2. Highly suitable for those with coexistent angina, not suitable for those with asthma
☐ 3. Highly suitable for those with coexistent heart failure or diabetic nephropathy, not suitable for those with hyperkalaemia
☐ 4. Highly suitable for elderly patients and those with peripheral vascular disease, not suitable for those with heart block or cardiac failure

☐ 5. Highly suitable for those with coexistent prostatic hypertrophy, not suitable for those with postural hypotension

54. THEME: RISK FACTORS FOR CARDIAC CONDITIONS

A   Constrictive pericarditis
B   Dilated cardiomyopathy
C   Hypertrophic cardiomyopathy
D   Right ventricular dysplasia
E   Myocarditis
F   Restrictive cardiomyopathy

For each of the following risk factors select the appropriate cardiac condition from the above list. The items may be used once or not at all.

☐ 1. Mutation in the β-cardiac myosin gene
☐ 2. Excessive alcohol consumption
☐ 3. Endomyocardial fibrosis
☐ 4. Acute *Trypanosoma cruzi* infection
☐ 5. Tuberculosis

55. THEME: UNCORRECTED CONGENITAL HEART DISEASE IN ADULTS

A   Ebstein's anomaly
B   Tricuspid atresia
C   Ostium secundum atrial septal defect
D   Eisenmenger syndrome
E   Eisenmenger complex secondary to persistent ductus arteriosus
F   Tetralogy of Fallot

For each of the following presentations in adults select the appropriate uncorrected congenital heart disease from the above list. The items may be used once or not at all.

☐ 1. Patient with clubbing and cyanosis, chest X-ray shows large right ventricle and large ascending aorta
☐ 2. Patient with clubbing and cyanosis, chest X-ray shows large pulmonary arteries with peripheral pruning
☐ 3. Patient with clubbing and cyanosis which is markedly more severe in the lower

limbs, chest X-ray shows small area of calcification above the left hilum
☐ 4. Patient who develops cyanosis after exercise, chest X-ray shows global cardiomegaly with a clear outline, underperfused lungs and a small aortic arch
☐ 5. Acyanotic patient with breathlessness on exertion, chest X-ray shows cardiomegaly, pulmonary plethora and a small aortic arch

56. THEME: INFECTIVE ENDOCARDITIS

A   Native mitral valve infection after vasectomy
B   Recent prosthetic valve replacement and now has endophthalmitis
C   Native mitral valve infection in a patient with recent change in bowel habit
D   Native mitral valve infection after dental extraction
E   Repeatedly culture-negative endocarditis
F   Native tricuspid valve infection in a young man

For each of the following organisms select the associated form of endocarditis from the above list. The items may be used once or not at all.

☐ 1. *Streptococcus sanguis*
☐ 2. *Streptococcus bovis*
☐ 3. *Staphylococcus aureus*
☐ 4. *Staphylococcus lugdunensis*
☐ 5. *Candida albicans*

PSYCHIATRY

57. THEME: DEFINITION OF TERMS

A Passivity phenomena
B Derealisation
C Hemisomatognosia
D Alien limb
E Phantom limb
F Depersonalisation

For each of the following descriptions select the appropriate symptom from the above list. The items may be used once or not at all.

☐ 1. Subjective feeling of detachment from one's own experiences and emotions
☐ 2. Subjective feeling that the external environment lacks true substance
☐ 3. Belief that one's own body, thoughts or actions are controlled by external forces
☐ 4. Belief that a limb is missing when it isn't
☐ 5. Limb movement occurring independently of voluntary control

58. THEME: 1983 UK MENTAL HEALTH ACT

A Section 5
B Section 3
C Section 4
D Section 2
E Section 37
F Section 7

For each of the following situations select the appropriate section of the 1983 UK Mental Health Act from the above list. The items may be used once or not at all.

☐ 1. Compulsory hospital admission for up to 28 days
☐ 2. Emergency order for compulsory admission to hospital for up to 72 hours
☐ 3. Temporary holding order for a patient already in hospital
☐ 4. Compulsory hospital inpatient treatment for up to 6 months
☐ 5. Guardianship of a patient in the community

59. THEME: PSYCHIATRIC THERAPY

A Cognitive therapy
B Implosion
C Dynamic interactional treatment
D Counter-transference
E Transference
F Desensitisation

For each of the following descriptions select the appropriate form of psychiatric therapy from the above list. The items may be used once or not at all.

☐ 1. A form of behavioural therapy where an exposure is gradually increased
☐ 2. Aims to identify and change negative ways of thinking
☐ 3. A form of behavioural therapy where patient imagines the exposure
☐ 4. Component of psychoanalysis used to develop insight into patient's problems
☐ 5. Form of group therapy using relationships formed by members to work through previous problems

MISCELLANEOUS

60. THEME: FAECAL INCONTINENCE

A Examination of a wet preparation of faeces
B Faecal fat estimation
C Proctoscopy
D Modified Ziehl-Neelsen stain on faeces
E Digital rectal examination
F Rigid sigmoidoscopy

For the diagnosis of each of the following conditions select the appropriate assessment of faecal incontinence from the above list. The items may be used once or not at all.

☐ 1. Lax anal sphincter
☐ 2. Haemorrhoids
☐ 3. Inflammatory bowel disease
☐ 4. *Trichuris trichiura* infection
☐ 5. Malabsorption syndrome

ANSWERS TO PAPER 4

The approximate difficulty rating for the answer to each question is given in brackets.

☆ (the majority of competent final year students will know the answer)

☆☆ (approximately 50% of final year students will be able to answer correctly)

☆☆☆ (only the better students will usually know the answer)

Q1. NITRIC OXIDE (☆☆☆)

1. E   2. C   3. A   4. B   5. F

NO is a transcellular messenger, previously known as endothelium-derived relaxant factor. Its diverse actions include vasodilatation, neurotransmission and inhibition of platelet aggregation. It is now realised that NO has an important role in the pathogenesis of many different conditions including septic shock, adult respiratory distress syndrome, Alzheimer's disease and myocardial infarction. NO is produced when NO synthase catalyses the conversion of the amino acid L-arginine to *N*-hydroxy-L-arginine, which is then converted to NO and citrulline. The local action of NO is mediated by activation of guanylate cyclase, which in turn activates the intracellular second messenger cGMP. There are three isoforms of NO synthase: endothelial and neuronal (constitutive) and macrophage (inducible). Release of endothelial and neuronal NO synthase depends on calcium and calmodulin regulation. Macrophage NO synthase production is stimulated by cytokines. Sodium nitroprusside is a synthetic nitrate used as a vasodilator to treat angina. It becomes active when converted into NO. Endothelin 1 is a potent vasoconstrictor produced in response to endothelial stress.

Q2. TISSUE INFLAMMATION AND REPAIR (☆☆☆)

1. F   2. C   3. D   4. E   5. A

Interleukin 1 is really a family of three related polypeptides: interleukin 1α, interleukin 1β and interleukin 1 receptor antagonist. Interleukin 1 potentiates local inflammatory changes by increasing gene expression for collagenases, phospholipases and cyclo-oxygenases. This is believed to be important in the pathogenesis of conditions such as rheumatoid arthritis. Tumour necrosis factor α is produced by macrophages, eosinophils and NK (natural killer) cells. It has a wide spectrum of actions including induction of granulocyte-monocyte colony-stimulating factor production. This leads to activation of monocytes and macrophages. Tumour necrosis factor α is produced in large quantities in septic shock and severe malaria and it can cause severe hypotension in these conditions. Chronic high levels of tumour necrosis factor α production are believed to contribute to cachexia in conditions such as AIDS wasting syndrome and tuberculosis. Specific inhibitors of tumour necrosis factor α (etanercept and infliximab) are used in the treatment of rheumatoid arthritis and Crohn's disease. Transforming growth factor β is released by platelets at the site of tissue injury. It induces monocytes to secrete fibroblast growth factor and induces the production of extracellular matrix proteins including collagen, fibronectin and proteoglycans. This leads to the development of fibrosis. Heat shock proteins are released in response to damaged intracellular protein as occurs after damage by heat, cytotoxic chemicals, radiation or free radicals. Heat shock proteins act as molecular chaperones, transporting proteins in and out of cells. Heat shock proteins also catalyse protein folding and unfolding and are involved in protein degradation. Free radicals are molecules or atoms that contain unpaired electrons. Those of physiological and pathological importance include the peroxide radical, the superoxide radical, the hydroxyl radical and nitric oxide. Natural scavengers for free radicals that are obtained from dietary sources include vitamins C and E, β-carotene and flavonoids. Superoxide dismutases convert superoxide into hydrogen peroxide, which is then removed by catalases and glutathione peroxide. It has been found that mutations in the copper-zinc superoxide dismutase 1 gene are the cause of some cases of familial motor neurone disease.

Q3. STATISTICAL TERMS (☆)

1. D   2. E   3. C   4. F   5. B

Incidence is the number of new cases of a disease occurring in a specified time interval per unit population size. It is usually quoted as number of new cases per 100,000 population per year but may be quoted as a figure for shorter periods of time for diseases characterised by epidemic spread where the situation may change rapidly, eg influenza. Incidence is used by epidemiologists to study changing patterns of disease and the effects of potential risk factors. Prevalence is the number of people who have a disease at a single point in time. Prevalence includes both recent and chronic cases of disease. It is less useful than incidence for studying the effects of risk factors in disease development as it is affected by case fatality and cure rates. Prevalence is widely used by health planners to estimate the burden of disease in a community so that appropriate resources can be allocated to it. Risk and rate are both measures of the chance that an outcome (eg a disease) will occur. Risk is a probability (eg one chance in 100 or 0.01), whereas rate is measured per unit of time (eg one per 100 person-years). The risk ratio is the probability of an outcome occurring in one group compared to another. Rate ratio is the relative probability of an outcome occurring in two groups per unit of time. For rare outcomes

risk ratio and rate ratio are the same, but for common outcomes they are different. Risk difference is the reciprocal of number needed to treat. Imagine 100 people are given a drug and 25 die, compared to 100 people who are given a placebo of whom 50 die. The risk difference between the drug and placebo is 25 per 100, which is 0.25 if expressed as a proportion. The reciprocal of 0.25 is four, therefore the number needed to treat to prevent one death is four.

Q4. COMPLEMENT (☆☆☆)

1. D   2. F   3. C   4. B   5. E

Hereditary angio-oedema is an autosomal dominant condition due to deficiency of C1 esterase inhibitor. C1 esterase controls activation of the classical pathway by inactivating the C1 complex. Patients develop non-pruritic oedema of subcutaneous tissues and of the bowel wall, which may cause acute abdominal pain. Laryngeal oedema is a relatively rare complication. C2 deficiency is present in approximately 1 in 10,000 Caucasians. Deficiency of the classical pathway components, C2 or C4, results in a systemic lupus erythematosus-like syndrome or other immune-complex-mediated disease. C3 deficiency is usually acquired and is caused by the production of an autoantibody such as C3 nephritic factor. C3 immune complex deposition in the renal mesangium produces membranoproliferative glomerulonephritis (type II) and the resulting C3 deficiency causes increased susceptibility to pyogenic infections. Deficiency of the alternative pathway components, properdin or factor D, or of the final common pathway components C6, C7, C8 or C9 results in increased susceptibility to recurrent infections with *Neisseria meningitidis*. C1q deficiency produces immune complex disease and severe skin infections. CD59 and C8-binding protein are complement receptors that are deficient in paroxysmal nocturnal haemoglobinuria.

Q5. COMPLEMENT RECEPTORS (☆☆☆)

1. B   2. A   3. E   4. D   5. C

CR1 is a ligand for C3b found on erythrocytes and monocytes. It is a cofactor for C3b cleavage and is involved in transport of immune complexes and phagocytosis. CR2 is a ligand for C3d that is present on B cells, renal podocytes and dendritic cells. It is involved in B lymphocyte differentiation and protects against immune complex deposition. CR3 is a ligand for iC3b found on neutrophils and monocytes that facilitates phagocytosis. CR4 is also a ligand for iC3b and is expressed on tissue macrophages. It enables macrophages to cross endothelium at sites of inflammation. C5aR binds C5a and is found on mast cells and neutrophils. It triggers mast cells to release inflammatory mediators and is therefore important in acute allergic reactions. C4b-binding protein promotes decay of C4b.

Q6. GENETIC SYNDROMES (☆☆☆)

1. E   2. D   3. A   4. F   5. C

Tuberous sclerosis is an autosomal dominant condition. However, due to incomplete penetrance and a high mutation rate, many cases appear to be sporadic. Two genes have been found which cause the condition on chromosomes 9 and 16. The cutaneous lesions include adenoma sebaceum (small fibromas in a butterfly facial distribution), depigmented patches and shagreen patches (elevated, roughened skin). Tuberous masses of glial cells and enlarged neurones occur in the brain, causing epilepsy and mental retardation. Retinal phakomas and cardiac rhabdomyomas also occur. In von Hippel-Lindau syndrome, haemangioblastomas develop in the cerebellum, retina and spinal cord. Occasionally hypernephromas or haemangioblastomas of the pancreas, kidneys or adrenals may develop. Neurofibromatosis type 1 (von Recklinghausen disease) is an autosomal dominant condition caused by defects in the neurofibromin gene on chromosome 17. This syndrome is characterised by multiple neurofibromas, café-au-lait spots, axillary/inguinal freckling, Lisch nodules (eye), phaeochromocytoma and astrocytomas of the optic nerve. Fabry disease is an X-linked condition where intralysosomal deposits of α-galactosyl-lactosyl-ceramide accumulate in blood vessel walls and reticuloendothelial cells. The cornea, kidney, myocardium, peripheral nerves and autonomic ganglia are all affected. Numerous red to blue-black telangiectases develop on the trunk and thighs, a condition known as angiokeratoma corpora diffusum. Patients suffer from severe paraesthesia, corneal and lens opacities, ischaemic heart disease and avascular necrosis of bone. Males are more severely affected than females and usually die from cardiovascular disease in middle age. Hexosaminidase A converts Gm_2-ganglioside to Gm_3-ganglioside and deficiency results in accumulation of Gm_2-ganglioside in the nervous system. The infant form of this condition is known as Tay-Sachs disease and affects 1 in 2000 Ashkenazi Jews. There are also juvenile and adult-onset forms. Patients develop ataxia, loss of speech, dystonias and optic atrophy with a cherry red spot at the macula. In the adult form retinal problems do not occur. Corneal clouding occurs in mucopolysaccharidosis type I, which is also known as Hurler syndrome.

Q7. FAMILIAL PATTERNS OF INHERITANCE (☆☆☆)

1. B   2. E   3. A   4. C   5. D

Large extended pedigrees showing classic autosomal recessive, autosomal dominant or X-linked inheritance are easy to recognise. Unfortunately, genetics is a complex subject and inheritance patterns in real families may be difficult to identify. Incomplete penetrance can result in a dominant gene mutation appearing to 'jump' a generation, affecting only child and grandparent. Autosomal recessive inheritance could also cause this pattern, but it would be unusual. Germline mosaicism occurs when a new mutation arises in the parental germline. It may be passed on to multiple offspring without being present in the parental somatic genome. If the gene defect is unknown the resulting pedigree, in which there are multiple affected siblings, resembles autosomal recessive inheritance. Anticipation occurs when successive generations exhibit progressively more severe symptoms or the onset is at a younger age. This arises in trinucleotide-repeat disorders such as myotonic dystrophy, where an unstable nucleotide triplet becomes longer with each generation. However, 'apparent anticipation' may also simply be due to bias if pedigrees of multiple cases are identified by screening older family members after identification of a severely affected younger case. Mitochondria show maternal inheritance so a father cannot pass on a mitochondrial mutation whereas a mother passes it to all of her children. A balanced translocation is the result of meiotic recombination between different chromosomes, eg 14 and 21. The carrier has an abnormal karyotype (eg including a 14^{21} fusion chromosome) but is phenotypically normal as there is no excess or loss of genetic material. However, if the fusion chromosome is passed on the offspring will be trisomic for that region (eg karyotype $46XX(14^{21})$). This can result in multiple offspring with the same trisomic disorder.

Q8. AUTONOMIC NERVE SUPPLY (☆☆)

1. E   2. A   3. F   4. B   5. D

The sympathetic nerve supply to the iris and levator palpebrae superioris is from T1 via the superior cervical sympathetic ganglion. The sympathetic supply causes dilation of the pupil and elevation of the eyelid. Damage to this supply results in Horner's syndrome, the combination of pupil constriction, drooping eyelid, enophthalmos, vasodilatation of cutaneous blood vessels and anhidrosis. The parasympathetic nerve supply to the iris is from the parasympathetic oculomotor (CN III) nucleus in the midbrain, via the oculomotor nerve and ciliary ganglion. This produces pupil constriction in response to light and accommodation. The sympathetic nerve supply

to the lungs is from T2-T4 via the 2nd to 5th thoracic sympathetic ganglia. This causes bronchodilation and vasoconstriction. The sympathetic supply to the stomach is from T5-T11 via the coeliac ganglion. This inhibits peristalsis and causes sphincter contraction slowing down movement of food through the gut. The parasympathetic supply to most of the thoracic and abdominal viscera is from the medulla via the vagus (CN X) nerve. The supply to the stomach is via the myenteric (Auerbach's) and submucosal (Meissner's) plexuses. The parasympathetic supply stimulates peristalsis and secretion and relaxes sphincters. Vagotomy can be performed to reduce stomach acid secretion in those with recurrent peptic ulcers, though this operation is performed much less frequently than previously.

Q9. NERVE ROOTS (☆)

1. D   2. A   3. C   4. E   5. B

The diaphragmatic muscles are supplied by C3-C5 via the phrenic nerve. Therefore, spinal cord transection will only cause diaphragmatic palsy if it occurs high in the cervical region. The long flexors and extensors of the fingers are predominantly supplied by C8. The muscles involved include flexor digitorum profundus, flexor digitorum superficialis, flexor pollicis longus, extensor pollicis longus, abductor pollicis longus and extensor digitorum. The nerve supply is via branches from the median, ulnar and radial nerves which arise from the brachial plexus. The intrinsic or small muscles of the hand are predominantly supplied by T1. These include the palmar and dorsal interossei (which respectively adduct and abduct the fingers) and the muscles of the thenar eminence (abductor and flexor pollicis brevis and opponens pollicis). The iliopsoas muscle produces flexion of the hip and the nerve root responsible is L1-L2. Iliopsoas is a large muscle and haemorrhage into it (eg in haemophilia) is potentially fatal. Extension of the knee is produced by quadriceps femoris. This powerful muscle is supplied by L2-L3 via the femoral nerve. Herniation of an intervertebral disc at this level causes weakness of knee extension and loss of the knee tendon stretch reflex. L4-L5 supplies the flexors of the knee.

Q10. HYPONATRAEMIA (✩✩)

1. C   2. E   3. A   4. F   5. D

In hyponatraemia it is essential to fully assess the patient in order to identify the likely cause and institute appropriate therapy. If the patient is dehydrated and the urine sodium is greater than 20 mmol/l then the problem is sodium and water loss from the kidney. Causes include the diuretic stage of renal failure, diuretic therapy, osmotic diuresis (eg with high blood glucose), nephrocalcinosis, medullary cystic kidney and Addison's disease. In the dehydrated patient with appropriate conservation of sodium by the kidney (urine sodium <20 mmol/l), the cause is sodium and water loss from somewhere other than the kidney. Causes include vomiting, diarrhoea, bowel fistulae, severe burns, villous adenoma of the rectum, excessive sweating and cystic fibrosis. If the patient is not dehydrated and shows evidence of fluid overload with peripheral oedema and/or ascites the likely causes are nephrotic syndrome, cardiac failure, cirrhosis or oliguric renal failure.

A hyponatraemic patient who is not oedematous and not dehydrated and who produces inappropriately concentrated urine (urine osmolality >500 mosmol/kg) has the syndrome of inappropriate antidiuretic hormone. This occurs in malignancy, central nervous system disease, chest disease, porphyria and with some drugs. If the patient is not dehydrated and not oedematous and is producing appropriately dilute urine, the cause is water overload. This most commonly occurs if the patient is given excessive intravenous fluid therapy, but may also be due to hypothyroidism or insufficient glucocorticoid production. In Conn's syndrome (primary hyperaldosteronism) there is usually hypernatraemia.

Q11. SERUM ENZYMES (✩)

1. C   2. F   3. B   4. A   5. E

Troponin I and troponin T are highly specific markers of myocardial damage. Levels rise rapidly after a myocardial infarction and are usually elevated within four hours of infarction facilitating early diagnosis. Levels remain elevated for up to two weeks. This enables the diagnosis of myocardial infarction to be made even when it has occurred several days before presentation. Total creatine kinase and/or aldolase are useful for diagnosis of skeletal muscle damage. Levels are elevated in myositis but can also be elevated following excessive exercise, a heavy fall or an intramuscular injection. Amylase is most frequently used in the diagnosis of acute pancreatitis. Amylase is also produced by the parotid glands and the level is therefore often elevated in acute parotitis as occurs in mumps. However, a normal amylase does not exclude the diagnosis of mumps, as many people do not produce salivary amylase. Alkaline phosphatase is elevated in conditions where there is increased bone turnover such as Paget's disease, fractures, osteomalacia, bone metastases, hyperparathyroidism and renal failure. Raised alkaline phosphatase is also elevated in cholestasis (due to the intestinal isoform) and pregnancy (due to the placental isoform). Alanine aminotransferase (ALT) is a specific marker of hepatocyte damage. Serum ALT is markedly elevated during acute hepatitis, which may be secondary to viral infection (eg hepatitis viruses A to E) or drugs (eg rifampicin or co-trimoxazole). Serum aspartate aminotransferase and lactate dehydrogenase (LDH) are also elevated following hepatocyte damage but these are less specific enzymes. LDH may be elevated in myocardial infarction, pulmonary embolism, haemolysis and tumour necrosis.

Q12. ELECTROLYTE ABNORMALITIES (☆☆)

1. C   2. F   3. D   4. E   5. B

Hyponatraemia has many causes. It may accompany water loss due to polyuric renal failure, diuretic therapy, diarrhoea, vomiting or an enteric fistula. In the oedematous patient it may be due to angiotensin-mediated water retention secondary to the nephrotic syndrome, liver cirrhosis or cardiac failure. Hyponatraemia with inappropriately concentrated urine suggests the syndrome of inappropriate antidiuretic hormone, which can be due to malignancy (eg small cell lung cancer), central nervous system disease (eg subarachnoid or subdural haemorrhage, stroke, meningoencephalitis or brain abscess), chest disease (eg tuberculosis, pneumonia or lung abscess) or drugs (eg chlorpropamide or psychotropics). Hypernatraemia may conversely be secondary to diabetes insipidus (DI), which is either due to failure of antidiuretic hormone production (cranial DI, eg due to pituitary disease) or renal resistance to its effects (renal DI, eg due to lithium). Hypernatraemia may also be due to dehydration with water loss in excess of salt loss, inappropriate intravenous fluid therapy or excessive mineralocorticoid production (in Conn's syndrome). Hyperkalaemia is commonly spurious due to haemolysis of the blood sample during phlebotomy. If hyperkalaemia is unexpected it should be confirmed before instituting therapy. Causes of genuine hyperkalaemia include drugs (eg potassium-sparing diuretics, angiotensin-converting enzyme inhibitors, suxamethonium), massive blood transfusion, rhabdomyolysis, tumour lysis syndrome and Addison's disease. Hypokalaemia can be caused by potassium loss by the kidneys (eg diuretic therapy, alkalosis, Conn's and Cushing's syndrome or steroid therapy), loss from the gut (eg diarrhoea, vomiting, villous adenoma, laxatives or enteric fistula) or when potassium is pushed inside cells (eg with an insulin infusion or in thyrotoxicosis). In the treatment of diabetic ketoacidosis the initially hyperkalaemic patient may rapidly become hypokalaemic following insulin therapy.

Hypercalcaemia may be caused by malignancy (eg myeloma, bone metastases, lymphoma), hyperparathyroidism, vitamin D excess or sarcoidosis. Hypocalcaemia may occur following parathyroidectomy (or thyroidectomy if the parathyroid blood supply is damaged), in renal failure, pancreatitis and pseudohypoparathyroidism.

Q13. BILIRUBIN METABOLIC PATHWAY (☆☆)

1. D   2. E   3. C   4. B   5. F

The bilirubin metabolic pathway commences with the breakdown of free haem to biliverdin, carbon monoxide and iron by the enzyme haem oxygenase. Haem oxygenase also catalyses the breakdown of a smaller quantity of haem from haemoglobin, cytochrome P450, catalase and carboxyhaemoglobin. Biliverdin is converted to bilirubin by biliverdin reductase. This reaction occurs rapidly at the site of haem breakdown so very little biliverdin is detectable in blood. Bilirubin is highly insoluble and is carried to the liver bound to albumin. This binding occurs to specific sites on the albumin molecule and bilirubin can be displaced by salicylates, sulphonamides, diazepam and vitamin K analogues. In neonatal jaundice these drugs increase the risk of kernicterus. In the liver bilirubin is conjugated with glucuronic acid by the enzyme uridine diphosphate glucuronyl transferase. This enzyme is deficient in Crigler-Najjar syndrome. Bilirubin diglucuronide is secreted into the bile ducts and is metabolised by gut bacteria to urobilinogen and other products. Urobilinogen is highly water soluble and is reabsorbed by the gut. It then undergoes excretion by the liver and shows extensive enterohepatic recirculation. If it escapes the liver it can be excreted by the kidneys and in cholestatic liver disease is detectable in increased quantities in the urine. In complete biliary tract obstruction, urine urobilinogen is decreased, as bilirubin diglucuronide does not enter the gut. Cholic acid is a primary bile acid, a breakdown product of cholesterol. It is not a part of the bilirubin metabolic pathway.

Q14. SITES OF COMPOUND PRODUCTION (☆)

1. D   2. A   3. C   4. B   5. F

Thrombopoietin is the hormone controlling megakaryopoeisis in the bone marrow. Thrombopoietin is produced by the liver and therefore a low platelet count frequently occurs in the cirrhotic patient. The kidney is the site of erythropoietin production. Erythropoietin is responsible for red cell formation. In renal failure anaemia frequently occurs and in renal cell carcinoma polycythaemia can result. Cholecalciferol is obtained in the diet and is produced in the skin from cholesterol. Cholecalciferol must be 1α-hydroxylated by the liver and 24-hydroxylated by the kidney to form the active vitamin D_3 metabolite 1,25-dihydroxycholecalciferol. Calcitonin is produced by the C cells in the thyroid. This hormone acts on osteoclasts to suppress bone remodelling. Glucagon is produced by the L-arginine α cells in the pancreas. This hormone raises serum glucose and amino acids and glucagon-secreting tumours can cause diabetes mellitus, amino-acidaemia, weight loss, anaemia, thromboembolism and an unusual rash called necrolytic migratory erythema. The stomach produces gastrin, which is a regulator of gastric acid production.

Q15. METHODS OF GLOMERULAR FILTRATION RATE MEASUREMENT (☆☆)

1. E   2. F   3. A   4. B   5. C

Inulin clearance provides the gold standard measure of glomerular filtration rate (GFR) because inulin is filtered entirely by the glomerulus, is not secreted or reabsorbed by the renal tubule and there is no extrarenal clearance. However, it is not widely used in practice because of technical difficulties in administration (must be heated to dissolve) and in measurement (requires expertise). Measurement of plasma urea and creatinine are convenient to perform and simple to measure in the laboratory. They are therefore the most widely used tests of renal function. The disadvantages of plasma urea are that it is influenced by dietary protein intake and catabolic rate and that urea clearance falls at low GFR (underestimating GFR). Plasma creatinine is dependent on muscle mass. Although an age and sex nomogram can be used to calculate creatinine clearance from plasma creatinine, there is still residual variation in body build. Creatinine undergoes very low secretion in the renal tubule and 24-hour urinary creatinine clearance is therefore a reasonable way to measure GFR. However, at low GFR, renal tubular secretion becomes increasingly important resulting in the overestimation of GFR by this method. An additional disadvantage is the need to collect an accurately timed, 24-hour urine collection with the bladder empty at the start and end of the time period. This instruction is not fully understood by every patient. Plasma β_2-microglobulin is produced at a fairly constant rate and its concentration is reliably linked to GFR. However, this test is not widely used to measure renal function because it requires an expensive immunoassay. Furthermore, in haematological malignancies and inflammatory conditions, β_2-microglobulin production is increased. Radioactively labelled DTPA provides a very accurate measure of GFR and is used to test whether GFR is normal in those with proteinuria or haematuria (eg for prognosis and insurance purposes). It is also used sequentially in transplant patients and those who have undergone surgical procedures. The disadvantages of this test are that it requires the administration of a radioisotope and it is unreliable at low GFR because extrarenal excretion becomes increasingly important.

Q16. RENAL STONES (☆☆)

1. E   2. A   3. F   4. C   5. D

Calcium oxalate stones are the commonest type of renal stones in men in the United Kingdom. Risk factors for their formation include hyperparathyroidism, hereditary hyperoxaluria, high dietary intake of oxalates (contained in rhubarb, spinach and tea), dehydration and idiopathic hypercalciuria. Calcium oxalate stones will often form around a small core of uric acid or calcium phosphate. Calcium oxalate stones have a spiky appearance and are often discoloured by altered blood. Magnesium ammonium phosphate stones are the commonest type of renal stones in women in the United Kingdom. These stones are associated with recurrent urinary tract infections, which explains why they are more common in women. Calcium phosphate calculi are also a common form of renal stones. These stones are smoother and larger than oxalate stones and are more friable. It is also common to have stones that are a mixture of calcium phosphate and oxalate. Uric acid stones are associated with gout and hyperuricaemia. Uric acid is the commonest cause of radiolucent renal stones. Acidic urine is a risk factor for their development (eg in patients losing alkaline fluid from nephrostomies or chronic diarrhoea). Cystine stones are common in patients with cystinuria, the commonest inherited amino-aciduria. Cystine stones are radiolucent and are pale yellow in appearance. Xanthine stones are a rare complication of treatment with allopurinol, a xanthine oxidase inhibitor. These radiolucent stones also occur in patients with hereditary xanthinuria, where there is deficiency of the enzyme xanthine dehydrogenase.

Q17. RENAL TOXICITY (☆☆☆)

1. D   2. C   3. B   4. F   5. A

Fanconi syndrome, distal renal tubular acidosis, nephrogenic diabetes insipidus and acute tubular necrosis usually occur as a result of dose-related renal toxicity. Acute interstitial nephritis is usually due to an allergic reaction and membranous nephropathy is mediated by immune complex deposition. Causes of Fanconi syndrome (glycosuria, phosphaturia, amino-aciduria and the proximal type of renal tubular acidosis) include acute lead poisoning and toxicity due to other heavy metals (eg cadmium). The distal type of renal tubular acidosis is a common complication of the

antifungal agent amphotericin B. The risk of this can be reduced by prehydration with normal saline before starting the infusion. Electrolytes and renal function must be monitored carefully during treatment with this drug. There is also a risk of acute tubular necrosis. Nephrogenic diabetes insipidus is a common complication of treatment with lithium. It may also be caused by fluoride and demeclocycline. Severe lithium poisoning may also result in acute tubular necrosis. This condition is also caused by aminoglycoside antibiotics, mercury poisoning, chronic lead poisoning, bismuth, thallium and ciclosporin. Acute interstitial nephritis is commonly caused by the penicillins. It was particularly common with methicillin, which is no longer available for clinical use. Diuretics, phenytoin, allopurinol and non-steroidal anti-inflammatory drugs also cause acute interstitial nephritis. There is often an accompanying rash, eosinophilia and raised circulating immunoglobulin E concentration. Immune-complex-mediated membranous nephropathy can be caused by penicillamine, gold and snake venom.

Q18. DRUG CHARACTERISTICS (☆☆)

1. F   2. A   3. D   4. C   5. B

Aspirin and other salicylates are organic acids that have increased excretion in alkaline urine. This is the basis for the use of forced alkaline diuresis in severe salicylate poisoning. Other inorganic acids are penicillins, cephalosporins, sulphonamides, fruosemide, thiazides, salicylates and probenecid. Vancomycin and the aminoglycosides are antibiotics that show marked potential for nephrotoxicity if given at too high a dose. Vancomycin is not significantly excreted by haemodialysis and may need very infrequent dosing in patients receiving renal replacement therapy. Usually a repeat dose is not given until trough levels have been checked and shown to be below 10 mg/l. Gentamicin and other aminoglycosides are excreted by haemodialysis. It is usually necessary to increase the dose for a given creatinine clearance by 50% when haemodialysis is performed and to give the dose after dialysis. Lithium is handled like a sodium ion by the kidney. Therefore, in hyponatraemia when the kidney is maximally reabsorbing sodium, lithium reabsorption is also increased. Tetracycline is excreted by the kidney and is antianabolic. In renal failure tetracycline may accumulate and cause worsening of uraemia because of its antianabolic effects. Quinine is excreted by the liver. It is not usually necessary to adjust the dose of quinine for treating malaria in renal failure unless the patient is completely anuric.

Q19. DISORDERS OF THYROID FUNCTION (☆☆)

1. F   2. C   3. A   4. B   5. D

Hashimoto's thyroiditis is an autoimmune disease that causes hypothyroidism and a goitre, which is usually though not invariably painless. On histology lymphocytic infiltration of the gland is seen. Although autoantibodies to thyroglobulin and thyroid peroxidase are found in the blood, they are not generally believed to be responsible for the disease. The other common cause of autoimmune thyroiditis is called atrophic thyroiditis. A goitre is not seen in this condition. Riedel's thyroiditis is an uncommon cause of hypothyroidism in which the thyroid feels very hard on palpation. Histology shows extensive fibrosis, which may also involve adjacent structures. There is an association with fibrosis in distant sites, eg retroperitoneal fibrosis. Although autoimmune diseases are the commonest cause of hypothyroidism in the UK, in many countries the principal cause is iodine deficiency. Graves' disease is the commonest cause of hyperthyroidism. Autoantibodies to the thyroid-stimulating hormone (TSH) receptor stimulate the thyroid to produce excess thyroid hormones and the gland becomes diffusely enlarged. The gland can be shown to be overactive with a radioiodine uptake scan. Patients may also develop thyroid eye disease and less commonly pretibial myxoedema. De Quervain's thyroiditis

is painful inflammation of the gland due to a viral infection. Mononuclear cells infiltrate and damage thyroid follicles causing release of thyroid hormones and temporary hyperthyroidism. This disease can be differentiated from autoimmune thyroiditis by the absence of TSH receptor antibodies and low uptake of radioactive iodine. In De Quervain's thyroiditis, hyperthyroidism may progress to hypothyroidism and eventual recovery.
A struma ovarii is a teratoma containing thyroid tissue, which secretes thyroid hormone. This is a rare cause of hyperthyroidism. Choriocarcinoma is a trophoblastic tissue that may cause hyperthyroidism because it produces excessive quantities of β-human chorionic gonadotrophin, which results in thyroid stimulation.

Q20. THYROID CANCER (☆☆)

1. D   2. C   3. F   4. A   5. E

Papillary carcinoma is the commonest type of thyroid cancer accounting for up to 75% of cases. It is associated with a previous history of exposure to radiation and usually occurs in young adults. There may be a solitary nodule or it may be multifocal and sometimes involves the whole of the thyroid gland. The treatment is with surgical lobectomy and preservation of the remaining thyroid tissue. If the patient develops metastases, these can be treated with radioactive iodine. The prognosis is excellent with over 95% survival. Follicular carcinoma is the second most common thyroid cancer and generally occurs in older patients than the papillary type. It is not multifocal but 20% will have metastases (usually in lung or bone) at the time of presentation. As the disease is more aggressive than papillary carcinoma treatment requires a total thyroidectomy and iodine-131 ablation of any thyroid remnant tissue (detected by a postoperative radioiodine uptake scan). For patients with metastases the five-year survival is around 40%. Anaplastic carcinoma is a poorly differentiated tumour that grows rapidly to invade local structures (eg trachea) and produce early metastases. It occurs in the elderly and has a median survival of only six months. Medullary carcinoma is a rare cancer that arises from the parafollicular or C cells. It secretes calcitonin and this is useful in making the diagnosis. Occasionally it arises as part of the multiple endocrine neoplasia syndrome (type 2). Lymphoma is an uncommon cause of thyroid malignancy. It can usually be treated with external radiotherapy alone but if there is mediastinal extension, chemotherapy is also administered. A Hürthle cell carcinoma is a form of follicular carcinoma that does not take up radioiodine. The survival is poorer than for follicular carcinoma with only a 20% five-year survival.

Q21. DISORDERS OF CALCIUM METABOLISM (☆☆☆)

1. D   2. A   3. E   4. F   5. C

Hyperparathyroidism is defined as an excess of circulating parathyroid hormone. Primary hyperparathyroidism is usually due to an autonomously functioning parathyroid adenoma of chief cell origin. In a small number of cases there are multiple adenomas or hyperplasia of the clear cells or chief cells. The serum calcium is high and the parathyroid hormone level is inappropriately high for the calcium level (ie it could be within the normal range). Treatment of primary hyperparathyroidism is surgical. Secondary hyperparathyroidism is parathyroid hyperplasia in response to hypocalcaemia (eg due to vitamin D deficiency or chronic renal failure). The parathyroid hormone level is high but is appropriate for the serum calcium level. All four parathyroid glands are usually enlarged. Treatment is management of the underlying disorder and correction of hypocalcaemia. The circulating parathyroid hormone levels then fall rapidly, but it may take several months for parathyroid gland hyperplasia to regress. If hypocalcaemia is present for a long time, prolonged stimulation of the parathyroid glands may eventually lead to autonomous functioning. The raised circulating parathyroid hormone may then produce hypercalcaemia. The commonest

cause of this is renal transplantation. Treatment involves both management of the underlying cause and surgical removal of the hypertrophied parathyroid glands. Pseudohyperparathyroidism is production of a parathyroid-like hormone by a small cell lung cancer or other tumour. Primary hypoparathyroidism is due to autoimmune destruction of the parathyroid glands. It is associated with Addison's disease, pernicious anaemia and the presence of anti-prathyroid antibodies. There is low serum calcium and low or undetectable circulating parathyroid hormone. Hypoparathyroidism can also be secondary to surgery or to failure of embryological development. Pseudohypoparathyroidism is a familial condition where there is peripheral resistance to the effects of parathyroid hormone. Serum calcium is low but circulating levels of parathyroid hormone are usually normal. Affected patients are usually of short stature, have a short neck and short metacarpals and metatarsals (often fourth and fifth only but sometimes all are affected).

Q22. ENDOCRINE DISORDERS (☆☆)

1. F   2. A   3. E   4. B   5. D

The features of Cushing's disease include weight gain due to central fat deposition, a plethoric moon-shaped face, muscle wasting, buffalo hump, menstrual irregularity, acne, cutaneous striae and easy bruising. Although ectopic ACTH syndrome might be expected to exhibit similar clinical features, patients are more likely to have weight loss than weight gain because of the underlying hormone-secreting carcinoma. The excess ACTH results in hyperpigmentation, which affects the sun-exposed areas, old scars, the axillae, the nipples, pressure points, the palmar creases and the mucosal membranes. Excess ACTH syndrome may be mistaken for Addison's disease, which also causes weight loss, fatigue and hyperpigmentation. However, patients with ectopic ACTH syndrome usually have hypokalaemic alkalosis secondary to excess mineralocorticoid production. They may also have glucose intolerance due to corticosteroid excess. In contrast, patients with Addison's disease have hyperkalaemia. ACTH deficiency results in secondary hypoaldosteronism. This causes the weight loss and fatigue seen in Addison's disease but without the hyperpigmentation. The patient will usually have deficiencies of other pituitary hormones and this produces accompanying symptoms such as hypoglycaemia and amenorrhoea. Conn's syndrome is excess mineralocorticoid production from an adrenal adenoma. This causes hypertension, hypokalaemia and alkalosis. Many patients do not complain of any symptoms but some will have muscle weakness and/or polyuria due to nephrogenic diabetes insipidus. Chinese patients may suffer from attacks of periodic paralysis in this condition. Hyporeninaemic hypoaldosteronism occurs predominantly in the elderly. Hyperkalaemic alkalosis occurs and this may lead to recurrent cardiac arrhythmias.

Q23. CONGENITAL PROBLEMS (☆)

1. B   2. F   3. A   4. D   5. C

Oesophageal atresia is often associated with the presence of a tracheo-oesophageal fistula and a history of polyhydramnios. The newborn infant presents with copious frothy saliva that cannot be swallowed. Unless this is suctioned frequently inhalation leads to choking, dyspnoea and cyanosis. A plain abdominal X-ray will reveal a complete absence of gas in the gastrointestinal tract unless a tracheo-oesophageal fistula is also present. Gastroschisis is a full-thickness defect in the abdominal wall adjacent to the umbilicus. The gastrointestinal tract herniates through this but other organs are rarely involved. In exomphalos the herniation is through the umbilical ring into the umbilical cord. Viscera other than the gut may be involved. Congenital pyloric stenosis presents between three and six weeks of age with projectile vomiting of milk feeds. The baby is alert and hungry, enabling distinction from a child vomiting due to systemic illness. The cause of pyloric stenosis is hypertrophy of the circular muscle of the

pylorus. Meckel's diverticulum is a vestigial remnant of the vitellointestinal duct. When this is lined with ectopic gastric mucosa it may produce ulceration of the adjacent small bowel and the consequent passage of bright red blood per rectum. Less commonly it may present with acute diverticulitis or obstruction caused by volvulus or intussusception. Diagnosis can be confirmed by a technetium-99m scan, which is taken up by the ectopic gastric mucosa. Meconium ileus is a feature of cystic fibrosis. It produces intestinal obstruction within 48 hours of birth. The infant presents with bile-stained vomiting, abdominal distension and failure to pass meconium. Hirschsprung's disease may present in the same way but the conditions can be distinguished by barium enema. In meconium ileus, the colon is small because of atrophy, whereas in Hirschsprung's the proximal colon is dilated.

Q24. GASTROINTESTINAL DISORDERS (☆☆)

1. B   2. A   3. C   4. F   5. E

Functional bowel disorders are frequent complaints. It is vital to perform a careful history and examination to enable discrimination from serious pathology and decide on whether further investigations are indicated. The Rome criteria define five types of functional bowel complaint: irritable bowel syndrome, functional constipation, functional abdominal bloating, functional diarrhoea and functional abdominal pain. Irritable bowel syndrome is defined as a greater than three-month history of abdominal pain relieved by defaecation associated with at least two of: altered stool frequency, altered stool consistency, altered ease of defaecation, passage of mucus or sensation of abdominal bloating. Functional constipation is defined as a greater than three-month history of two or more of: straining at defaecation on at least one in four occasions, passing lumpy or hard stools on at least one in four occasions, sensation of incomplete evacuation or passage of two or fewer stools per week. Prolonged laxative abuse can also cause constipation. The diagnosis is suggested by the finding of pigmented rectal mucosa on sigmoidoscopy (called melanosis coli). Recent change of bowel habit (constipation or diarrhoea), passage of blood per rectum and/or weight loss should make one suspicious of serious pathology. Rectal carcinoma frequently causes the passage of blood mixed in with the stool. Blood that is found only on the toilet paper is suggestive of anal conditions such as haemorrhoids. If a barium enema is normal the cause of bleeding per rectum may be angiodysplasia. This may be detected by colonoscopy but on occasions angiography is required to find the source of bleeding. Diverticular disease is often blamed as a cause of rectal bleeding. Although it may present with a single episode of bleeding it does not usually cause regular passage of blood.

Q25. VIRAL HEPATITIS (☆☆)

1. C   2. A   3. D   4. B   5. E

Hepatitis A virus is an enterally transmitted picornavirus. It usually causes mild infection and the case fatality rate is very low. Hepatitis A infection does not lead to chronic disease. Hepatitis B virus is transmitted by body fluids, needles, blood transfusions, etc. It is a hepadnavirus and it often causes severe acute hepatitis. When acquired as an adult fewer than 5% of those infected become chronic carriers. However, if infected at birth there is a greater than 90% probability of becoming a chronic carrier. Hepatitis C virus is a parenterally transmitted flavivirus. It rarely causes jaundice during acute infection but it does cause transaminitis. The majority of those infected become chronic carriers. Hepatitis D virus requires hepatitis B envelope proteins in order to replicate and infect other cells. This parenterally transmitted RNA virus may be acquired at the same time as hepatitis B infection (produces low carriage rate) or later (produces high carriage rate). Chronic infection with hepatitis B virus (and hepatitis D virus co-infection) or hepatitis C virus can lead to the development of cirrhosis and hepatocellular

carcinoma. Hepatitis E virus is an enterally transmitted calicivirus. This virus often causes acute jaundice and in pregnancy it has a high mortality. Cytomegalovirus is a common cause of hepatitis in the immunocompromised. This herpes virus causes a glandular-fever-like illness in the general population. It lies dormant in the body and can reactivate many years later if severe immunosuppression occurs.

Q26. INFECTIONS (☆☆)

1. E   2. A   3. F   4. B   5. D

Enterotoxigenic *Escherichia coli* (ETEC) is the commonest cause of diarrhoea in travellers to tropical countries, accounting for approximately 50% of cases. ETEC produces watery diarrhoea because it produces heat-labile and heat-stable enterotoxins that promote active secretion of water into the intestinal lumen. The heat-labile enterotoxin is similar to that of *Vibrio cholerae*. *E. coli* O157:H7 causes haemorrhagic colitis which is sometimes complicated by haemolytic uraemic syndrome. Food-borne outbreaks of this organism have received widespread publicity but it is probably more commonly acquired by contact with animals. *Cryptosporidium parvum* is a coccidian protozoon that produces spores resistant to some water treatment processes. It is therefore intermittently found in domestic water supplies and has caused several water-borne outbreaks of gastroenteritis. In healthy people it causes transient diarrhoea but in the immunocompromised it causes severe prolonged diarrhoea and substantial weight loss. Unfortunately there is no treatment that can effectively cure cryptosporidiosis. It is because of this organism that the UK Government advises all immunocompromised people to boil their drinking water. *Clostridium difficile* is a major cause of diarrhoea in patients taking broad-spectrum antibiotics. Epidemic spread of this bacterium may occur among hospital patients and the residents of institutions. *Clostridium difficile* causes pseudomembranous colitis due to the production of an enterotoxin. *Clostridium perfringens* also causes diarrhoea because of enterotoxin production. In Papua New Guinea, *C. perfringens* infection causes necrotising enterocolitis among children who have been fed undercooked pork. This frequently fatal condition is known as 'pig bel'. *Campylobacter jejuni* is a common cause of gastroenteritis in the UK. Recovery may be complicated by the development of autoimmune conditions such as Guillain-Barré or Reiter's syndrome.

Q27. NEUROLOGICAL FINDINGS (☆☆)

1. E   2. B   3. F   4. C   5. D

Subacute combined degeneration of the cord is caused by vitamin B_{12} deficiency. The commonest underlying cause is pernicious anaemia, which usually presents in middle-aged or elderly adults. Typical features include peripheral paraesthesia (often unpleasant), loss of proprioception (Romberg's test is positive), absent ankle deep tendon reflexes and extensor plantar responses. Syringomyelia presents in young adults who usually have an underlying Arnold-Chiari malformation (herniation of the cerebellar tonsils). The onset of symptoms is insidious with initial involvement of the upper limbs. There is a dissociated sensory loss with marked loss of pain and temperature sensation but preservation of fine touch and proprioception. This may lead to painless burns and Charcot's arthropathy. The wasting affects muscles supplied by multiple nerves and different nerve roots. In transverse myelitis there is a painless acute onset of paraplegia and sensory loss below the affected dermatomal level. There may also be accompanying bowel and bladder sphincter involvement. Causes include inflammation following viral infections and multiple sclerosis. The classic triad of Guillain-Barré syndrome is back pain, peripheral paraesthesia and a lower motor neurone facial palsy (unilateral or bilateral). An ascending paralysis occurs which can lead to respiratory muscle paralysis and the need for mechanical ventilation. Botulism is caused by a toxin which blocks acetylcholine release at the neuromuscular junction, autonomic ganglia and parasympathetic nerve terminals. The

diagnosis is easily missed or mistaken for Guillain-Barré syndrome, myasthenia gravis or other cause of paralysis. In botulism there is invariably cranial nerve involvement and the paralysis is a descending one. There are no sensory symptoms or signs and the patient has a clear sensorium. Extrinsic compression of the cervical spinal cord initially causes painful paraesthesia in the ipsilateral arm followed by muscle weakness initially affecting the ipsilateral arm, then the ipsilateral leg, then the contralateral leg and finally the contralateral arm. There may be sparing of sacral sensation but this sign is not diagnostic.

Q28. NARCOLEPSY (☆☆☆)

1. F   2. A   3. D   4. C   5. E

Narcolepsy is a bizarre disorder characterised by sleep attacks, cataplexy, sleep paralysis, hypnagogic hallucinations and automatic behaviours. Nocturnal hypersomnia (excessive total duration of sleeping) is not a feature of narcolepsy. Sleep attacks are the commonest presenting symptom. The patient may suddenly drop off to sleep in unexpected situations such as the middle of a conversation or during a meal. There is loss of consciousness and failure to recall the event. The patient will usually awake within ten to 30 minutes. Cataplexy is an abrupt reversible paralysis precipitated by emotional events. The patient may collapse to the ground but consciousness and recollection of the event are preserved. The attack usually only lasts a few seconds but it may occur many times each day. Sleep paralysis is a total inability to perform voluntary movements (including speech and even opening eyes), despite being awake and aware of surroundings. The attacks can be very frightening and the sufferer may be convinced he/she is dying. They sometimes occur on falling asleep and usually last less than ten minutes. Hypnagogic hallucinations also occur on falling asleep and may accompany sleep attacks. They are usually visual and are perceived as real images by the sufferer. Hypnopompic hallucinations occur on awakening and are common in those who do not have narcolepsy. Automatic behaviours are fugue-like states where the patient is awake and able to perform basic tasks and answer simple questions. However, the patient will not be able to answer questions requiring careful consideration and may give bizarre or illogical answers. This phenomenon is reminiscent of sleepwalking and the patient usually has amnesia for the event.

Q29. GLASGOW COMA SCALE (☆)

1. D   2. F   3. C   4. E   5. A

The Glasgow coma scale of Jeanett and Teasdale is a reliable method for monitoring changes in conscious level. The maximum 15 points are awarded for eye opening, best verbal response and best motor response as follows:

Eye opening:

Eyes open spontaneously	4
Eyes open to speech	3
Eyes open to painful stimulus	2
Eyes remain closed	1

Best verbal response (after painful stimulus if needed)

Orientated in time and place	5
Confused but speech is intelligible	4
Makes inappropriate but recognisable words	3
Makes incomprehensible sounds	2
Makes no verbal response	1

Best motor response

Obeys commands	6
Localizes to pain (eg moves arm towards pressure on sternum)	5

If above fails exert pressure on nail bed and assess response:

Withdrawal reaction	4
Flexion without withdrawal	3
Extension	2
No response	1

Note that even no response elicits one point and the minimum total score is therefore three not zero.

Q30. DEMENTIA (☆☆)

1. C   2. F   3. E   4. A   5. B

Dementia is global impairment of cognitive function. Alzheimer's disease is the commonest form, accounting for around 50–70% of cases. Alzheimer's disease is associated with inheritance of the apolipoprotein E_4 allele. Histopathology demonstrates neurofibrillary tangles and plaques containing a core of amyloid protein and aluminium silicate deposits. Sufferers develop memory impairment, loss of word-finding ability, comprehension difficulties, visuospatial difficulties and loss of insight into their problem. Pick's disease is focal lobar atrophy usually affecting the frontal lobe. Cerebral computed tomography or magnetic resonance imaging reveals that atrophy is restricted to one lobe with preservation of the rest of the brain tissue. Histology may demonstrate Pick bodies (argyrophilic intracytoplasmic inclusions) and Pick cells (diffusely staining ballooned neurones) but these are not invariably present. The peak age of onset (45 to 60 years) is younger than for Alzheimer's. Patients develop changes in personality, behaviour and social functioning and there is progressive reduction in speech. In contrast to patients with Alzheimer's, patients with Pick's disease may perform well on mini-mental state examination. Multi-infarct dementia produces a characteristic stepwise deterioration in function. There may be focal neurological symptoms or signs due to previous strokes and the patient may have hypertension or vascular bruits. Creutzfeldt-Jakob disease (CJD) is a spongiform encephalopathy due to the accumulation of abnormal prion protein. The usual onset is aged 45 to 75 years but the hereditary and iatrogenic (from human growth hormone treatment) forms may present much earlier, as may new variant CJD. The condition progresses rapidly and death may occur within two to three months. Patients develop dementia, myoclonus, extrapyramidal signs and ataxia. In Lewy body disease there are intraneuronal inclusions widely distributed throughout the cortical and subcortical structures. There is a combination of dementia and Parkinson's disease. These patients are at marked risk of severe extrapyramidal reactions if given antipsychotics even at low doses. Wilson's disease (hepatolenticular degeneration) is due to widespread copper deposition because of caeruloplasmin deficiency. An akinetic-rigid syndrome and cirrhosis usually develop in childhood.

Q31. ATYPICAL PNEUMONIA (☆☆)

1. E   2. A   3. B   4. F   5. C

Chlamydia psittaci causes malaise, lethargy, arthralgia and bronchopneumonia. Diagnosis is by serology. This organism is acquired from infected parrots, poultry and pigeons. It should not be confused with pigeon-fancier's lung, which is a form of extrinsic allergic alveolitis. *Chlamydia pneumoniae* is spread from person to person and may be a much commoner cause of pneumonia than has previously been realised. The serology is non-specific and this has hampered epidemiological studies. Infected patients develop pharyngitis, a hoarse voice, otitis and pneumonia. *Mycoplasma pneumoniae* is also spread from person to person and causes epidemics approximately every four years. The diagnosis is suggested by the presence of cold agglutinins in a patient with bronchopneumonia. A rise in specific antibody titre is diagnostic but this can only be used to make a retrospective diagnosis. Patients may develop immune reactions such as erythema multiforme, erythema nodosum, haemolytic crises or Guillain-Barré syndrome. In rare cases severe meningoencephalitis occurs. *Legionella pneumophila* multiplies in warm still water as occurs in air-conditioning systems. Patients often give a recent history of staying in a hotel in a warm climate. Infection usually occurs by aerosol inhalation but some hospital-acquired cases have been caused by aspiration. Patients with *Legionella* infection may develop a severe pneumonia and mortality is high. Diagnosis is by culture or serology but the latter is often negative early in the disease course. Rapid

diagnosis can be made by specific antigen detection from urine. However, this test only detects serogroup I (the commonest) and therefore a negative test does not exclude the diagnosis. *Pneumocystis carinii* is the commonest AIDS-defining illness in the developed world. Diagnosis is by silver-staining or immunofluorescence of bronchoalveolar lavage fluid or sputum induced by hypertonic saline. *Coxiella burnetii* is the cause of Q fever. This disease usually occurs in those with contact with farm animals (eg farmers and abattoir workers). It may present as a pyrexia of unknown origin or an atypical pneumonia. Diagnosis is by serology. Phase I antigens indicate previous infection and phase II antigens indicate acute disease.

Q32. LUNG TUMOURS (☆☆)

1. E   2. A   3. C   4. F   5. B

Squamous cell carcinoma is the commonest histological type of bronchial malignancy accounting for 35% of total cases. It is composed of flattened, stratified neoplastic cells which produce keratin. It often presents as an obstructive lesion with a distal pneumonia or lung abscess. Adenocarcinoma is composed of granular or acinar structures and may be mucus-producing. It is often located peripherally and may present as a pleural effusion. It accounts for around 21% of cases of lung cancer and it shows the least association with tobacco smoking. Large cell carcinoma is a highly malignant tumour, which shows little or no evidence of differentiation. Surgery may be effective if the disease is diagnosed early but radiotherapy is of little benefit. Large cell carcinoma makes up around 19% of total bronchial carcinomas. Small cell (also known as oat cell) carcinoma consists of highly malignant cells with dark nuclei and scanty cytoplasm. It metastasises early and often presents with advanced disease. In approximately 10% of cases secretion of hormones such as antidiuretic hormone, adrenocorticotrophic hormone or parathyroid-related hormone occurs. This tumour accounts for approximately 24% of lung cancers and it may respond to chemotherapy. Carcinoid tumour is a slow-growing tumour that arises from APUD cells (amine precursor uptake and decarboxylation). The majority of these tumours arise in the gastrointestinal tract but 10% occur in the lung. Secretion of serotonin ($5HT_1$) causes acute episodes of facial flushing, tachycardia and hypertension. Mesothelioma is a malignancy arising from the pleura.

Q33. CHEST X-RAYS (☆)

1. C   2. A   3. E   4. F   5. B

The posteroanterior (PA) film is the standard view for a patient who is able to stand upright. The film is placed in front of the chest and the arms should be abducted to rotate the scapulae out of the way. This view provides the maximal information on the lung fields but one-third of the lungs are still partially obscured by the mediastinum, diaphragm or ribs. The anteroposterior (AP) film is used in place of the PA film if the patient is unable to stand upright. The film is placed behind the sitting (or supine) patient and the X-rays traverse the chest from front to back. As there is lung between the heart and the film in this view, the apparent heart size is magnified. The AP film is therefore less useful than the PA film for accurately assessing the size of the heart. The lateral film is used to complement the standard PA view. This projection enables abnormalities that are hidden behind the heart on the PA film to be seen. It also enables the position of abnormalities seen on the PA film to be determined. The lateral decubitus film is taken with the patient lying on the side of interest. The X-ray beam traverses the patient horizontally from anterior to posterior. This enables detection of small pleural effusions, which are not clearly seen on the PA film. Fluoroscopy allows real-time imaging of the patient throughout the respiratory cycle. Diaphragmatic movement can be studied, enabling the diagnosis of diaphragmatic palsy to be confirmed. It is also used to detect air-trapping in children who are suspected of having inhaled a foreign body. Apical views provide clearer images of the lung apices than the standard PA film. In modern practice these views have largely been replaced by computed tomography which provides better quality images. However, in resource-poor countries apical views are still widely used particularly in the investigation of suspected tuberculosis.

Q34. COLLAGEN VASCULAR DISEASE (☆☆☆)

1. E   2. A   3. B   4. F   5. D

The respiratory complications that occur in rheumatoid arthritis include cricoarytenoid arthritis, pleural disease, necrobiotic nodules, Caplan's syndrome (usually associated with pneumoconiosis), fibrosing alveolitis and bronchiolitis obliterans with or without organising pneumonia. Alveolar haemorrhage complicates systemic lupus erythematosus (SLE) more often than other connective tissue disease. Alveolar haemorrhage also commonly occurs in Goodpasture's syndrome and Wegener's granulomatosis. SLE is also associated with pleuritis and pleural effusion, shrinking lung syndrome (loss of lung volume of uncertain aetiology), opportunistic infections and lupus pneumonitis. Pulmonary embolism may occur in the variant of lupus known as antiphospholipid syndrome. Systemic sclerosis frequently causes oesophageal dysmotility leading to recurrent aspiration pneumonia. Other complications include pulmonary hypertension, pleuritis, pneumothorax and occasionally pulmonary haemorrhage. Adult-onset dermatomyositis is associated with underlying malignancy including bronchial carcinoma. It is also associated with chronic hypoventilation, aspiration pneumonia and fibrosing alveolitis. Ankylosing spondylitis is associated with upper zone fibrosis and cavitation. This may become complicated by infection with *Aspergillus* species or non-tuberculous mycobacteria. Sjögren's syndrome produces drying of secretions which may lead to a persistent dry cough. Affected patients may also develop interstitial lymphocytic pneumonitis and lymphoma.

Q35. INFECTIOUS AETIOLOGY OF RHEUMATIC DISEASE (☆☆)

1. D   2. A   3. F   4. B   5. C

Lyme disease is caused by the spirochaete *Borrelia burgdorferi*. This infection is acquired from the bite of an infected ixodid tick (*Ixodes ricinus* in Europe). The characteristic rash of erythema chronicum migrans may be followed by acute arthritis. Recurrent attacks of arthritis may then occur. Parvovirus B19 is the cause of erythema infectiosum (fifth disease). This acute febrile illness is often accompanied by marked facial erythema, which has resulted in the disease being nicknamed 'slapped cheek syndrome'. A symmetrical polyarthropathy affecting the small joints of the hands and feet is a common occurrence. *Sporothrix schenckii* is a fungus that can cause a cutaneous infection following skin penetration by a rose thorn or other plant. In some cases local lymphangitis occurs followed by inflammation of the large joints. Strict aseptic technique is required when injecting steroids into painful joints to avoid introducing infections. Worsening arthritis due to atypical mycobacterial infection is a not uncommon complication of intra-articular steroid injections. *Staphylococcus aureus* is the commonest cause of monoarticular septic arthritis in most age groups. This organism is blood-borne and most easily infects joints that are already damaged. When a patient with rheumatoid arthritis develops an acutely swollen joint the possibility of bacterial infection should always be considered. Gonococcal arthritis is a common cause of septic arthritis in previously healthy, sexually active young adults.

Q36. AUTOANTIBODIES AND CONNECTIVE TISSUE DISEASE/VASCULITIDES (☆☆☆)

1. F   2. B   3. E   4. C   5. D

The connective tissue diseases are often associated with particular autoantibodies. However, several autoantibodies are not specific to a single disease and history and examination should be used to establish a diagnosis rather than relying on the autoantibody tests alone. There are also many patients with overlap syndromes that do not easily fit into the definition of a single connective tissue disease. Systemic lupus erythematosus (SLE) is a multisystem disorder affecting the skin, joints, kidneys, brain, heart and lungs. Antibodies are produced to double-stranded DNA (highly specific) and extractable nuclear antigen phospholipids. These antinuclear antibodies show a rim or homogeneous staining pattern in SLE. Polymyositis and dermatomyositis predominantly affect muscle and skin. Anti-Jo1 antibodies are characteristically found in these conditions. Anti-Scl-70 and anticentromere antibodies are typical of scleroderma, which predominantly affects skin, the smooth muscle of the gut and the lungs. There is a nucleolar pattern of staining for antinuclear antibodies. Sjögren's syndrome shows a speckled pattern of antinuclear antibody, as does mixed connective tissue disease. Anti-Ro and anti-La antibodies are typically found in Sjögren's syndrome, which is a disease affecting the exocrine glands. Salivary and lacrimal glands are particularly affected, producing dry eyes and a dry mouth. pANCA is not specific to Churg-Strauss syndrome and is also positive in other vasculitides including microscopic polyangiitis, Henoch-Schönlein purpura and vasculitis associated with rheumatoid arthritis.

Q37. PHOTODERMATOSES (☆☆☆)

1. E   2. C   3. B   4. D   5. A

Polymorphic light eruption is generally a mild reaction to ultraviolet (UV) A and/or B. Pruritic papules, vesicles or other morphological variants occur within a few hours of sunlight exposure. This reaction is very common and may affect 10–20% of the population. Actinic prurigo is an uncommon disease that usually begins in the first decade of life. Persistent and pruritic papules and nodules develop and the eruption may be severe. Actinic reticuloid syndrome is a variant of photosensitive dermatitis that occurs most commonly in elderly males. This pseudolymphomatous state may require treatment with azathioprine or ciclosporin. Solar urticaria is a UV-A-induced type I hypersensitivity reaction which can often be suppressed with antihistamines. In severe cases systemic symptoms, including anaphylactic shock, may occur. Xeroderma pigmentosum is a group of inherited defects of DNA repair enzymes. Patients develop delayed-onset, persistent sunburn and have a high risk of developing skin tumours. Hydroa vaccineforme is a sunlight-induced, blistering reaction that occurs in children.

Q38. SKIN TUMOURS (☆☆)

1. A   2. E   3. B   4. D   5. F

Malignant melanoma is the most aggressive form of skin cancer and metastases occur early. It is associated with excessive sunlight exposure, atypical mole syndrome, giant congenital melanocytic naevi and lentigo maligna. Melanomas are clinically differentiated from benign moles by looking for **a**symmetry, **b**order irregularity, **c**olour variation and **d**iameter greater than 6 cm. Basal cell carcinoma is the most common skin tumour. It occurs predominantly in sunlight-exposed sites. The initial nodule ulcerates as it enlarges and it develops a pearly edge with telangiectasia. It is slow growing and locally destructive but does not metastasise. Squamous cell carcinomas are rapidly growing nodules that ulcerate and can metastasise. They are sunlight related and arise in solar keratoses and areas of chronic inflammation. Immunosuppression can result in the development of multiple tumours. Past use of arsenic is now an uncommon predisposing factor. Keratoacanthoma is a rapidly growing epidermal tumour that shows central ulceration. These lesions occur in sunlight-exposed areas. They grow up to 2–3 cm in diameter and then resolve over a few months. They resemble squamous cell carcinomas and are therefore usually excised to exclude this condition. Pyogenic granuloma is a rapidly growing benign proliferation of blood vessels

that arises following local trauma. The appearance is of a pinkish-red nodule that has a tendency to bleed. It is easily confused with an amelanotic malignant melanoma and is usually excised to exclude this. Basal cell papilloma is also known as a seborrhoeic wart. This extremely common benign overgrowth of basal cells can be flesh-coloured, brown or even black. It has a characteristic greasy appearance with tiny keratin cysts on its irregular surface. It is usually clinically distinguishable from potentially malignant tumours and does not require excision.

Q39. ANAEMIA (☆)

1. D   2. E   3. C   4. A   5. F

Iron deficiency is due to iron loss/demands in excess of intake. This can occur with any cause of gastrointestinal blood loss such as occult colon cancer, peptic ulcer or hookworm infection or with menstruation in excess of 100 ml per month. It can also occur with poor diet or increased demands (eg frequent pregnancies). Coeliac disease is a not uncommon cause of iron deficiency (due to malabsorption) and antiendomyseal antibody measurement should be performed for patients without another identifiable cause. B_{12} and folate deficiency cause megaloblastic anaemia. Causes of B_{12} deficiency include pernicious anaemia, vegan diet, gastrectomy, congenital intrinsic factor deficiency and terminal ileal disease. Folate deficiency can be due to poor intake or increased requirements, eg in pregnancy or premature infants, or in association with increased red cell turnover. Folate antagonists such as phenytoin, methotrexate and pyrimethamine can also cause folic acid deficiency. Long-term use of pyrimethamine requires folinic acid supplements. Sideroblastic anaemia can be inherited (X-linked) or secondary to lead poisoning, drugs (eg isoniazid), myelodysplasia, myeloproliferative diseases or alcohol. Aplastic anaemia may be congenital (eg Fanconi syndrome), autoimmune, due to chemicals (eg benzene), drugs (eg cytotoxic chemotherapy), infections (eg parvovirus B19, HIV, tuberculosis) or paroxysmal nocturnal haemoglobinuria. Haemolysis can be due to inherited red cell membrane defects, enzyme deficiency (eg glucose-6-phosphate dehydrogenase) or haemoglobinopathies. It can also be caused by drugs, mechanical trauma (mechanical heart valves), renal or liver failure, malaria, burns or hypersplenism.

Q40. HAEMOGLOBIN (✰✰)

1. F   2. E   3. A   4. B   5. C

Haemoglobin is composed of four globin chains and a haem molecule. In normal adults 92% of haemoglobin is $\alpha_2\beta_2$, known as HbA_1. Glycosylated haemoglobin, known as HbA_{1c} has the formula $\alpha_2\beta_2$-NH-glucose. This constitutes less than 5% of the total haemoglobin in non-diabetic adults. Levels of HbA_{1c} are a reflection of the prevailing blood sugar during the lifespan of red blood cells (up to three months). Levels of HbA_{1c} are elevated in poorly controlled diabetics and this assay is therefore used to monitor the effectiveness of diabetic treatment. However, it is important to realise that HbA_{1c} is reduced if red blood cell survival is decreased and it can then provide falsely reassuring values. $\alpha_2\delta_2$, known as HbA_2, makes up only 2% of haemoglobin in normal adults, but this level is increased in β-thalassaemia. $\alpha_2\gamma_2$, known as HbF, is the predominant haemoglobin found in the fetus but makes up less than 1% of haemoglobin in normal adults. HbF levels are increased in β-thalassaemia. β_4, known as HbH, is found in adults with α-thalassaemia, where the number of β-globin chains produced exceeds that for α-globin. HbH is not capable of carrying oxygen. γ_4, known as HbBarts, is the non-functional haemoglobin found in the fatal condition of α-thalassaemia major. Three other forms of haemoglobin, $\zeta_2\epsilon_2$, $\alpha_2\epsilon_2$ and $\zeta_2\gamma_2$, known respectively as Gower1, Gower2 and Portland, are found in the developing embryo.

Q41. CLOTTING FACTORS (✰✰)

1. A   2. E   3. D   4. F   5. B

The common coagulation pathway includes factors X (Stuart-Prower factor), V (proaccelerin), II (prothrombin), I (fibrinogen) and XIII (fibrin stabilising factor). This pathway can be initiated by the intrinsic or extrinsic pathways, which cause the activation of factor X. Activated factor X, in the presence of factor V, causes the activation of prothrombin to thrombin. This then leads to the conversion of fibrinogen to fibrin monomer, which is stabilised by factor XIII and forms a polymer that traps platelets, producing a blood clot. The intrinsic pathway includes factors XII (Hageman factor), XI (plasma thromboplastin antecedent), IX (Christmas factor or antihaemophilic factor B) and VIII (antihaemophilic factor A). The extrinsic pathway includes tissue factor, calcium ions (sometimes called factor IV), factor III (tissue thromboplastin) and factor VII (proconvertin). Factor III is produced by most tissues and factor VIII is produced by megakaryocytes. The other clotting factors is all produced by the liver but only factors II, VII, IX and X are dependent on vitamin K. Congenital deficiency of clotting factors is well known. The commonest is deficiency of factor VIII called haemophilia A. This X-linked condition can lead to severe haemorrhage, haemarthroses and ecchymoses. The activated partial thromboplastin time (APTT) is prolonged but the bleeding time and prothrombin time (PT) are normal. Haemophilia B is a clinically similar but less common condition due to deficiency of factor IX. Patients with a variant of factor V (called V-Leiden) and those with factor XII deficiency (Hageman trait) have an increased risk of thromboses.

Q42. VIRAL DISEASE (✰✰)

1. B   2. D   3. A   4. C   5. F

Subacute sclerosing panencephalitis is a rare sequela of measles infection, occurring in approximately 1 in 100,000 cases, several years after the initial infection. Progressive multifocal leukoencephalopathy is a demyelinating disease that occurs in HIV patients. JC polyoma virus is a member of the DNA papovaviridae, which is named after a patient and is not related to Creutzfeldt-Jakob. Guillain-Barré syndrome is frequently preceded by infection. The most reliable associations are with cytomegalovirus and *Campylobacter jejuni*. Bell's palsy is a lower motor neurone seventh nerve palsy for which there is no obvious cause. Serological studies suggest it is due to herpes simplex 1 infection and many experts recommend treatment with aciclovir. Bell's palsy may also be caused by *Borrelia burgdorferi*, the agent of Lyme disease. Erythema infectiosum, or fifth disease, is a common childhood infection that presents with a characteristic 'slapped cheek' appearance. The causative virus, parvovirus B19, also causes transient bone marrow suppression which may produce anaemia in those with increased red cell turnover and it causes fetal hydrops in the last trimester of pregnancy. Adenoviruses cause conjunctivitis and respiratory tract infections.

Q43. STREPTOCOCCI (☆☆)

1. E   2. A   3. F   4. B   5. C

Streptococcus milleri is really a group of several related microaerophilic streptococci. They frequently cause abscesses and pulmonary empyema. *S. pneumoniae* is the commonest cause of community-acquired pneumonia and also frequently causes sinusitis and otitis media. Peritonitis is most frequently caused by coliforms but *S. pneumoniae* causes an estimated 15% of non-dialysis-associated primary peritonitis. The natural habitat of *S. mutans* is the teeth. Low pH facilitates its proliferation and the development of dental caries. The gastrointestinal tract is the normal habitat of *S. agalactiae*. However, it can colonise the vagina and cause neonatal infection during parturition. This can result in neonatal meningitis and septicaemia with a very high mortality. *S. pyogenes* causes many infections including acute pharyngitis and cellulitis. Serious immune-complex-related

sequelae include post-streptococcal glomerulonephritis and rheumatic fever. *S. bovis* is a bowel organism that can cause bacteraemia and endocarditis. *S. bovis* and *Enterococcus faecalis* more commonly cause bacteraemia in older people and underlying colonic pathology, eg a carcinoma, should be looked for.

Q44. RISK FACTORS FOR INFECTION (☆☆)

1. E   2. C   3. B   4. D   5. F

Cryptococcus neoformans is a yeast that commonly causes meningitis in patients with advanced AIDS. *Babesia divergens* is a coccidian protozoon that causes the rare European form of babesiosis. This febrile illness is caused by parasitisation of red blood cells and occurs following a tick bite. Approximately 50% of reported cases have occurred in asplenic subjects. Treatment is difficult, involving exchange transfusion, clindamycin and quinine. *Burkholderia pseudomallei* is the cause of melioidosis, a disease frequently seen in diabetics. This soil-borne organism causes local or systemic infections in those who work in agricultural fields in South East Asia. In the septicaemic cases mortality is very high. *Burkholderia cepacia* is a less common cause of pneumonia in cystic fibrosis patients than is *Pseudomonas aeruginosa*. However, this organism is important because it is frequently impossible to eradicate and infection results in a significantly poorer long-term prognosis. *Vibrio cholerae* is killed by gastric acid. In gastric achlorydria a smaller infective dose can establish symptomatic disease. Cirrhosis is an established risk factor for spontaneous bacterial peritonitis and for invasive infection following ingestion of non-cholera vibrios such as *V. vulnificus* (an occasional cause of severe bullous cellulitis).

Q45. BACTERIAL TAXONOMY (☆☆)

1. D   2. A   3. B   4. F   5. E

Bacterial taxonomy appears dull but is important because Gram stain results are usually available 24 hours before culture results. Knowledge of the appearance of bacteria facilitates the most appropriate choice of empirical treatment. *Listeria monocytogenes* can be acquired from ingestion of unpasteurised cheeses and characteristically causes a rhombencephalitis in the immunocompromised. *Acinetobacter baumannii* is a cause of nosocomial infections particularly in those given multiple broad-spectrum antibiotics in intensive care units. It is often highly antibiotic resistant and strains that are only sensitive to polymyxins are not uncommon. *Neisseria gonorrhoea* causes urethritis in males and may cause pelvic inflammatory disease or be asymptomatic in females. Systemic dissemination is not uncommon and may cause arthritis, pustular skin eruptions and peri-hepatitis (Fitz-Hugh-Curtis syndrome, which can also be caused by *Chlamydia trachomatis*). *Bacteroides* species are a major part of the bowel flora. They are opportunistic pathogens and cause disease following colonic ischaemia, perforation or other gastrointestinal pathology. *Nocardia asteroides* is most frequently acquired by inhalation and causes pneumonia usually in the immunocompromised. In 50% of cases the infection metastasises to brain and routine brain imaging is therefore essential. The related species *N. brasiliensis* is a cause of mycetoma. Spirochaetes include *Treponema pallidum*, the cause of syphilis, *Borrelia recurrentis*, the cause of relapsing fever, and *Leptospira icterohaemorrhagiae*, the cause of Weil's disease.

Q46. ANTIMICROBIAL THERAPY IN AIDS (☆☆☆)

1. F   2. A   3. B   4. C   5. E

Cerebral toxoplasmosis causes ring-enhancing lesions that are most often located in the basal ganglia. The standard treatment is pyrimethamine and sulphadiazine, although co-trimoxazole or pyrimethamine and clindamycin can be used as alternatives. If there is no response to empirical treatment within seven to 10 days a brain biopsy is performed. *Cyclospora cayetanensis* is an intestinal protozoon that produces outbreaks of acute watery diarrhoea in the immunocompetent population. Among AIDS patients chronic diarrhoea and severe weight loss can occur. Seven days of co-trimoxazole treatment is given for immunocompetent patients but a more prolonged course is usually required in AIDS. *Cryptococcus neoformans* is a yeast infection that infects the lungs and has a marked tropism for the meninges. *C. neoformans* var. *neoformans* is strongly associated with AIDS but *C. neoformans* var. *gattii* occurs in previously healthy subjects. Combination treatment with amphotericin B and flucytosine is more effective at clearing fungus from CSF than amphotericin B alone. *Babesia microti* is a coccidian parasite acquired following tick bites. In the USA it has been found to be HIV associated, whereas in Europe infection with the related species, *Babesia divergens*, is associated with splenectomy. Quinine plus clindamycin is the treatment of choice for both species. Those infected with *B. divergens* may also require exchange transfusion. Microsporidia are classified with protozoa although they are phylogenetically very different lacking mitochondria, peroxisomes and Golgi apparatus and reproducing by the production of multiple spores. Albendazole is the recommended treatment for both intestinal and extra-intestinal disease. Pentamidine is used for treatment and prophylaxis of *Pneumocystis carinii* pneumonia in people with co-trimoxazole allergy.

Q47. ANTIARRYTHMIC DRUGS (☆☆☆)

1. E   2. D   3. B   4. A   5. F

Class I agents are those which inhibit the rapid sodium current during depolarisation. Class Ia drugs increase the duration of the action potential (eg quinidine), Ib drugs decrease it (eg lignocaine) and Ic drugs do not alter it (eg flecainide). Class II drugs are defined as those that antagonise the effects of arrhythmogenic catecholamines. These drugs are β-blockers (including atenolol) and they act on nodal and non-nodal tissue. Class III agents increase the duration of the action potential and thus the effective refractory period. No pure class III agents exist in current clinical practice. Although amiodarone is sometimes described as a class III agent, it exerts complex class I, II, III and IV activities. Class IV drugs decrease the inward calcium current at the sinoatrial and atrioventricular nodes. Verapamil and diltiazem are class IV drugs. Adenosine and digoxin do not really fit into the Vaughan-Williams classification.

Q48. ANTIFUNGAL AGENTS (☆☆)

1. F   2. A   3. B   4. E   5. C

Amorolfine and terbinafine are allylamine antifungals that are licensed for treatment of skin and nail infections. Amorolfine is available as a cream for application to skin and as a lacquer to apply to nails. Fingernails require 6 months of treatment and toenails require nine to 12 months. Terbinafine is administered orally and can cause severe cholestatic jaundice. Its use should be restricted to microscopically proven infections that fail to respond to other treatments. Amphotericin B is a broad-spectrum polyene antifungal with activity against many yeasts and moulds. It is not absorbed orally and intravenous administration requires slow infusion and premedication with paracetamol and antihistamines because of the high incidence of reactions. It is nephrotoxic but colloid and lipid preparations are also available which cause less renal impairment. The related drug nystatin is too toxic for systemic use. It is not absorbed from the gastrointestinal tract and can be given orally to prevent and treat intestinal candidiasis. Fluconazole and itraconazole are both triazole drugs. Fluconazole is more effective in cryptococcal meningitis but it is not active against *Aspergillus* species. Itraconazole has a broader spectrum of activity, which includes *Aspergillus* and it can also be used against fluconazole-resistant *Candida*.

Q49. ANTIBIOTIC PROPHYLAXIS (☆☆)

1. B   2. F   3. D   4. C   5. A

Suitable antibiotic prophylaxis for a close contact (usually defined as a household or kissing contact) of a patient with meningococcal disease is a single dose of ciprofloxacin 500 mg or rifampicin 600 mg bd for two days. If the contact is pregnant, a single 250 mg dose of intramuscular ceftriaxone is the recommended alternative. Following splenectomy there is a high risk of infection with encapsulated organisms. Patients should be vaccinated against pneumococcus and *Haemophilus influenzae* group B and should receive long-term prophylaxis with phenoxymethylpenicillin 500 mg bd. In patients with valvular heart disease undergoing dental work, amoxicillin is given as it is better absorbed than phenoxymethylpenicillin and provides broader-spectrum cover. Clindamycin is an alternative if patients have received penicillin in the previous month or if penicillin allergic. If the patient is at very high risk because of a past history of endocarditis or has a prosthetic valve, then gentamicin is also given for its synergistic activity. Dental prophylaxis may also be supplemented by use of chlorhexidine mouthwash before the procedure. Hindquarter amputations require five days of prophylaxis with intravenous benzylpenicillin to prevent gas gangrene. Metronidazole is an alternative for those with penicillin allergy. There is no evidence of increased risk of prosthetic joint infection following dental treatment and therefore antibiotic prophylaxis should not be given.

Q50. DRUG SIDE-EFFECTS (☆☆)

1. C   2. E   3. A   4. F   5. B

When giving patients new medications it is important to warn them about common or serious side-effects. For the drugs listed above the *British National Formulary* specifies warnings that should be given to the patient. Following the use of prazosin severe first-dose hypotension may lead to collapse. This can be avoided if the patient takes the first dose at bedtime and lies down if symptoms occur. The patient should be warned to remain lying down until the symptoms have resolved completely. Grapefruit juice inhibits the first-pass metabolism of ciclosporin and can lead to increased serum levels of this drug. Quinolones such as ciprofloxacin can cause tendon damage and patients should stop the drug immediately if symptoms occur. Aminosalicylates such as mesalazine, olsalazine and sulfasalazine are used in induction and maintenance of remission in ulcerative colitis. These drugs occasionally cause serious blood dyscrasias and patients should be warned to seek medical attention if suggestive symptoms develop. High strength pancreatin may cause fibrosing colonopathy leading to large bowel stricture. It is believed that dehydration may be a risk factor for development of this condition. When warnings are given to patients they should preferably also be written down for the patient to refer to later. Patients given rifampicin should be warned that urine, sweat and tears will become stained orange, to avoid causing alarm.

Q51. DRUGS USED TO TREAT MALIGNANCY (☆☆)

1. A   2. E   3. B   4. C   5. D

The oral alkylating agent melphalan is frequently used to treat myeloma and occasionally used for lymphoma and solid tumours. It is given for four to six days and repeated every four to eight weeks after marrow recovery. Kaposi's sarcoma is most frequently seen in HIV patients. Both the HIV- and non-HIV-related types are associated with the presence of human herpesvirus 8. Liposomal daunorubicin is licensed for treatment of advanced HIV-related Kaposi's sarcoma. Interferon α is also used for treatment of this condition. Fludarabine is an antimetabolite that is used in the treatment of B cell chronic

lymphatic leukaemia after failure of first-line therapy. Fludarabine causes marked myelo- and immunosuppression. Carboplatin is a derivative of cisplatin that causes less nephro-, neuro- and ototoxicity, although it is more myelosuppressive. It is used in the treatment of ovarian cancer and small cell cancer of the lung. Hydroxyurea is used orally in the treatment of chronic myeloid leukaemia and occasionally in polycythaemia rubra vera or essential thrombocythaemia. It is also used in 'salvage therapy' for HIV patients with drug-resistant virus. Ciclosporin is a potent immunosuppressive agent used to prevent rejection of organ transplants.

Q52. INFLAMMATORY BOWEL DISEASE (☆☆)

1. D   2. A   3. C   4. F   5. E

Treatment of mild to moderate colitis involves the use of 5-aminosalicylic acid (5-ASA). Sulfasalazine was the first preparation developed for delivery of 5-ASA. It consists of 5-ASA linked to a sulfapyridine molecule. This prevents absorption of 5-ASA by the small intestine. In the colon bacteria break down the conjugate molecule and release the 5-ASA, which exerts a local anti-inflammatory effect. The disadvantage of this preparation is that the sulfapyridine molecule may produce allergic reactions or other side-effects. Other systems have since been developed for delivery of 5-ASA to the colon. Mesalazine is an enteric-coated modified-release preparation and olsalazine is a dimer consisting of two 5-ASA molecules joined together. Oral steroids are used in the treatment of terminal ileitis (in Crohn's disease) and in colitis that does not respond to 5-ASA alone. As steroids have significant systemic side-effects, preparations have been developed to deliver the maximal amount of drug to the site of inflammation. Budesonide is a corticosteroid available in a modified release form that is claimed to have fewer systemic side-effects than oral prednisolone. Long-term use should still be avoided if possible. Patients with distal colitis and proctitis can be treated with prednisolone enemas. Severe colitis usually requires hospital admission for intravenous steroid treatment. Infliximab is a monoclonal antibody to tumour necrosis factor α that is used to treat Crohn's disease when it is not responding to steroids or when there are chronic fistulae. Immune-suppressants such as azathioprine are also used in the maintenance of remission in inflammatory bowel disease.

Q53. HYPERTENSION (☆)

1. C   2. A   3. B   4. E   5. F

There are six main classes of drugs used in the treatment of hypertension. There are also a few other agents that are occasionally used (eg centrally acting agents). β-blockers and thiazide diuretics are cheap and have the most supporting evidence for their effectiveness in terms of reducing morbidity and mortality. These agents should preferably be used first for patients who do not have a compelling indication to use a different class of drug. Thiazide diuretics are highly suitable for those with coexistent heart failure, systolic hypertension or diabetes and for the elderly. They are contraindicated in gout and are probably unsuitable for those with dyslipidaemia and for sexually active males. β-blockers are highly suitable for those with coexistent ischaemic heart disease or tachyarrhythmias. They are contraindicated in asthma and heart block and are probably unsuitable for those with dyslipidaemia or peripheral vascular disease and for highly active patients. Used with caution they may be beneficial for those with coexistent cardiac failure. Angiotensin-converting enzyme (ACE) inhibitors are being increasingly used despite their cost because they are beneficial for those with coexistent cardiac failure or left ventricular dysfunction (on echocardiography), after myocardial infarction and those with diabetic nephropathy. They are contraindicated in pregnancy and for those with hyperkalaemia or bilateral renal artery stenosis. Calcium channel blockers are suitable for the elderly and those with isolated systolic hypertension, angina or

peripheral vascular disease. Diltiazem and verapamil are contraindicated in heart block and should probably be avoided in cardiac failure. α-blockers are useful for those with coexistent prostatic hypertrophy and may also be useful for those with dyslipidaemia or glucose intolerance. They are unsuitable for patients with postural hypotension. Angiotensin II receptor antagonists are relatively new drugs with limited available information. They are generally reserved for those in whom an ACE inhibitor is indicated but who have suffered side-effects with these drugs (eg cough).

Q54. RISK FACTORS FOR CARDIAC CONDITIONS (☆☆)

1. C   2. B   3. F   4. E   5. A

The term cardiomyopathy implies that the cause of the cardiac disease is unknown. When the cause is known to be secondary to a systemic disease the condition is referred to as a specific heart muscle disorder (eg diabetic heart disease). Hypertrophic cardiomyopathy and right ventricular dysplasia are familial conditions with autosomal dominant inheritance. Sporadic cases are also seen perhaps due to incomplete penetrance or new mutations. Hypertrophic cardiomyopathy can be caused by mutations in several different genes including β-cardiac myosin, α-tropomyosin and cardiac troponin T. This condition is a common cause of sudden, unexpected death in young people during exercise. The dilated form is the commonest type of cardiomyopathy. By definition the underlying cause is unknown or uncertain. In many cases it is likely to have been caused by previous viral myocarditis or unidentified excessive alcohol intake. Similar specific heart muscle disorders may be caused by prolonged hypertension, ischaemic heart disease, metabolic disorders (eg diabetes mellitus), infiltrative disorders (eg amyloid), malignancy, drug abuse, vasculitis and neuromuscular diseases. The restrictive form is the least common cardiomyopathy. In this condition there is restriction of ventricle filling during diastole. Endomyocardial fibrosis is a not uncommon cause in the tropics. This disease is associated with eosinophilia and is probably due to chronic infection with the filarial worm *Loa loa*. A similar pattern of cardiac disease can be seen in infiltrative diseases (eg amyloid and sarcoid), glycogen storage disorders, metastatic cancer, carcinoid syndrome and following radiation or doxorubicin treatment. Myocarditis is an acute inflammation of the heart. It is often suspected clinically but only occasionally undergoes biopsy to fulfil the Dallas' diagnostic criteria. Acute myocarditis in South America is often due to *Trypanosoma cruzi*, the cause of Chagas disease. In Europe or North America the cause is more likely to be Coxsackie B virus infection. Constrictive pericarditis can be caused by tuberculosis, systemic lupus erythematosus, rheumatoid arthritis and malignancy.

Q55. UNCORRECTED CONGENITAL HEART DISEASE IN ADULTS (☆☆☆)

1. F   2. D   3. E   4. A   5. C

Congenital heart disease often presents in childhood particularly for the most severe conditions. However, even patients with cyanotic heart disease may occasionally survive to adulthood without the diagnosis being made. Tetralogy of Fallot is the combination of a large ventricular septal defect, pulmonary infundibular stenosis, right ventricular hypertrophy and an overriding aorta. The patient has a lifelong right to left shunt causing central cyanosis and clubbing. Affected children learn that they can ease symptoms of breathlessness by adopting a squatting posture, which decreases the volume of blood passing through the shunt. On examination there is a parasternal heave, single second heart sound, a pulmonary ejection systolic murmur but no murmur associated with the ventricular septal defect. The chest X-ray shows a large right ventricle and large ascending aorta. A large ventricular septal defect with a left to right

shunt eventually leads to pulmonary hypertension, right ventricular hypertrophy and a reversal of the shunt. Once the right to left shunt is established the patient has Eisenmenger syndrome. When a similar sequence of events occurs with other cardiac defects initially causing a left to right shunt, the condition is called Eisenmenger complex. Patients with Eisenmenger syndrome have cyanosis, a loud pulmonary component of the second heart sound, a pulmonary ejection systolic click and tricuspid regurgitation. Chest X-ray shows large pulmonary arteries with peripheral pruning secondary to longstanding pulmonary hypertension. In the Eisenmenger complex secondary to a patent ductus arteriosus, the lower body receives a larger proportion of blood passing through the shunt than the upper body. Cyanosis and clubbing are therefore more marked in the feet than the hands. The chest X-ray confirms the diagnosis as the calcified duct is usually easily seen. Ebstein's anomaly is where the tricuspid valve originates from below the atrioventricular ring. The myocardium of the inflow of the right ventricle is thinner and weaker than usual resulting in impaired right ventricular contraction. There is usually an associated patent foramen ovale or true atrial septal defect. Most patients are not cyanosed at rest but may become so after exercise. The prognosis is variable but some patients survive to an advanced age. The chest X-ray shows global cardiomegaly with a sharp outline, underperfused lungs and a small aortic knuckle. Ostium secundum atrial septal defects (ASD) do not border the atrioventricular valves whereas the more severe ostium primum defects do. Fewer than 10% of patients with an ostium secundum ASD develop pulmonary hypertension and cyanotic heart disease. The majority of ASDs lead to symptoms over the age of 40 years due to congestive cardiac failure and arrhythmias. There is wide splitting of the second heart sound and this does not usually vary with respiration. The chest X-ray shows cardiomegaly, pulmonary plethora and a small aorta. Tricuspid atresia (failure of valve development) does not usually allow survival to adulthood without surgical correction.

Q56. INFECTIVE ENDOCARDITIS (☆☆)

1. D   2. C   3. F   4. A   5. B

The commonest organisms causing native valve endocarditis are viridans group streptococci, enterococci, *Staphylococcus aureus* and HACEK organisms (**H**aemophilus, **A**ctinobacillus, **C**ardiobacterium, **E**ikenella and **K**ingella). Many patients have preceding valvular abnormalities. *Streptococcus sanguis* and other viridans streptococcal species inhabiting the mouth are a frequent cause of endocarditis after dental manipulation. *S. bovis, S. salivarius* and enterococci are bowel flora and endocarditis due to these organisms should prompt a search for colon pathology. *Staphylococcus aureus* is the most likely cause of endocarditis in an intravenous drug user and frequently affects the right side of the heart. *S. lugdunensis* is a virulent coagulase-negative staphylococcus which behaves like *S. aureus*. Many recent cases of endocarditis with this organism have been linked to breaches of the perineal skin. A large number of organisms can cause endocarditis following mechanical prosthetic valve insertion including *S. epidermidis, S. aureus*, viridans streptococci, *Enterococcus* species, coliforms and *Candida* species. Endophthalmitis is a frequent complication of candidaemia and often requires surgical vitrectomy. *Candida* species, *S. aureus* and *S. lugdunensis* cause particularly aggressive valve destruction and early valve replacement reduces mortality. Repeatedly negative cultures may occur in endocarditis when the patient has been given antibiotics, when the cause is not an infection (eg marantic endocarditis in malignancy or Libman-Sachs endocarditis in systemic lupus erythematosus) or if the organism is difficult to culture (eg *Coxiella burnetii, Bartonella henselae*, fungi, etc).

Q57. DEFINITION OF TERMS (☆)

1. F   2. B   3. A   4. C   5. D

Depersonalisation is the feeling of being detached from one's own experiences. Patients complain that they are no longer able to feel real emotions. Derealisation is a feeling that the external world is not real. Patients complain that it seems as though things have no real life or substance. Both derealisation and depersonalisation are distressing symptoms. They do not necessarily indicate mental illness and may be found in people who are tired or as reactions to stress. Passivity phenomena include thought withdrawal, where the patient believes his/her thoughts are stolen from his/her mind, thought insertion where ideas are implanted and thought broadcasting where they are made known to others. The belief that one's body movements or actions are controlled by others is also a passivity phenomenon. Hemisomatognosia is the belief that one of one's limbs is missing when it is not. This is different to neglect where the patient ignores the limb. Insight may be preserved so that the patient knows the limb is present but just feels it is not there. In other cases the patient may be convinced that the limb is really absent. An alien limb moves independently of voluntary control. This may occur secondary to damage to the basal ganglia. A phantom limb is the feeling that an amputated limb is still present. The patient may feel normal sensations from the limb (including troublesome pain) but is almost always aware that the limb is not present.

Q58. 1983 UK MENTAL HEALTH ACT (☆☆☆)

1. D   2. C   3. A   4. B   5. F

Section 2 of the Mental Health Act covers application for compulsory admission to hospital for assessment and treatment for up to 28 days. This requires application by the patient's next of kin or social worker and recommendation by two doctors, one of whom must be approved under the Mental Health Act.

Section 4 is an emergency order which is valid for only 72 hours. If further detention is felt necessary for the safety of the patient or others this should be converted to a Section 2 or 3 order rather than renewed. The process requires the request of a social worker or the nearest relative and the approval of one doctor. Section 5 covers holding orders for a patient who is already in hospital. This requires the recommendation of the doctor in charge of the patient's care or his or her delegated deputy. The order lapses after 72 hours, as for a Section 4 order. A nurse's holding order is a similar procedure, which allows a nurse to hold a patient for up to 6 hours, until he or she can be assessed by a doctor. Section 3 of the Mental Health Act covers long-term hospital admission and treatment of a patient with a diagnosed mental illness. The doctors must specify the diagnosis and verify that the patient requires treatment for his/her own health and safety or for that of others. Section 7 covers application for guardianship. Usually it is the Social Services Department who are the guardians and they can then direct the patient as to appointments, which must be attended, and to other restrictions. Section 37 deals with the criteria for a Court to commit an offender to a hospital. The patient/offender is then bound by similar terms as a patient held under Section 3 of the Act.

Q59. PSYCHIATRIC THERAPY (☆)

1. F   2. A   3. B   4. E   5. C

Behavioural therapy attempts to modify a person's behaviour by working through problems. It is not essential for the patient to develop insight into the nature of the problem. Exposure therapy is a form of behavioural therapy used to treat phobias. The exposure can be given in practice (eg walking into a crowded place in agoraphobia) or in imagination. Desensitisation is where the exposure is increased gradually with the patient moving into increasingly stressful situations once he/she is comfortable in the earlier stage. Flooding is where the patient is immediately taken to the most stressful situation and kept there until anxiety subsides. Implosion is the term used for flooding by imagination. Cognitive therapy is a psychological treatment that aims to identify and adapt negative ways of thinking. This is particularly useful in anxiety states and in depression. For example, a patient may suffer depression which leads to negative thoughts about self-worth, which then leads to worsening of the depression. Cognitive therapy can be used to recognise this cycle and to interrupt it by encouraging positive thoughts. Psychoanalysis uses the transference of the patient's earlier thoughts and emotions onto the analyst to enable interpretation and working through of problems. The aim is to eventually develop the patient's insight into the cause of his or her problems. Counter-transference is the term used to describe feelings that the analyst has towards the patient. These feelings are believed to interfere with the psychoanalytic process so the analyst should try to maintain neutral emotions. Dynamic interactional treatment is a form of group therapy that enables the previous relationship problems of group members to be expressed in a non-hostile environment. The group's participants benefit from the development of cohesiveness, mutual support and increased self-respect and by learning that others have similar problems to themselves and that these can be overcome.

Q60. FAECAL INCONTINENCE (☆)

1. E   2. C   3. F   4. A   5. B

Faecal incontinence is a distressing problem that can be caused by loose stools or by conditions affecting the anus. Digital examination of the rectum is an essential aspect of assessment of all patients with faecal incontinence. This may reveal faecal impaction, a distal rectal tumour, weakness of the external anal sphincter or pelvic floor muscles or a palpable fissure. Digital examination will fail to detect lesions that are not palpable such as haemorrhoids and small anal fistulae. Proctoscopy allows an adequate view of the anus to diagnose these conditions. Sigmoidoscopy does not provide a view of the anal mucosa but does allow visualisation of mucosa up to about 15 cm. This is useful for the identification of rectal tumours, rectal ulcers and for diagnosis of inflammatory bowel disease by visualisation and biopsy of the rectal mucosa. Examination of a wet preparation of faeces allows identification of ova, cysts and parasites. This is performed to diagnose intestinal protozoa (eg *Entamoeba histolytica* and *Giardia lamblia*) and helminth infections. *Trichuris trichiura* attaches to the colonic mucosa and can cause faecal incontinence and even rectal prolapse. Faecal fat estimation is useful to identify steatorrhoea in patients with malabsorption. The modified Ziehl-Neelsen stain is used to diagnose cryptosporidia, cyclospora and isospora infections.

CELLULAR AND MOLECULAR BIOLOGY

1. THEME: INTERCELLULAR ADHESION MOLECULES

A E-selectin
B L-selectin
C Intercellular adhesion molecule 1
D CD4
E $\alpha_{IIb}\beta$-integrin
F Cadherins

For each of the following descriptions select the appropriate intercellular adhesion molecule from the list above. The items may be used once or not at all.

☐ 1. Member of immunoglobulin superfamily which binds to lymphocyte function associated molecule 1
☐ 2. Involved in interaction between muscle and nerve in the developing embryo
☐ 3. Cofactor for antigen presentation on T lymphocytes
☐ 4. Integrin which functions as the platelet receptor for fibrinogen
☐ 5. Expressed on leukocytes to facilitate adhesion to endothelium

2. THEME: RECEPTOR TYPES

A Vitamin D receptor
B Nicotinic acetylcholine receptor
C Muscarinic acetylcholine receptor
D TATA box
E Insulin receptor
F p53

For each of the following receptor types select the receptor which belongs to this group from the list above. The items may be used once or not at all.

☐ 1. Ligand-gated ion channel
☐ 2. Protein-tyrosine-kinase-mediated receptor
☐ 3. G-protein-coupled receptor
☐ 4. Nuclear hormone receptor
☐ 5. Gene promoter element

STATISTICS AND EPIDEMIOLOGY

3. THEME: SCREENING TESTS

A Sensitivity
B Positive predictive value
C Precision
D Validity
E Specificity
F Negative predictive value

For each of the following descriptions related to screening tests select the appropriate term from the list above. The items may be used once or not at all.

☐ 1. Proportion of positive test results where the subject has the condition tested for
☐ 2. Proportion of negative test results where the subject does not have the condition tested for
☐ 3. Proportion of subjects with the disease who have a positive result on testing
☐ 4. Proportion of subjects who do not have the disease who have a negative result on testing
☐ 5. Ability to replicate a result on repeated testing

IMMUNOLOGY

4. THEME: MONOCYTE-DERIVED CELLS

A Microglial cell
B Dendritic cell
C Langhans' giant cell
D Osteoclast
E Kupffer cell
F Mast cell

For each of the following descriptions select the appropriate monocyte-derived cell from the list above. The items may be used once or not at all.

☐ 1. A multinucleate cell found in granulomas
☐ 2. Resident macrophage in the liver
☐ 3. Potent antigen-presenting cell capable of stimulating a primary immune response
☐ 4. Resident macrophage of central nervous system parenchyma
☐ 5. Not a descendant of the monocyte cell lineage

5. THEME: MACROPHAGE MEMBRANE RECEPTORS

A TNF receptor
B Interleukin 10 receptor
C Chemokine receptor 5
D FcR
E MHC class I
F Interferon γ receptor

For each of the following descriptions select the appropriate macrophage membrane receptor from the list above. The items may be used once or not at all.

☐ 1. Important for opsonic phagocytosis
☐ 2. Stimulation results in macrophage deactivation
☐ 3. A co-receptor for HIV entry
☐ 4. Stimulation results in increased expression of MHC class II
☐ 5. Stimulation produces granuloma formation

CLINICAL GENETICS

6. THEME: INHERITED DISEASE

A Myotonic dystrophy
B Fragile X syndrome
C Hereditary motor and sensory neuropathy type Ia
D DiGeorge syndrome
E Huntington's chorea
F Haemophilia A

For each of the following genetic abnormalities select the associated disease from the list above. The items may be used once or not at all.

☐ 1. Two-megabase duplication at chromosome 17p11.2
☐ 2. Chromosomal inversion on Xq
☐ 3. Microdeletion of 22q11.2
☐ 4. Expansion of CGG repeat at Xq27.3
☐ 5. Expansion of CTG repeat on chromosome 19

7. THEME: PROBLEMS ASSOCIATED WITH INBORN ERRORS OF METABOLISM

A Refsum's disease
B Phenylketonuria
C Acid maltase deficiency
D Myophosphorylase deficiency
E Hunter syndrome
F Hurler syndrome

For each of the following problems select the appropriate inborn error of metabolism from the list above. The items may be used once or not at all.

☐ 1. Type II respiratory failure
☐ 2. Exercise-induced muscle cramps
☐ 3. Hepatosplenomegaly, skeletal deformity, characteristic facies and corneal clouding
☐ 4. Hepatosplenomegaly, skeletal deformity and characteristic facies without corneal clouding
☐ 5. Retinitis pigmentosa, deafness and peripheral neuropathy

NEUROANATOMY

8. THEME: NERVE SUPPLY

A Median nerve
B Radial nerve
C Accessory nerve
D Axillary nerve
E Phrenic nerve
F Ulnar nerve

For each of the following muscles select the appropriate nerve supply from the list above. The items may be used once or not at all.

- 1. Deltoid
- 2. Trapezius
- 3. First dorsal interosseus
- 4. Brachioradialis
- 5. First lumbrical

9. THEME: CEREBRAL CORTEX

A Lateral surface of postcentral gyrus of parietal lobe
B Medial surface of postcentral gyrus of parietal lobe
C Calcarine sulcus of occipital lobe
D Superior temporal gyrus and adjacent parietal region
E Posterior part of inferior gyrus of frontal lobe
F Lateral sulcus of temporal lobe

For each of the following functional areas of the cerebral cortex select the associated anatomical area from the list above. The items may be used once or not at all.

- 1. Primary visual area
- 2. Primary somaesthetic area for the foot
- 3. Primary somaesthetic area for the tongue
- 4. Primary auditory area
- 5. Sensory speech area of Wernicke

PHYSIOLOGY, BIOCHEMISTRY AND METABOLISM

10. THEME: BILE

A Chenodeoxycholic acid
B Deoxycholic acid
C Lipoprotein lipase
D Phospholipase
E Cholesterol 7α-hydroxylase
F Hydroxymethylglutaryl coA reductase

For each of the following descriptions related to the metabolism of bile constituents select the appropriate term from the list above. The items may be used once or not at all.

- 1. Rate-limiting enzyme in cholesterol synthesis
- 2. Rate-limiting enzyme in primary bile acid synthesis
- 3. A primary bile acid
- 4. A secondary bile acid
- 5. The enzyme which metabolises lecithin

11. THEME: BODY WATER

A 60 kg
B 45 kg
C 30 kg
D 15 kg
E 10 kg
F 5 kg

For each of the following body compartments in a 75 kg, healthy, non-obese adult male select the associated weight of body water it contains from the list above. The items may be used once or not at all.

- 1. Intracellular compartment
- 2. Extracellular compartment
- 3. Total body water
- 4. Blood
- 5. Interstitial space

12. THEME: HORMONAL REGULATION OF SALT AND WATER HOMEOSTASIS

A   Adrenocorticotrophic hormone
B   Renin
C   Aldosterone
D   Antidiuretic hormone
E   Angiotensin II
F   Human α-atrial natriuretic peptide

For each of the following actions related to salt and water homeostasis select the appropriate hormone from the list above. The items may be used once or not at all.

☐ 1. Stimulates urine concentration by the collecting ducts
☐ 2. Stimulates conversion of angiotensinogen to angiotensin I
☐ 3. Stimulates aldosterone secretion
☐ 4. Stimulates sodium reabsorption in the distal nephron
☐ 5. Stimulates sodium loss

13. THEME: PHYSIOLOGY OF BONE

A   1,25-dihydroxyvitamin D_3
B   Parathyroid hormone
C   Alkaline phosphatase
D   Hydroxyproline
E   Type I collagen
F   Calcitonin

For each of the following descriptions related to the physiology of bone select the appropriate compound from the list above. The items may be used once or not at all.

☐ 1. Decreases bone resorption by suppressing osteoclast activity
☐ 2. Increases bone resorption
☐ 3. Increases intestinal calcium absorption
☐ 4. A serum marker of increased osteoblast activity
☐ 5. A marker of increased osteoclast activity

14. THEME: REGULATION OF CORONARY BLOOD FLOW

A   α-adrenergic receptor
B   β-adrenergic receptor
C   Nitric oxide
D   Endothelin 1
E   Coronary vasculature oxygen concentration
F   Coronary vasculature carbon dioxide concentration

For each of the following descriptions related to the regulation of coronary blood flow select the appropriate term from the list above. The items may be used once or not at all.

☐ 1. Decrease results in coronary arteriole vasodilatation
☐ 2. Mediates the neurohumeral control of coronary artery vasoconstriction
☐ 3. Mediates the neurohumeral control of coronary artery vasodilatation
☐ 4. Powerful vasoconstrictor released locally
☐ 5. Powerful vasodilator released locally

RENAL MEDICINE

15. THEME: FIRST-TIME PRESENTATION OF RENAL FAILURE

A   Acute glomerulonephritis
B   Pre-renal failure
C   Myeloma
D   Acute tubular necrosis
E   Acute urinary tract obstruction
F   Chronic renal failure

For each of the following findings in a patient presenting with renal failure for the first time select the appropriate diagnosis from the list above. The items may be used once or not at all.

☐ 1. Bilateral small kidneys on ultrasound
☐ 2. Bilateral dilated renal calyces on ultrasound
☐ 3. Large numbers of red cell casts on urine microscopy

4. Normal appearance of kidneys on ultrasound, urinary sodium less than 20 mmol/l, urine osmolality greater than 500 mosmol/kg, urine-to-plasma creatinine ratio of greater than 40

5. Bence Jones protein in urine

16. THEME: RISK FACTORS FOR ACUTE RENAL FAILURE

A   Myoglobinuria
B   Haemoglobinuria
C   Acute cortical necrosis
D   Acute interstitial nephritis
E   Acute glomerulonephritis
F   Uric acid nephropathy

For each of the following risk factors select the appropriate cause of acute renal failure from the list above. The items may be used once or not at all.

1. Malaria
2. Neuroleptic malignant syndrome
3. Induction chemotherapy for acute leukaemia
4. Recent group A streptococcal pharyngitis
5. Postpartum haemorrhage

17. THEME: RENAL REPLACEMENT THERAPY

A   Intermittent peritoneal dialysis
B   Continuous cyclic peritoneal dialysis
C   Continuous ambulatory peritoneal dialysis
D   Haemofiltration
E   Haemodialysis
F   Tidal intermittent peritoneal dialysis

For each of the following descriptions select the appropriate form of renal replacement therapy from the list above. The items may be used once or not at all.

1. Form of peritoneal dialysis where fluid is changed manually every few hours
2. Form of peritoneal dialysis where a cycler machine performs up to 40 exchanges in one day

3. Requires vascular access, solute is then removed from blood by diffusion across a semipermeable membrane
4. Form of peritoneal dialysis where fluid is left in the abdomen all day and then exchanged four to five times by a cycler machine during the night
5. Requires vascular access and places less strain on the cardiovascular system than membrane-diffusion method

18. THEME: REVERSIBLE RENAL FAILURE

A   Skull X-ray
B   Anti-dsDNA antibodies
C   Rectal biopsy
D   Renal angiography
E   cANCA
F   Renal ultrasound

For each of the following potentially reversible causes of renal failure select the most useful test from the list above. The items may be used once or not at all.

1. Urinary tract obstruction
2. Systemic amyloidosis
3. Multiple myeloma
4. Systemic lupus erythematosus
5. Polyarteritis nodosa

ENDOCRINOLOGY AND DIABETES

19. THEME: ENDOCRINE DISEASE

A   Primary hyperaldosteronism
B   Mineralocorticoid deficiency without corticosteroid deficiency
C   Ectopic ACTH syndrome
D   Cushing's disease
E   Primary adrenal failure
F   Secondary adrenal failure

For each of the following diseases select the associated condition from the list above. The items may be used once or not at all.

- [ ] 1. Pituitary adenoma derived from corticotroph cells
- [ ] 2. Bronchial carcinoid tumour
- [ ] 3. Tuberculosis
- [ ] 4. Craniopharyngioma
- [ ] 5. Congenital adrenal hyperplasia

20. THEME: CUSHING'S SYNDROME

A   Serum ACTH measurement
B   Serum potassium
C   Twenty-four-hour urinary free cortisol excretion
D   High-dose dexamethasone suppression test
E   Adrenal computed tomography
F   Adrenal scintigraphy scan

For each of the following statements related to the diagnosis and differential diagnosis of Cushing's syndrome select the appropriate test from the list above. The items may be used once or not at all.

- [ ] 1. Useful outpatient screening test for diagnosis of Cushing's syndrome
- [ ] 2. Useful to differentiate adrenal adenomas from Cushing's disease; not generally useful to differentiate between Cushing's disease and ectopic ACTH syndrome
- [ ] 3. Useful to differentiate ectopic ACTH syndrome from Cushing's disease; not generally useful to differentiate between Cushing's disease and adrenal adenomas
- [ ] 4. Useful to differentiate ectopic ACTH syndrome from Cushing's disease; not generally useful to differentiate between ectopic ACTH syndrome and adrenal adenomas
- [ ] 5. Most useful test to distinguish asymmetrical adrenal nodular hyperplasia from an adrenal adenoma

21. THEME: ENDOCRINE PROBLEMS CAUSED BY DRUGS AND DISEASE

A   Haemochromatosis
B   Mesothelioma
C   AIDS
D   Amiodarone
E   Ketoconazole
F   Sarcoidosis

For each of the following endocrine problems select the causative drug or disease from the list above. The items may be used once or not at all.

- [ ] 1. Diabetes insipidus
- [ ] 2. Hypoadrenalism
- [ ] 3. Thyrotoxicosis
- [ ] 4. Diabetes mellitus
- [ ] 5. Hypoglycaemia

22. THEME: INTERSEX DISORDERS

A   17α-hydroxylase deficiency
B   Testicular feminisation syndrome
C   XY gonadal dysgenesis
D   Maternal androgen-secreting adrenal adenoma
E   21-hydroxylase deficiency
F   XX male syndrome

For each of the following statements select the appropriate intersex disorder from the list above. The items may be used once or not at all.

- [ ] 1. Commonest cause of female pseudohermaphroditism
- [ ] 2. Rare cause of female pseudohermaphroditism
- [ ] 3. Causes male pseudohermaphroditism due to impaired production of androgens

☐ 4. Causes male pseudohermaphroditism due to androgen insensitivity

☐ 5. Causes male pseudohermaphroditism due to incomplete differentiation of testes

GASTROENTEROLOGY

23. THEME: GASTROINTESTINAL DISORDERS

A   Pneumatosis cystoides intestinalis
B   Budd-Chiari syndrome
C   Microvesicular steatosis
D   Peliosis hepatis
E   Ménétrier's disease
F   Malakoplakia

For each of the following descriptions select the appropriate condition from the list above. The items may be used once or not at all.

☐ 1. Presence of blood-filled cavities in the liver

☐ 2. Lipid droplets distributed throughout the liver

☐ 3. Multiple gas-filled cysts in the wall of the colon

☐ 4. Granulomatous disease of urinary tract and/or colon

☐ 5. Gastric disease causing marked protein loss

24. THEME: JAUNDICE

A   Crigler-Najjar syndrome
B   Rotor's syndrome
C   Primary biliary cirrhosis
D   Gilbert's disease
E   Dubin-Johnson syndrome
F   Primary sclerosing cholangitis

For each of the following descriptions related to jaundice select the appropriate condition from the list above. The items may be used once or not at all.

☐ 1. Unconjugated hyperbilirubinaemia causing jaundice during episodes of fasting

☐ 2. Unconjugated hyperbilirubinaemia causing fatal jaundice in neonates

☐ 3. Conjugated hyperbilirubinaemia with non-visualisation of the gallbladder on cholecystography

☐ 4. Conjugated hyperbilirubinaemia with raised total urinary coproporphyrins

☐ 5. Conjugated hyperbilirubinaemia with strictures and dilatations of the biliary tree

25. THEME: SYSTEMIC CONDITIONS

A   Systemic sclerosis
B   Osler-Weber-Rendu syndrome
C   Angiodysplasia
D   Familial Mediterranean fever
E   Henoch-Schönlein disease
F   Polyarteritis nodosa

For each of the following findings select the appropriate systemic condition from the list above. The items may be used once or not at all.

☐ 1. Recurrent abdominal pain and multiple aneurysms on mesenteric angiography

☐ 2. Recurrent attacks of peritonitis with no surgical cause found

☐ 3. Progressive dysphagia and accompanying malabsorption

☐ 4. Bleeding per rectum, abdominal pain, arthritis and a vasculitic rash

☐ 5. Bleeding per rectum and facial telangiectases

26. THEME: CIRRHOSIS

A   Wilson's disease
B   Autoimmune hepatitis
C   Budd-Chiari syndrome
D   Haemochromatosis
E   Primary biliary cirrhosis
F α_1-antitrypsin deficiency

For each of the following findings select the appropriate cause of cirrhosis from the list above. The items may be used once or not at all.

☐ 1. Presence of anti-smooth muscle antibody
☐ 2. Presence of antimitochondrial antibody
☐ 3. Presence of Kayser-Fleischer ring
☐ 4. Markedly raised serum ferritin
☐ 5. History of onset of emphysema at an early age

NEUROLOGY

27. THEME: HEREDITARY NEUROLOGICAL CONDITIONS

A   Adrenoleucodystrophy
B   Adult-onset Gaucher's disease
C   Neurofibromatosis type 2
D   Lesch-Nyhan syndrome
E   Friedreich's ataxia
F   Fabry's disease

For each of the following descriptions select the appropriate hereditary neurological condition from the list above. The items may be used once or not at all.

☐ 1. Development of progressive cerebellar problems, upper motor neurone weakness, extensor plantars and absent ankle reflexes
☐ 2. Widespread cerebral demyelination causing dementia, cortical blindness, ataxia and spastic weakness
☐ 3. Presents with painful paraesthesia, followed by peripheral neuropathy, cerebral infarcts, corneal opacities and cutaneous telangiectasia

☐ 4. Bilateral acoustic neuromas characteristically occur
☐ 5. Increased uric acid production, mental retardation, self-mutilation, choreoathetosis and limb spasticity

28. THEME: SIGNS OF BRAIN LESIONS

A   Frontal lobe
B   Midbrain
C   Temporal lobe
D   Cerebellum
E   Parietal lobe
F   Occipital lobe

For each of the following effects caused by space-occupying brain lesions select the appropriate anatomical region in the brain from the list above. The items may be used once or not at all.

☐ 1. Contralateral upper quadrantanopia
☐ 2. Contralateral lower quadrantanopia
☐ 3. Contralateral homonymous hemianopia
☐ 4. Failure of downgaze
☐ 5. Past-pointing on finger-nose test

29. THEME: INTRACRANIAL BRAIN TUMOURS

A   Meningioma
B   Glioblastoma multiforme
C   Medulloblastoma
D   Schwannoma
E   Ependymoma
F   Craniopharyngioma

For each of the following descriptions select the appropriate intracranial tumour from the list above. The items may be used once or not at all.

☐ 1. Rapidly growing tumour arising from astrocytes
☐ 2. Usually benign tumour arising from the arachnoid cells of the dura
☐ 3. Generally benign tumour most frequently located in the cerebellopontine angle
☐ 4. Usually benign tumour of epithelial cells which may compress the optic chiasm

5. Highly malignant tumour usually occurring in children which may metastasise outside the central nervous system

30. THEME: RISK FACTORS FOR NEUROPATHY

A Lead poisoning
B Cisplatin treatment
C Pelvic cancer
D Acromegaly
E Vitamin B_{12} deficiency
F Diabetes mellitus

For each of the following types of neuropathy select the appropriate risk factor from the list above. The items may be used once or not at all.

1. Median nerve palsy
2. Obturator nerve palsy
3. Third cranial nerve palsy with pupil sparing
4. Peripheral motor neuropathy
5. Eighth cranial nerve palsy

RESPIRATORY MEDICINE

31. THEME: RESPIRATORY CONDITIONS

A Behçet's syndrome
B Churg-Strauss syndrome
C Hughes-Stovin syndrome
D Necrotising sarcoid granulomatosis
E Bronchocentric granulomatosis
F Wegener's granulomatosis

For each of the following problems select the causative condition from the list above. The items may be used once or not at all.

1. Asthma, peripheral eosinophilia and systemic vasculitis
2. Upper and lower respiratory tract granulomas
3. Multiple miliary nodules and hilar lymphadenopathy
4. An upper lobe alveolar infiltrate without hilar lymphadenopathy

5. Haemoptysis due to rupture of a pulmonary artery aneurysm

32. THEME: HAEMOPTYSIS

A Idiopathic pulmonary haemosiderosis
B Systemic lupus erythematosus
C Hereditary haemorrhagic telangiectasia
D Goodpasture's syndrome
E Haemophilia
F Mitral stenosis

For each of the following presentations related to haemoptysis select the most likely cause from the list above. The items may be used once or not at all.

1. Acute severe haemoptysis in a patient with glomerulonephritis and antibodies to the α3-chain of type IV collagen
2. Recurrent small volume haemoptysis in a young adult with progressive breathlessness and iron-deficiency anaemia
3. Acute severe haemoptysis in an elderly patient with a malar flush
4. Acute severe haemoptysis in a young patient with facial telangiectasia and glomerulonephritis
5. Acute severe haemoptysis in a patient with facial telangiectasia and a history of recurrent gastrointestinal haemorrhage and epistaxis

33. THEME: RESPIRATORY DISEASE IN FARMERS

A   Cryptogenic fibrosing alveolitis
B   Acute extrinsic allergic alveolitis
C   Organic dust toxic syndrome
D   Paraquat poisoning
E   Nitrogen dioxide pneumonitis
F   Q fever

For each of the following findings in a farmer presenting with respiratory symptoms select the most likely diagnosis from the list above. The items may be used once or not at all.

- ☐ 1. Brief history of cough and breathlessness beginning hours after working in a silo: the patient admits to having had previous attacks which improved with corticosteroids
- ☐ 2. Brief history of cough and breathlessness beginning a few hours after working in a silo: the patient is very unwell and is found to have methaemoglobinaemia
- ☐ 3. Brief history of cough and breathlessness beginning a few hours after working in a silo: fungal hyphae are found on bronchoalveolar lavage
- ☐ 4. Two-day history of progressive breathlessness. Painful ulcers are present on the tongue and oropharynx
- ☐ 5. Two-day history of cough, chest pain, breathlessness and severe headache. Routine investigations demonstrate transaminitis and a thrombocytosis of 800×10^9 per litre

34. THEME: RESPIRATORY SIDE-EFFECTS OF DRUGS

A   Hydrochlorothiazide
B   Lisinopril
C   Methysergide
D   Propranolol
E   Amiodarone
F   Co-trimoxazole

For each of the following respiratory problems select the drug most likely to have caused them from the list above. The items may be used once or not at all.

- ☐ 1. Acute pulmonary oedema
- ☐ 2. Alveolitis
- ☐ 3. Pulmonary eosinophilia
- ☐ 4. Pleural fibrosis
- ☐ 5. Asthma

RHEUMATOLOGY

35. THEME: VASCULITIDES

A   Scleroderma
B   Churg-Strauss syndrome
C   Takayasu's arteritis
D   Polyarteritis nodosa
E   Henoch-Schönlein purpura
F   Microscopic polyangiitis

For each of the following histological appearances select the appropriate type of vasculitides from the list above. The items may be used once or not at all.

- ☐ 1. Large vessel vasculitis with granulomas
- ☐ 2. Medium-sized vessel vasculitis without granulomas
- ☐ 3. Small vessel vasculitis with granulomas
- ☐ 4. Small vessel vasculitis without granulomas or immunoglobulin A deposition
- ☐ 5. Small vessel vasculitis with immunoglobulin A deposition and without granulomas

36. THEME: DRUG THERAPY IN RHEUMATIC DISEASE

A   Rheumatoid arthritis
B   Chronic gouty arthritis (prevention of attacks)
C   Osteoarthritis
D   Acute gout
E   Whipple's disease
F   Giant cell arteritis

For each of the following drug treatments select the condition it is used for from the list above. The items may be used once or not at all.

1. Allopurinol
2. Colchicine
3. Penicillamine
4. Penicillin
5. Prednisolone

DERMATOLOGY

37. THEME: BLISTERING CONDITIONS

A Junctional epidermolysis bullosa
B Dermatitis herpetiformis
C Epidermolysis bullosa simplex
D Pemphigus vulgaris
E Necrolytic migratory erythema
F Bullous pemphigoid

For each of the following biopsy findings select the appropriate blistering condition from the list above. The items may be used once or not at all.

1. Subepidermal split with linear immunoglobulin G at basement membrane
2. Intraepidermal split with intercellular immunoglobulin G
3. Subepidermal split with no antibodies demonstrable
4. Subepidermal split with patchy granular immunoglobulin A
5. Split in lamina lucida with no antibodies demonstrable

38. THEME: HISTOLOGY OF SKIN DISEASE

A Liquefaction
B Acantholysis
C Hyperkeratosis
D Parakeratosis
E Necrobiosis
F Spongiosis

For each of the following skin diseases select the characteristic histological feature from the list above. The items may be used once or not at all.

1. Acne vulgaris
2. Psoriasis
3. Eczema
4. Pemphigus vulgaris
5. Erythema multiforme

HAEMATOLOGY

39. THEME: PARAPROTEINAEMIAS

A Multiple myeloma
B Heavy chain disease
C Cryoglobulinaemia
D Primary amyloidosis
E Waldenström's macroglobulinaemia
F Monoclonal gammopathy of undetermined significance

For each of the following findings select the appropriate paraproteinaemia from the list above. The items may be used once or not at all.

1. Excess monoclonal immunoglobulin M in serum
2. Excess monoclonal immunoglobulin G in serum and Bence Jones proteinuria
3. Excess heavy chains in serum
4. Excess monoclonal immunoglobulin G in serum and no Bence Jones proteinuria
5. Patient with nephrotic syndrome and immunoglobulin light chains in serum

40. THEME: BLOOD DISORDERS

A   Disseminated intravascular coagulation
B   Thrombotic thrombocytopaenic purpura
C   Liver failure
D   Renal failure
E   Evans' syndrome
F   Haemolytic uraemic syndrome

For each of the following descriptions select the appropriate condition from the list above. The items may be used once or not at all.

☐ 1. Microangiopathic haemolytic anaemia often associated with *Escherichia coli* O157 infection
☐ 2. Microangiopathic haemolytic anaemia with neurological abnormalities in the majority of cases
☐ 3. Intravascular thrombosis producing coagulation factor depletion and activation of the fibrinolytic system
☐ 4. Coagulation factor depletion due to decreased production of clotting factors
☐ 5. Coombs' positive autoimmune haemolytic anaemia and thrombocytopenia

41. THEME: BLOOD FILM ABNORMALITIES

A   Basophilia
B   Neutropenia
C   Neutrophilia
D   Lymphocytosis
E   Eosinophilia
F   Monocytosis

For each of the following conditions select the associated blood film abnormality from the list above. The items may be used once or not at all.

☐ 1. Polyarteritis nodosa
☐ 2. Urticaria pigmentosa
☐ 3. Acute myeloid leukaemia type M5
☐ 4. Pneumococcal pneumonia without bacteraemia
☐ 5. Typhoid fever

INFECTIOUS DISEASES AND TROPICAL MEDICINE

42. THEME: HUMAN PATHOGENS

A   A cause of granulomatous amoebic encephalitis
B   A gastrointestinal flagellate
C   A ciliate causing occasional gastrointestinal infection
D   A yeast causing meningitis in patients with AIDS
E   A coccidian causing outbreaks of diarrhoea
F   A flagellate which can be diagnosed by buffy coat smear

For each of the following potential human pathogens select the appropriate description from the list above. The items may be used once or not at all.

☐ 1. *Balamuthia mandrillaris*
☐ 2. *Cyclospora cayetanensis*
☐ 3. *Leishmania donovani*
☐ 4. *Balantidium coli*
☐ 5. *Dientamoeba fragilis*

43. THEME: HUMAN HERPES VIRUSES

A   Herpes simplex virus type 1
B   Herpes zoster virus
C   Epstein-Barr virus
D   Cytomegalovirus
E   Human herpes virus 6
F   Human herpes virus 8

For each of the following conditions select the appropriate causative human herpes virus from the list above. The items may be used once or not at all.

☐ 1. Endemic Burkitt's lymphoma
☐ 2. Acute necrotising encephalitis
☐ 3. Pneumonitis after a bone marrow transplant
☐ 4. Acute retinal necrosis in the immunocompetent
☐ 5. Roseola infantum

44. THEME: VIRUSES

A   Cytomegalovirus
B   Ebola virus
C   Human immunodeficiency virus
D   Human papilloma virus
E   Norwalk virus
F   Poliovirus

For each of the following descriptions select the appropriate virus from the list above. The items may be used once or not at all.

☐ 1. RNA-containing, unenveloped, icosahedral picornavirus
☐ 2. DNA-containing, enveloped, icosahedral herpes virus
☐ 3. RNA-containing, unenveloped, icosahedral calicivirus
☐ 4. RNA-containing, enveloped, helical filovirus
☐ 5. DNA-containing, unenveloped, icosahedral papovavirus

45. THEME: ROUTES OF ACQUISITION OF PLATYHELMINTH INFECTION

A   Mosquito bite
B   Penetration of intact skin by cercariae
C   Ingestion of metacercariae in uncooked crabs and crayfish
D   Ingestion of metacercariae on water chestnuts
E   Ingestion of metacercariae on watercress
F   Ingestion of metacercariae in uncooked freshwater fish

For infection with each of the following platyhelminths (trematodes) select the appropriate route of acquisition from the list above. The items may be used once or not at all.

☐ 1. *Paragonimus westermani*
☐ 2. *Fasciola hepatica*
☐ 3. *Fasciolopsis buski*
☐ 4. *Clonorchis sinensis*
☐ 5. *Schistosoma haematobium*

GENITOURINARY MEDICINE

46. THEME: ANTIBIOTIC THERAPY

A   Ceftriaxone plus doxycycline
B   Doxycycline
C   Co-trimoxazole
D   Ceftriaxone
E   Single dose of ciprofloxacin
F   Metronidazole

For each of the following clinical situations select the appropriate antibiotic from the list above. The items may be used once or not at all.

☐ 1. Traveller returning from India with watery diarrhoea
☐ 2. Epididymo-orchitis in a 20-year-old heterosexual man
☐ 3. HIV-positive patient with a six-week history of cough and progressive breathlessness and perihilar infiltrates on chest X-ray
☐ 4. Twenty-five-year-old man with a purulent urethral discharge but no Gram-negative diplococci on Gram stain
☐ 5. Acute epiglottitis in a fully vaccinated child

CLINICAL PHARMACOLOGY

47. THEME: TOPICAL EYE PREPARATIONS

A   A mydriatic which decreases aqueous humour production and increases trabecular drainage
B   A miotic which increases trabecular drainage
C   A mydriatic used in iridocyclitis
D   A local anaesthetic used before procedures on the eye
E   A mast cell stabiliser
F   A β-blocker which reduces production of aqueous humour

For each of the following topical eye preparations select the appropriate description from the list above. The items may be used once or not at all.

☐ 1. Pilocarpine
☐ 2. Dipivefrine
☐ 3. Timolol
☐ 4. Atropine
☐ 5. Nedocromil sodium

48. THEME: ANTINAUSEA DRUGS

A   Dexamethasone
B   Hyoscine
C   Nabilone
D   Ondansetron
E   Prochlorperazine
F   Cyclizine

For each of the following descriptions select the appropriate antinausea drug from the list above. The items may be used once or not at all.

☐ 1. A phenothiazine which acts on the chemoreceptor trigger zone
☐ 2. A synthetic cannabinoid
☐ 3. A $5HT_3$ receptor antagonist
☐ 4. An antimuscarinic available as a skin patch
☐ 5. An antihistamine which acts on the emetic centre

49. THEME: HYPNOTIC/ANXIOLYTIC DRUGS

A   Zopiclone
B   Diazepam
C   Chlormethiazole
D   Buspirone
E   Temazepam
F   Sodium amytal

For each of the following descriptions select the appropriate hypnotic/anxiolytic drug from the list above. The items may be used once or not at all.

☐ 1. A benzodiazepine with a relatively short duration of action
☐ 2. A benzodiazepine with a relatively long duration of action
☐ 3. A hypnotic licensed for treatment of insomnia only in the elderly
☐ 4. A cyclopyrrolone used for insomnia
☐ 5. A serotonin partial agonist acting on $5HT_1$ receptors

50. THEME: β-ADRENOCEPTOR BLOCKERS

A   Propranolol
B   Oxprenolol
C   Sotalol
D   Labetalol
E   Esmolol
F   Atenolol

For each of the following properties select the appropriate β-adrenoceptor blocker from the list above. The items may be used once or not at all.

☐ 1. Relatively water soluble and β_1-selective (cardiac receptors) so fewer side-effects
☐ 2. Relatively lipid soluble and non-β_1-selective
☐ 3. Intrinsic sympathomimetic activity producing less coldness of extremities
☐ 4. Very short duration of action so useful in situations with potential need to reverse effects rapidly

□ 5. Non-cardioselective action and additional class III anti-arrhythmic activity

51. THEME: SIDE-EFFECTS OF RESPIRATORY DRUGS

A   Development of Churg-Strauss syndrome
B   Acute glaucoma
C   Hypoglycaemia
D   Hypokalaemia
E   Feeling of perineal warmth
F   Bronchoconstriction

For each of the following respiratory drugs select the appropriate adverse event from the list above. The items may be used once or not at all.

□ 1. Nebulised ipratropium
□ 2. Oral salbutamol
□ 3. Doxapram
□ 4. Nebulised pentamidine
□ 5. Montelukast

52. THEME: ACUTE POISONING

A   Paraquat
B   Ethylene glycol
C   Carbon monoxide
D   Iron
E   Theophylline
F   Quinine

For each of the following adverse effects related to acute poisoning select the appropriate compound from the list above. The items may be used once or not at all.

□ 1. Severe metabolic acidosis
□ 2. Blindness
□ 3. Hepatocellular necrosis
□ 4. Cerebral oedema
□ 5. Proliferative alveolitis

CARDIOVASCULAR MEDICINE

53. THEME: BACTERIAL ENDOCARDITIS

A   Long PR interval on ECG
B   Janeway lesions
C   Early diastolic murmur
D   Roth spots
E   Splinter haemorrhages
F   Osler's nodes

For each of the following descriptions select the appropriate feature of bacterial endocarditis from the list above. The items may be used once or not at all.

□ 1. Fundal haemorrhages with a central pale area
□ 2. Circumscribed, erythematous, tender nodules on the fingers and toes
□ 3. Transient, non-tender macules on the palms and soles
□ 4. Petechial lesions under the nail bed
□ 5. A finding which is suggestive of aortic root abscess

54. THEME: HEART SOUNDS

A   First heart sound
B   Second heart sound
C   Third heart sound
D   Fourth heart sound
E   Ejection click
F   Opening snap

For each of the following occurrences select the appropriate heart sound from the list above. The items may be used once or not at all.

□ 1. Atrial contraction
□ 2. Aortic and pulmonary valve closure
□ 3. Mitral and tricuspid valve closure
□ 4. Aortic valve opening
□ 5. Mitral valve opening

55. THEME: PULMONARY OEDEMA

A   Decreased interstitial tissue pressure
B   Increased endothelial permeability
C   Decreased plasma colloid osmotic pressure
D   Decreased lymphatic drainage
E   Increased capillary hydrostatic pressure
F   Increased interstitial colloid osmotic pressure

For each of the following conditions select the mechanism primarily responsible for pulmonary oedema from the list above. The items may be used once or not at all.

☐ 1. Mitral stenosis
☐ 2. Obstructive sleep apnoea
☐ 3. Hypoproteinaemia
☐ 4. Goodpasture's syndrome
☐ 5. Immediate postoperative period in lung transplantation

56. THEME: FUNDOSCOPY

A   Chronic open-angle glaucoma
B   Diabetic retinopathy
C   Grade I hypertensive retinopathy
D   Grade II hypertensive retinopathy
E   Grade III hypertensive retinopathy
F   Grade IV hypertensive retinopathy

For each of the following fundoscopic findings select the appropriate condition from the list above. The items may be used once or not at all.

☐ 1. Increased light reflex from the arterial wall
☐ 2. Flame-shaped haemorrhages
☐ 3. Papilloedema and retinal oedema
☐ 4. Arteriovenous nipping
☐ 5. New vessel formation at the optic disc

PSYCHIATRY

57. THEME: SCHIZOPHRENIA

A   Delusional paranoid disorder
B   Simple schizophrenia
C   Hebephrenic schizophrenia
D   Paranoid schizophrenia
E   Catatonic schizophrenia
F   Residual schizophrenia

For each of the following descriptions select the appropriate type of schizophrenia from the list above. The items may be used once or not at all.

☐ 1. Predominant bizarre delusions with some passivity phenomena
☐ 2. Predominant affective symptoms causing childish behaviour and prominent thought disorder
☐ 3. Predominant motor abnormalities including posturing and waxy flexibility
☐ 4. Predominant social withdrawal, odd behaviour and emotional blunting without preceding hallucinations
☐ 5. Predominant social withdrawal with a previous history of marked hallucinations and delusions

58. THEME: ANTIDEPRESSANTS

A   Venlafaxine
B   Mirtazapine
C   Lofepramine
D   Imipramine
E   Paroxetine
F   Amitriptyline

For each of the following descriptions select the appropriate antidepressant from the list above. The items may be used once or not at all.

☐ 1. Well-established, tricyclic antidepressant with moderate sedating, antimuscarinic and cardiac side-effects
☐ 2. Well-established, tricyclic antidepressant with moderate antimuscarinic and cardiac side-effects but fewer sedative effects
☐ 3. Tricyclic antidepressant with fewer sedative, antimuscarinic and cardiac side-effects
☐ 4. Serotonin and noradrenaline reuptake inhibitor
☐ 5. Selective serotonin reuptake inhibitor

59. THEME: PSYCHIATRIC PROBLEMS RELATED TO PREGNANCY

A   Couvade syndrome
B   Puerperal psychosis
C   Maternity blues
D   Puerperal depression
E   De Clerambault's syndrome
F   Pseudocyesis

For each of the following descriptions related to psychiatric problems in pregnancy select the appropriate condition from the list above. The items may be used once or not at all.

- [ ] 1. A woman becomes convinced she is pregnant and develops symptoms suggestive of this
- [ ] 2. A man experiences symptoms of pregnancy similar to his partner's
- [ ] 3. Very common lability of mood experienced three to four days postpartum
- [ ] 4. An acute psychiatric illness occurring in the first two weeks after delivery
- [ ] 5. A common illness occurring more than two weeks after delivery

MISCELLANEOUS

60. THEME: URINARY INCONTINENCE

A   Neurogenic
B   Functional incontinence
C   Retention with overflow
D   Vesico-vaginal fistula
E   Urge incontinence
F   Stress incontinence

For each of the following findings select the matching type of urinary incontinence from the list above. The items may be used once or not at all.

- [ ] 1. Bladder calculus
- [ ] 2. Childbirth
- [ ] 3. Dementia
- [ ] 4. Imipramine use
- [ ] 5. Diabetes mellitus

ANSWERS TO PAPER 5

The approximate difficulty rating for the answer to each question is given in brackets.

☆ (the majority of competent final year students will know the answer)

☆☆ (approximately 50% of final year students will be able to answer correctly)

☆☆☆ (only the better students will usually know the answer)

Q1. INTERCELLULAR ADHESION MOLECULES (☆☆☆)

1. C   2. F   3. D   4. E   5. B

There are four families of intercellular adhesion molecules: the immunoglobulin superfamily, integrins, selectins and cadherins. Intercellular adhesion molecule 1 (ICAM1) is a member of the immunoglobulin superfamily expressed on epithelial and endothelial cells. Expression is induced by interleukin 1 and tumour necrosis factor α. ICAM1 binds to the integrin lymphocyte function associated molecule 1 to facilitate leukocyte migration to sites of inflammation. CD4 is a member of the immunoglobulin superfamily expressed on T helper lymphocytes that acts as a cofactor for recognition of antigens presented in conjunction with major histocompatibility complex class II molecules. Cadherins are a superfamily involved in the interaction between muscle and nerve cells in the developing embryo. The integrin $\alpha_{IIb}\beta$ is the platelet receptor for fibrinogen. Antibodies and other molecules that can block this receptor are now being used to treat non-ST segment elevation myocardial infarcts and unstable angina. L-selectin is found on neutrophils, monocytes and lymphocytes. It enables these cells to adhere to endothelium, facilitating migration to sites of inflammation. E-selectin and P-selectin occur on endothelium (P-selectin also on platelets) and are probably the binding sites for L-selectin.

Q2. RECEPTOR TYPES (☆☆☆)

1. B   2. E   3. C   4. A   5. D

Receptors are mediators of cell signalling. Receptors may be bound to the cell membrane (eg ligand gated ion channels, protein-tyrosine-kinase-mediated receptors, G-protein-coupled receptors) or may be able to migrate to the nucleus. Cell-membrane-bound receptors exert their effects via second messengers, whereas those that migrate to the nucleus usually affect gene expression directly. The nicotinic acetylcholine receptor consists of five non-covalently bound subunits that form a channel for sodium ions at the postsynaptic neuromuscular junction. When acetylcholine binds to the α-subunit, the complex undergoes conformational change and sodium ions pass into the cell causing depolarisation. The muscarinic acetylcholine receptor is a G-protein-coupled receptor consisting of three non-covalently bound subunits. In the resting state GDP is bound to the α-subunit. Following ligand binding and G protein activation, the α-subunit dissociates from the complex, allowing the β- and γ-subunits to interact with second messengers (eg cGMP). The α- and β-adrenergic receptors are also of this type. The insulin receptor is a protein-tyrosine-kinase-mediated receptor. The binding of insulin causes dimerisation of the receptor and autophosphorylation of the tyrosine residue. The resultant activation of tyrosine kinase activity phosphorylates cytoplasmic proteins, initiating an intracellular cascade leading to alterations in cell metabolism. Several growth factor receptors (eg IGF1) are of this type. Steroid hormone receptors bind corticosteroids, androgens, oestrogens, progesterone, vitamin D_3 and retinoic acid. The steroid hormone binds to an intracellular receptor and the hormone-receptor complex migrates to the nucleus. Here it binds to hormone response elements on DNA, altering the transcription of specific genes. Gene promoter elements can be thought of as receptors for transcription factors. The TATA box is a promoter element located 25 to 30 base pairs 5′ (upstream) of the start of transcription that binds RNA polymerase II. Transcription factors are proteins that bind to specific sequences of DNA. The tumour suppressor, p53, is a transcription factor.

Q3. SCREENING TESTS (☆☆)

1. B   2. F   3. A   4. E   5. C

The sensitivity of a test is its ability to correctly identify those with the disease. For example, a screening test for breast cancer that has a sensitivity of 90% will produce a negative test result in 10% of those with the disease. Specificity is the ability to correctly identify those who do not have the disease. If a test for breast cancer has a specificity of 90% then 10% of those who do not have disease will have a positive test result. Specificity and sensitivity are properties of the test itself and do not depend on the population prevalence of the disease. Positive predictive value (PPV) is the percentage of people who have a positive test result who have the disease. Negative predictive value (NPV) is the percentage of people who have a negative test who do not have the disease. These are more useful figures to know when interpreting the significance of an individual's test result. PPV and NPV are dependent on the prevalence of the disease in the population being tested. Imagine breast cancer is present in only one person per thousand being screened. After testing 1000 people approximately 100 subjects without breast cancer will have a positive result if the test specificity is 90%. The one person with

breast cancer in the total group has a 90% chance of testing positive. Among the approximately 101 positive results only one has breast cancer; therefore the PPV is <1%. PPV will be greater if the population disease prevalence is higher or if a test with greater specificity is used. Precision and validity are relevant to the measurements of quantitative variables. Precision is the ability to replicate a result on repeat testing. The result may not necessarily be correct however. For example, a machine measuring blood pressure may produce the same reading on a patient on three occasions but this may be consistently less than the true blood pressure. Validity is the ability to produce a correct result though there may be some variability in the measurement. For example, the blood pressure machine may record several different values on the same subject but the mean of these may be correct.

Q4. MONOCYTE-DERIVED CELLS (☆)

1. C   2. E   3. B   4. A   5. F

The monocyte/macrophage cell lineage includes a diverse group of circulating and tissue phagocytic cells. Langhans' giant cells result from fusion of macrophages. These large multinucleate cells are found in tuberculosis and other granulomatous conditions. Kupffer cells are the resident tissue macrophages lining the liver sinusoids. Microglia are highly specialised monocyte derivatives located in the parenchyma of the central nervous system. They have many structural differences from other macrophages. Dendritic cells are derivatives of Langerhan's cells found in lymph nodes and other tissues. They are potent antigen-presenting cells that can stimulate a primary immune response by interaction with naive T lymphocytes. Osteoclasts are multinucleate derivatives of mononuclear phagocytes that are important in bone resorption. Mast cells are polymorphonuclear cells and are not derivatives of the mononuclear/macrophage cell lineage.

Q5. MACROPHAGE MEMBRANE RECEPTORS (☆☆☆)

1. D   2. B   3. C   4. F   5. A

The FcR is a member of the immunoglobulin superfamily that binds to IgG and IgE constant regions. This enables opsonic phagocytosis of antibody-coated pathogens. The interleukin 10 receptor binds the cytokine IL 10, which is produced by T helper (Th$_2$) lymphocytes. IL 10 is anti-inflammatory and deactivates macrophages. Chemokine receptor 5 and CD4 are both required for entry of M-tropic strains of HIV into macrophages and dendritic cells. Syncytium-forming, T-tropic HIV enters T lymphocytes using CXCR4 and CD4. The normal function of these chemokine receptors is to bind intercellular messengers such as RANTES and monocyte chemotactic protein 1, which recruit monocytes to sites of inflammation. Stimulation of the interferon γ receptor produces increased expression of MHC class II and induces the nitric oxide respiratory burst (via inducible nitric oxide synthase, iNOS). Abnormalities of the interferon γ or interferon γ receptor genes result in increased susceptibility to atypical mycobacteria and *Salmonella* infections. Tumour necrosis factor (TNF) has widespread systemic effects including fever and shock as well as local effects on tissue macrophages. Stimulation of the macrophage TNF receptor results in granuloma formation, which is essential in controlling mycobacterial and other infections. MHC class I is ubiquitously expressed (ie not limited to cells of the immune system) and enables foreign antigens to be presented to cytotoxic T lymphocytes.

Q6. INHERITED DISEASE (☆☆)

1. C   2. F   3. D   4. B   5. A

Myotonic dystrophy and fragile X syndrome are due to expansion of trinucleotide repeat sequences affecting the *DM* and *FMR1* genes respectively. Why expansion of these repeats occurs is unknown. Hereditary motor and sensory neuropathy (HMSN) is also known as

Charcot-Marie-Tooth disease. HMSN type Ia is due to a 2-Mb duplication at 17p11.2, a region which includes the peripheral myelin protein 22 gene. Affected people develop pes cavus, clawed toes, foot drop and wasting of peroneal muscles producing a 'stork leg' appearance. HMSN I is a demyelinating disease and HMSN II is an axonal degeneration. Microdeletion of 22q11.2 can cause the DiGeorge syndrome or isolated cardiac malformations. DiGeorge syndrome is due to developmental malformation of the third and fourth branchial arches resulting in facial abnormalities, cardiac malformation, thymic aplasia and absence of the parathyroids (causing neonatal hypocalcaemia). Fifty per cent of cases of haemophilia A are due to chromosomal inversion of Xq. The breakpoint occurs within the haemophilia A gene, disrupting its function. A DNA sequence within intron 22 of the haemophilia A gene is similar to a sequence on the tip of Xq. Mispairing between these sequences at meiosis with the resultant formation of a chromosomal inversion occurs in 1 in 40,000 males born. Huntington's chorea is caused by a triplet repeat expansion on chromosome 4p.

Q7. PROBLEMS ASSOCIATED WITH INBORN ERRORS OF METABOLISM (☆☆☆)

1. C   2. D   3. F   4. E   5. A

Refsum's disease is a non-lysosomal storage disease in which phytanic acid accumulates due to deficiency of the peroxisomal enzyme, phytanic acid 2-hydroxylase. Symptoms commonly begin in the teenage years and include motor and sensory neuropathy, retinitis pigmentosa, nerve deafness, ichthyosis, cardiomyopathy and epiphysial dysplasia. Treatment is a chlorophyll-free diet. Acid maltase deficiency and myophosphorylase deficiency are glycogenoses types II and V respectively. The infantile form of deficiency of the lysosomal enzyme, acid maltase, is known as Pompe's disease and is usually fatal by age two years. There are also milder juvenile and adult-onset varieties. Presentation is with a progressive proximal myopathy and respiratory failure occurs secondary to diaphragmatic weakness. In glycogenosis type V, known as McArdle's disease, there is a failure to produce lactate in muscles. Patients usually have relatively mild symptoms such as exercise-induced muscle cramps but may develop myoglobinuria on strenuous exercise. Muscle biopsy and enzyme assay can be used to diagnose both of these glycogenoses. Hurler and Hunter syndromes are mucopolysaccharidosis types I and II respectively. The clinical features are very similar though the features are usually less severe in Hunter compared to Hurler syndrome. Children present with mental retardation and hydrocephalus, characteristic coarse facies with bushy eyebrows, a flat nasal bridge, broadly spaced teeth and hypertrichosis, hepatosplenomegaly and skeletal deformities. One distinguishing feature is that Hurler patients have corneal clouding and Hunter patients do not. The enzyme defect is alpha-L-iduronidase in Hurler and iduronate sulphate sulphatase in Hunter. In both conditions heparan and dermatan sulphate are found in the urine. All of the above inborn errors of metabolism are autosomal recessive except Hunter syndrome which is X-linked recessive. Phenylketonuria causes mental retardation and albinism.

Q8. NERVE SUPPLY (☆)

1. D   2. C   3. F   4. B   5. A

Deltoid is supplied by the axillary nerve. This nerve may be damaged by pressure in the axilla as used to occur with badly fitting crutches. Deltoid produces abduction of the shoulder. Trapezius and sternocleidomastoid are supplied by the accessory nerve (CN XI). Trapezius elevates the shoulder as occurs when shrugging the shoulders. All of the dorsal and palmar interossei and the third and fourth lumbricals are supplied by the ulnar nerve. The first and second lumbricals are supplied by the median nerve. Opponens pollicis and abductor pollicis

brevis are also supplied by the median nerve and flexor pollicis brevis receives innervation from both the median and ulnar nerves. The palmar interossei adduct the fingers and the dorsal interossei abduct them. The lumbricals produce flexion at the metacarpophalangeal joints with extension at the proximal interphalangeal joints. Brachioradialis is supplied by the radial nerve. It produces supination of the forearm when the elbow is flexed. The phrenic nerve supplies the diaphragm.

Q9. CEREBRAL CORTEX (☆)

1. C   2. B   3. A   4. F   5. D

The primary visual area is located in the posterior part of the calcarine sulcus of the occipital lobe. This receives afferent fibres from the lateral geniculate body via the optic radiation. The secondary visual area supplies the primary visual area and receives fibres from other parts of the cortex. This area relates visual images to past experiences enabling visual recognition. The postcentral gyrus of the parietal lobe is the primary somaesthetic area. The foot, leg and thigh are located on the most medial part and the pharynx, tongue and jaw on the most lateral part. The primary auditory area is the inferior wall of the lateral sulcus of the temporal lobe. Afferent fibres are received from the medial geniculate body via the auditory radiation of the internal capsule. The sensory speech area of Wernicke is located in the superior temporal gyrus and extends to the posterior end of the lateral sulcus and into the adjacent parietal region. It connects to Broca's motor area of speech (the posterior part of the inferior gyrus of the frontal lobe) by the arcuate fasciculus.

Q10. BILE (☆☆☆)

1. F   2. E   3. A   4. B   5. D

The principal components of bile are the primary bile acids (chenodeoxycholic acid and cholic acid), phospholipids and free cholesterol (non-esterified). Gallstones can be formed from bile acids or cholesterol. The rate-limiting enzyme in cholesterol synthesis is hydroxymethylglutaryl coA reductase, inhibitors of which (known as 'statins') are used to lower serum cholesterol. Primary bile acids are formed in the liver from the metabolism of cholesterol. The rate-limiting enzyme in this process is cholesterol 7α-hydroxylase. Primary bile acids are secreted into the bile and 95% re-circulate to the liver following reabsorption from the terminal ileum. The remainder pass into the colon and are metabolised by bacteria to the secondary bile acids deoxycholic and lithocholic acid. Lecithin is the principal phospholipid in bile. It is converted to lysolecithin in the small intestine by pancreatic phospholipase and is then reabsorbed. Lipoprotein lipase is involved in the metabolism of chylomicrons and very low density lipoproteins (VLDLs) not the constituents of bile. It progressively removes triglycerides from chylomicrons and VLDLs by hydrolysing them to fatty acids and glycerol.

Q11. BODY WATER (☆)

1. C   2. D   3. B   4. F   5. E

A non-obese, healthy, adult male is made up of approximately 60% water. A 75-kg male therefore contains around 45 kg of water in total. Two-thirds of this water is intracellular (30 kg) and one-third is extracellular (15 kg). Two-thirds of the extracellular component is found in the interstitial space (10 kg) and one-third in the blood (5 kg). Third space fluid (eg peritoneal or pleural fluid) contains a very small amount of water in the healthy subject but this may be markedly increased in disease states (eg cirrhosis, cardiac failure, nephrotic syndrome). Cell membranes are freely permeable to water and the osmolality of intracellular and extracellular fluid is the same (normally 290 mosmol/kg). The electrolyte composition of blood and interstitial fluid is similar but the intracellular compartment is very different. Sodium is the main extracellular cation, followed by calcium and potassium ions. Potassium is the main intracellular cation,

followed by magnesium and sodium. The main extracellular anion is chloride followed by bicarbonate and phosphate. The main intracellular anion is phosphate followed by bicarbonate and negatively charged proteins. It is important to remember these differences when examining blood results. A low serum potassium may represent a substantial total body depletion which may persist despite apparent initial correction of the serum value.

Q12. HORMONAL REGULATION OF SALT AND WATER HOMEOSTASIS (☆)

1. D   2. B   3. E   4. C   5. F

Humans have an extremely sensitive mechanism for maintaining sodium and water homeostasis. Sodium load is regulated most carefully with body water following changes in body sodium. In states of salt retention body water will usually rise to maintain a normal serum osmolality (290 mosmol/kg). The renin-angiotensin-aldosterone system works to retain sodium. Renin is released by the juxtaglomerular cells when the macula densa in the thick ascending limb detects a fall in sodium within the nephron. Renin catalyses the conversion of angiotensinogen to angiotensin I, which is then converted to angiotensin II by angiotensin-converting enzyme. Angiotensin II is a potent vasoconstrictor that increases blood pressure and stimulates aldosterone secretion from the zona glomerulosa cells of the adrenal glands. Aldosterone promotes sodium retention and potassium loss in the distal nephron. Human α-atrial natriuretic peptide (ANP) is released by the atria in response to atrial muscle distension. ANP decreases renin activity and thus decreases the circulating aldosterone concentration. This promotes sodium loss by the nephron. Antidiuretic hormone (ADH) is produced in the supraoptic and paraventricular nuclei in the hypothalamus and stored in the posterior pituitary. In response to a fall in intravascular volume ADH is released into the systemic circulation. It binds to the V_2 receptor in the renal collecting duct and stimulates concentration of urine to promote water retention. Adrenocorticotrophic hormone stimulates the release of corticosteroids from the adrenal glands. It is not directly involved in salt and water homeostasis although corticosteroids can cause salt and water retention.

Q13. PHYSIOLOGY OF BONE (☆☆)

1. F   2. B   3. A   4. C   5. D

Despite its inert and rigid appearance bone is a metabolically active tissue which undergoes continuous remodelling. The osteoblast synthesises type I collagen and other proteins such as osteocalcin, sialoproteins and phosphoproteins. The multinucleate osteoclast breaks down bone using Howship's resorption lacunae. Bone turnover is regulated by hormones and mechanical stresses. Calcitonin is produced by the C cells in the thyroid gland. It decreases bone resorption by suppressing osteoclast activity. Calcitonin's function may be to protect the skeleton from physiological stresses such as pregnancy and the adolescent growth spurt. Parathyroid hormone (PTH) increases bone resorption via indirect effects on the osteoblast. PTH also stimulates the conversion of 1α-hydroxyvitamin D_3 to 1,25-dihydroxyvitamin D_3 and increases calcium reabsorption from the kidney. 1,25-dihydroxyvitamin D_3 increases calcium absorption from the gut but its direct effects on bone physiology are poorly understood. The vitamin D receptor is expressed in many tissues and it may have widespread effects on cell growth and on regulation of the immune system. Alkaline phosphatase is produced by osteoblasts. Raised serum levels suggest increased osteoblast activity. However, alkaline phosphatase is also produced from the intestines and the placenta. Raised levels of alkaline phosphatase occur in pregnancy and liver disease. If there is uncertainty about the source of an elevated alkaline phosphatase the individual isoforms can be subtyped. Hydroxyproline is liberated during bone resorption and can be used as a marker of increased osteoclast activity. Levels are measured in urine and may be markedly elevated in conditions such as Paget's disease.

Q14. REGULATION OF CORONARY BLOOD FLOW (☆☆☆)

1. E   2. A   3. B   4. D   5. C

Coronary blood flow is matched to myocardial oxygen requirements by a complex interaction between metabolic, neurohumeral and local endothelial-cell-regulated control. This ensures adequate coronary arterial blood flow and consequent oxygen supply despite changes in aortic pressure and myocardial wall tension. Local coronary hypoxia results in coronary arteriole vasodilatation. An increase in carbon dioxide concentration has a similar effect. α-adrenergic and β-adrenergic receptors respectively mediate vasoconstriction and vasodilatation in the coronary circulation. Imbalance between these stimuli may be responsible for the coronary artery spasm which causes Prinzmetal's angina. Parasympathetic fibres may also be involved in the neurohumeral control of the coronary circulation. Endothelin 1 is a peptide containing 21 amino acids that stimulates vasoconstriction. Endothelin 1 release from endothelial cells is inhibited by nitric oxide and stimulated by angiotensin II, vasopressin and thrombin. Nitric oxide (formerly called endothelium-derived relaxing factor) is produced when endothelial nitric oxide synthase (eNOS) catalyses the conversion of L-arginine to L-citrulline. This occurs in response to increased shear stress on the vessel wall. Nitric oxide is a potent vasodilator, which is believed to be particularly important in the reflex vasodilatation that occurs after reperfusion. Regulators of nitric oxide are a subject of much current research in the hope that they could be used to limit the damage caused by myocardial infarction.

Q15. FIRST-TIME PRESENTATION OF RENAL FAILURE (☆☆)

1. F   2. E   3. A   4. B   5. C

Bilateral small kidneys on ultrasound scan suggest that renal failure is likely to be of chronic duration. In this situation renal biopsy is technically more difficult and unlikely to produce useful information to guide treatment. If renal osteodystrophy is present this also indicates that renal failure is chronic but this is rarely found at initial presentation. Anaemia, hypocalcaemia and hyperphosphataemia should not be regarded as evidence of chronic renal failure as they can also develop after renal failure of just a few days duration. Dilated renal calyces and ureters on ultrasound indicate urinary tract obstruction. This must be treated urgently (eg by bladder catheterisation or percutaneous nephrostomy) to avoid further renal damage. The presence of numerous red cell casts on urine microscopy is a typical finding in rapidly progressive glomerulonephritis. However, this is not diagnostic as red cell casts may also be seen in renal vasculitis, malignant hypertension and occasionally interstitial nephritis. In severe dehydration, hypotension or hepatorenal syndrome, oliguria/anuria is said to have a pre-renal cause. If the concentrating function of the kidneys is preserved, the urinary sodium is less than 20 mmol/l, urine osmolality is greater than 500 mosmol/kg and the urine-to-plasma creatinine ratio is greater than 40. In contrast once acute tubular necrosis has developed the urinary sodium is typically greater than 40 mmol/l, the urine osmolality is less than 350 mosmol/kg and the urine-to-plasma ratio is less than 20. Bence Jones protein is made up of immunoglobulin light chains. The finding of Bence Jones protein in the urine is suggestive of myeloma. This condition causes tubulointerstitial nephritis. Renal failure may also occur in myeloma because of hypercalcaemia and dehydration.

Q16. RISK FACTORS FOR ACUTE RENAL FAILURE (☆☆)

1. B   2. A   3. F   4. E   5. C

Haemoglobinuria can cause renal failure following acute intravascular haemolysis. This occurs in falciparum malaria, mismatched blood transfusions, severe burns and haemolytic crises in glucose-6-phosphate dehydrogenase deficiency. Myoglobinuria may occur following severe muscle damage. This can occur because of direct trauma to muscle, compression or occlusion of the blood supply, pressure on muscles in coma, uncontrolled contractions in status epilepticus, strenuous exercise (eg marathon running), polymyositis and neuroleptic malignant syndrome. Acute renal failure due to uric acid nephropathy occurs when massive cell death results in large amounts of uric acid release. This may occur when induction treatment is given for lymphoma, leukaemia, myeloma or other tumours with a very rapid turnover. The xanthine oxidase inhibitor allopurinol is usually given before commencement of treatment to try to prevent this. Following pharyngitis with certain serotypes of group A β-haemolytic streptococci, immunological reactions such as acute glomerulonephritis and rheumatic fever may occur. These conditions are now much less common in developed nations but remain a major cause of morbidity in resource-poor countries. Glomerulonephritis may also occur following cellulitis due to group A streptococci but rheumatic fever is not associated with this infection. Acute glomerulonephritis also occurs in association with antiglomerular basement membrane antibody disease, microscopic polyarteritis, Wegener's granulomatosis, infective endocarditis and ventriculoatrial cerebrospinal fluid shunts. Acute cortical necrosis is a rare cause of acute renal failure that is associated with several obstetric complications (eg postpartum haemorrhage, abruptio placentae, eclampsia and septic abortion), disseminated intravascular coagulation, Gram-negative septicaemia and pancreatitis. Acute interstitial nephritis is usually caused by drugs such as penicillins, sulphonamides, rifampicin, non-steroidal anti-inflammatory drugs and diuretics, septicaemia and sarcoidosis.

Q17. RENAL REPLACEMENT THERAPY (☆☆)

1. C   2. A   3. E   4. B   5. D

Continuous ambulatory peritoneal dialysis (CAPD) involves the manual exchange of 2 litres of dialysis fluid four or five times per day. Each replacement is performed approximately every four hours and is left unchanged for around eight hours at night. The fluid is hypertonic and removes around 1.5 litres of excess fluid from the body by an osmotic effect. This method gives patients great freedom from hospitals but does necessitate frequent exchanges, which some patients find inconvenient. Alternative methods of peritoneal dialysis have been developed using cycler machines that perform more rapid fluid exchanges. In continuous cyclic peritoneal dialysis the patient does not change the dialysis fluid during the day. At night the cycler exchanges fluid every one to two hours so that the same number of total exchanges can be achieved as in CAPD. In tidal intermittent peritoneal dialysis no dialysis is performed during the day and at night the cycler exchanges fluid very rapidly around 25 times in total. Intermittent peritoneal dialysis is performed in hospital over a 24-hour period usually only if home dialysis is not practicable. A cycler machine performs up to 40 exchanges over this time. This process requires repeating three times each week and places marked restrictions on the patient's lifestyle. Haemodialysis is performed on patients when peritoneal dialysis is impractical (eg in inflammatory bowel disease) or when there have been problems with peritonitis. Haemodialysis can be performed in a dialysis centre or in the patient's home. It is performed for four to eight hours, three times each week. Solute transfer is achieved by dialysis across a semipermeable, cellulose or synthetic membrane. Excess fluid is removed from the body by negative transmembrane pressure. Haemofiltration removes solute by filtration rather than diffusion and avoids contact with dialysis fluid. This method causes less cardiovascular strain than haemodialysis but is not as widely used because it is more expensive. Although it can be carried out intermittently like haemodialysis, it is most often used continuously in patients with acute renal failure on intensive care units.

Q18. REVERSIBLE RENAL FAILURE (☆)

1. F   2. C   3. A   4. B   5. D

In a patient with renal failure it is essential to identify any underlying reversible cause before further damage occurs. Several screening tests should be performed in all patients with renal failure of unknown aetiology, including blood glucose, autoantibody screen and renal ultrasound. Other more specialised tests (eg renal angiography) should be reserved for patients in whom there is a clinical suspicion of a particular disease. Ultrasound is useful to identify renal tract obstruction. This requires urgent intervention (eg by bladder catheterisation, ureteric stenting or percutaneous nephrostomy). Anti-dsDNA antibodies are a specific test for systemic lupus erythematosus, which can be treated with corticosteroids and immune-suppressants. cANCA is positive in patients with Wegener's granulomatosis, which may cause rapidly progressive glomerulonephritis. In polyarteritis nodosa, pANCA is more likely to be positive. Antiproteinase 3 antibodies are found in Wegener's and antimyeloperoxidase antibodies in polyarteritis nodosa. Polyarteritis nodosa affecting the kidneys may also be diagnosed by angiography by finding multiple aneurysms affecting the medium-sized renal and/or mesenteric arteries. Renal angiography is also useful to identify renal artery stenosis. Amyloidosis can be diagnosed by rectal or renal biopsy. Myeloma is diagnosed by the demonstration of a monoclonal band on serum protein electrophoresis and the presence of Bence Jones proteinuria. Skull X-rays may show multiple osteolytic lesions which are sometimes described as a 'pepperpot skull'.

Q19. ENDOCRINE DISEASE (☆☆)

1. D   2. C   3. E   4. F   5. B

Cushing's disease is adrenal hyperplasia and corticosteroid excess secondary to an ACTH-secreting pituitary tumour of corticotroph cells. Cushing's syndrome is corticosteroid excess from any cause. It can be caused by Cushing's disease, an adrenal adenoma or ectopic ACTH production. The commonest tumour producing ACTH is a malignant small cell carcinoma of the lung. Bronchial carcinoids produce serotonin (5HT) but occasionally produce ACTH. Primary adrenal failure is insufficient corticosteroid production despite adequate ACTH. The commonest cause in the developed world is autoimmune Addison's disease but worldwide it is tuberculosis. Many AIDS-related opportunistic infections can also result in adrenal failure. Less common causes of adrenal failure include lymphoma, amyloid, meningococcaemia, metastases, haemochromatosis and the rare hereditary conditions, adrenoleukodystrophy and adrenomyeloneuropathy. Secondary adrenal insufficiency is failure of the adrenal glands due to insufficient ACTH production. This can occur following a head injury, pituitary surgery, pituitary irradiation or postpartum pituitary infarction (Sheehan's syndrome). It may also be caused by a pituitary tumour, craniopharyngioma, metastases (eg from bronchial carcinoma), or granulomatous diseases (eg tuberculosis, sarcoid or histiocytosis X). Mineralocorticoid deficiency without corticosteroid deficiency can be produced by congenital adrenal hyperplasia, hyporeninaemic hypoaldosteronism or be secondary to angiotensin-converting enzyme inhibitors. Primary hyperaldosteronism is excess mineralocorticoid production by an adrenal adenoma (Conn's syndrome), primary adrenal hyperplasia, an aldosterone-producing adrenal carcinoma or the familial condition, glucocorticoid-suppressible hyperaldosteronism.

Q20. CUSHING'S SYNDROME (☆☆☆)

1. C   2. A   3. B   4. D   5. F

The 24-hour urinary cortisol test is a useful outpatient investigation for patients with suspected Cushing's syndrome. The disadvantage of this test is that the collection must be correctly timed and the instructions for this are not followed by all patients. An alternative test is the overnight dexamethasone suppression test. This test has high sensitivity but low specificity and should be confirmed by the 48-hour, inpatient, low-dose dexamethasone suppression test. In normal subjects administration of dexamethasone inhibits cortisol production and urinary free cortisol excretion but in patients with Cushing's syndrome it does not. Establishing the cause of Cushing's syndrome requires further tests. In ectopic ACTH syndrome and Cushing's disease, ACTH levels are inappropriately high for the simultaneously measured serum cortisol. In an adrenal adenoma ACTH is usually undetectable. Potassium levels are low in over 90% of patients with ectopic ACTH because there is increased mineralocorticoid production. Potassium is elevated in fewer than 10% of patients with Cushing's disease and is not elevated in those with corticosteroid-producing adrenal adenomas. The high-dose dexamethasone suppression test results in decreased production of cortisol and decreased excretion of urinary free cortisol in patients with Cushing's disease. Suppression of cortisol production does not occur with ectopic ACTH syndrome or an adrenal adenoma. Adrenal computed tomography can often identify adenomas but they may be mistaken for asymmetrical adrenal nodular hyperplasia in Cushing's disease. Adrenal scintigraphy distinguishes these conditions. An adrenal adenoma appears as a single hot nodule and there is no uptake by the contralateral suppressed adrenal. In nodular hyperplasia both adrenal glands show isotope uptake.

Q21. ENDOCRINE PROBLEMS CAUSED BY DRUGS AND DISEASE (☆☆☆)

1. F   2. C   3. D   4. A   5. B

Sarcoidosis can cause diabetes insipidus and/or hyperprolactinaemia when it affects the hypothalamus. It may also cause hypercalcaemia due to increased production of 1,25-dihydroxyvitamin D_3 by alveolar macrophages. This mechanism is also responsible for the hypercalcaemia that is occasionally seen in pulmonary tuberculosis, histoplasmosis and coccidioidomycosis. Hypoadrenalism is often seen in patients living with AIDS. This is probably due to damage by opportunistic infections such as cytomegalovirus, tuberculosis, other mycobacteria and fungal infections (eg *Cryptococcus neoformans*). Ketoconazole is a weak inhibitor of the adrenal enzyme 11β-hydroxylase. In those with low adrenal reserve it may precipitate hypoadrenalism but it is not a sufficient cause in those with normal adrenal function. AIDS patients also frequently suffer from low testosterone but the cause of this is uncertain. Amiodarone contains iodine and this can affect the thyroid in several different ways. Some patients treated with the drug become thyrotoxic, others become hypothyroid and some patients remain clinically euthyroid but have abnormal thyroid function test results (eg raised T_4). Haemochromatosis causes diabetes mellitus due to iron deposition in the pancreas. It also causes increased skin pigmentation, cardiac failure, cirrhosis and arthritis. Other secondary causes of diabetes mellitus include drugs (eg steroids and sympathomimetics) and genetic syndromes (eg acute intermittent porphyria and glycogen storage diseases). Hypoglycaemia can be caused by mesothelioma and other tumours derived from mesenchymal tissues (eg fibrosarcoma and leiomyosarcoma). It is believed to be caused by tumour production of insulin-like growth factor 2.

Q22. INTERSEX DISORDERS (☆☆☆)

1. E   2. D   3. A   4. B   5. C

The definition of a female pseudohermaphrodite is an individual with a 46XX genotype, normal ovaries and müllerian structures but virilisation of the external genitalia. 21-hydroxylase deficiency is the commonest cause of female pseudohermaphroditism, accounting for approximately 90% of cases. Salt depletion also occurs due to mineralocorticoid deficiency. An androgen-secreting adrenal adenoma in the mother (or fetus) can also cause severe virilisation of a female fetus but this is a rare cause. Male pseudohermaphroditism is defined as a 46XY genotype with the presence of testes but failure of development of external male genitalia. 17α-hydroxylase deficiency causes failure of the normal development of male external genitalia due to a lack of androgen production by the Leydig cells and adrenals. Males with 3β-hydroxysteroid dehydrogenase deficiency or Leydig cell hypoplasia have failure of external genitalia development for the same reason. 21-hydroxylase deficiency, 17α-hydroxylase deficiency and 3β-hydroxysteroid dehydrogenase deficiency are all forms of congenital adrenal hyperplasia. Male pseudohermaphroditism can also be caused by androgen insensitivity. In testicular feminisation syndrome this occurs because of defects in the androgen receptor and in 5α-reductase deficiency it is caused by a lack of dihydrotestosterone. In complete testicular feminisation syndrome the male pseudohermaphrodite may have the external appearance of a normal female. XY gonadal dysgenesis is caused by defective expression of the testicular determining factor gene carried on the Y chromosome. This produces a male pseudohermaphrodite with incomplete differentiation of the testes and consequent deficient production of testosterone and anti-müllerian hormone. The XX male syndrome does not fulfil the definition of pseudohermaphroditism. Affected individuals appear male but they may develop gynaecomastia and poor secondary sexual characteristics.

Q23. GASTROINTESTINAL DISORDERS (☆☆)

1. D   2. C   3. A   4. F   5. E

Peliosis hepatis is the presence of blood-filled cavities (sometimes called venous lakes) in the liver. These cavities are bordered by histiocytes and they can be drug-induced (eg anabolic steroids, azathioprine) or due to infection (*Bartonella henselae* or tuberculosis). Microvesicular steatosis is the presence of small lipid droplets throughout the liver. This may be accompanied by hepatitis, pancreatitis and renal failure. It is believed that the cause is inhibition of mitochondrial β-oxidation of fatty acids. Drugs that can cause this reaction include sodium valproate and tetracyclines. Pneumatosis cystoides intestinalis is the presence of multiple gas-filled cysts in the colon and occasionally the small intestine. It is associated with chronic obstructive lung disease, pyloric obstruction, mesenteric thrombosis and Whipple's disease. It is also seen in HIV patients with cryptosporidiosis. This condition may cause abdominal pain, diarrhoea and rectal bleeding. Malakoplakia is a rare, granulomatous disease affecting the urinary tract and occasionally the colon. Histology shows the presence of numerous periodic acid-Schiff (PAS)-positive histiocytes. The disorder is believed to be due to an inability of macrophages to destroy phagocytosed bacteria. When it affects the colon this condition presents with fever and diarrhoea. Ménétrier's disease is a severe protein-losing enteropathy with giant rugae in the gastric mucosa. Budd-Chiari syndrome is thrombosis of the hepatic vein. This can be caused by myeloproliferative disease or drugs (eg doxorubicin or the oral contraceptive).

Q24. JAUNDICE (☆☆☆)

1. D   2. A   3. E   4. B   5. F

Unconjugated hyperbilirubinaemia occurs if there is decreased uptake of bilirubin by the liver or decreased conjugation by uridine diphosphate glucuronyl transferase (UDPGT).

Conjugated hyperbilirubinaemia occurs if there is abnormal excretion of conjugated bilirubin or if there is biliary tract obstruction. Gilbert's syndrome is unconjugated hyperbilirubinaemia due to decreased hepatocyte uptake of bilirubin in the absence of liver disease or overt haemolysis. Characteristically the plasma bilirubin rises with fasting or after a diagnostic test dose of intravenous nicotinic acid. Crigler-Najjar syndrome is inherited deficiency of UDPGT. In type I Crigler-Najjar syndrome there is severe enzyme deficiency, which may cause fatal neonatal jaundice or severe kernicterus. Type II is a more variable condition that includes some cases resembling Gilbert's syndrome. Dubin-Johnson syndrome causes conjugated hyperbilirubinaemia and non-visualisation of the gallbladder on cholecystography. On the bromsulphthalein test there is a late peak at 90 minutes due to reflux of glutathione-conjugated bromsulphthalein. Liver biopsy shows pigment deposition and the urinary I:III coproporphyrin ratio is increased (total levels normal). Rotor's syndrome also causes conjugated hyperbilirubinaemia. The gallbladder can be visualised on cholecystography and there is no excess pigment in the liver. The bromsulphthalein test shows slow initial clearance but no late peak. Total urinary coproporphyrins are elevated and the I:III ratio is increased. In primary sclerosing cholangitis there are multiple strictures and bead-like dilatations of the intrahepatic and extrahepatic bile ducts. In primary biliary cirrhosis the bile ducts appear normal on endoscopic retrograde cholangiopancreatography.

Q25. SYSTEMIC CONDITIONS (☆☆)

1. F   2. D   3. A   4. E   5. B

Polyarteritis nodosa affects medium-sized blood vessels and classically causes aneurysms of the mesenteric and renal arteries. Mesenteric ischaemia leads to recurrent attacks of abdominal pain. Typically ischaemic pain occurs approximately two hours after a meal. Other features of polyarteritis nodosa include cutaneous vasculitic purpuric nodules, hypertension, renal failure and eosinophilia. Familial Mediterranean fever causes recurrent episodes of abdominal pain due to peritoneal inflammation. Patients may have had operations for a suspected acute abdomen without a cause being determined. Episodes of chest pain due to pleural inflammation and arthritis may also occur. Systemic sclerosis frequently affects the oesophagus, leading to progressive dysphagia, and the small intestine, leading to bacterial overgrowth and malabsorption. Henoch-Schönlein purpura (HSP) is an acute immunoglobulin A-mediated, autoimmune vasculitis which causes palpable purpura, glomerulonephropathy, polyarthritis and abdominal pain. Colonic intramural haematomas are a common feature of HSP and may cause bleeding per rectum or less commonly may lead to intussusception, bowel perforation or infarction. HSP usually resolves after a few days. Osler-Weber-Rendu syndrome is also known as hereditary haemorrhagic telangiectasia, an autosomal dominant condition. Recurrent gastrointestinal bleeds occur because telangiectases are found throughout the gastrointestinal tract. The diagnosis is usually suspected clinically because patients also have facial telangiectasia.

Q26. CIRRHOSIS (☆)

1. B   2. E   3. A   4. D   5. F

A large number of diseases can lead to cirrhosis. The detection of anti-smooth muscle antibodies suggests the diagnosis of autoimmune hepatitis (formerly called chronic active hepatitis). Antibodies against soluble liver antigen and double-stranded DNA may also be detected. Primary biliary cirrhosis is an autoimmune disease in which antimitochondrial antibodies are present. In particular the M2, M4, M8 and M9 types are found. This disease usually produces raised serum alkaline phosphatase and γ-glutamyl transferase. In Wilson's disease there is excess copper deposition due to deficiency of the serum copper transporter, caeruloplasmin. Copper

deposition predominantly affects the liver, causing cirrhosis, and the basal ganglia, causing an akinetic-rigid syndrome. The Kayser-Fleischer ring is caused by the deposition of copper in Descemet's membrane of the eye. Haemochromatosis is an abnormality of iron metabolism in which there is excess serum ferritin and excess iron deposition in the liver. α_1-antitrypsin deficiency affects the liver and the lungs. Severe emphysema may occur at an early age even in non-smokers. The Budd-Chiari syndrome is the name given to hepatic vein thrombosis. This can present suddenly with abdominal distension and pain.

Q27. HEREDITARY NEUROLOGICAL CONDITIONS (☆☆☆)

1. E   2. A   3. F   4. C   5. D

Friedreich's ataxia is an autosomal recessive condition that presents with progressive ataxia, upper motor neurone leg weakness, extensor plantar responses, depressed or absent deep tendon reflexes and loss of joint position sense. It presents in the second decade of life and after many years produces severe disability. Adrenoleukodystrophy is an X-linked condition causing widespread cerebral demyelination and adrenal hypofunction. Affected males develop dementia, cortical blindness, ataxia and spastic weakness. Fabry's disease is an X-linked recessive condition caused by lack of α-galactosidase. Presentation is usually with severe painful paraesthesia and mild peripheral neuropathy. Other neurological complications include cerebral infarcts and cerebral haemorrhage. There are widespread cutaneous telangiectases (angiokeratoma corporis diffusum) particularly around the lower part of the trunk and the thighs. Neurofibromatosis type 2 is an autosomal dominant condition that frequently causes bilateral acoustic neuromas. There may also be other cranial nerve tumours or tumours affecting the spinal nerve roots. Lesch-Nyhan syndrome is an X-linked condition caused by lack of hypoxanthine guanine phosphoribosyl transferase. This results in increased uric acid production, mental retardation, self-mutilation, choreoathetosis, limb spasticity and eventually death from renal failure. The adult-onset form of Gaucher's disease (glucocerebrosidase deficiency) causes hepatosplenomegaly and fractured neck of femur but it does not affect the nervous system.

Q28. SIGNS OF BRAIN LESIONS (☆)

1. C   2. E   3. F   4. B   5. D

Space-occupying lesions in the temporal lobe can lead to seizures that produce unusual hallucinatory symptoms affecting smell, taste, sound or the powerful impressions of déjà vu. Temporal lobe epilepsy is also associated with fugue states, psychosis, bouts of illogical fear and/or rage and hypersexuality. The classic field defect in temporal lobe lesions is a contralateral upper quadrantanopia. In contrast parietal lobe lesions characteristically produce a contralateral lower quadrantanopia. In addition there may be hemisensory loss, failure of two-point discrimination, astereognosis (inability to recognise objects by touch), sensory inattention and occasionally Gerstmann's syndrome. This eponym refers to the association of finger agnosia, right/left disorientation, dysgraphia and acalculia. In the occipital lobe the fibres of the optic radiation which have passed through the temporal and parietal lobes come together. A space-occupying lesion of the occipital lobe therefore produces a contralateral homonymous hemianopia. Midbrain lesions produce pupillary abnormalities and failure of downgaze. There may also be somnolence and loss of short-term memory with confabulation. Cerebellar lesions produce nystagmus, ataxia, dysdiadochokinesis, intention tremor and past-pointing on the finger-nose test.

Q29. INTRACRANIAL BRAIN TUMOURS (☆☆)

1. B   2. A   3. D   4. F   5. C

The commonest intracranial tumours are astrocytomas. These tumours may arise in the cerebral hemispheres, cerebellum or brainstem. Glioblastoma multiforme is the most rapidly growing form of astrocytoma and the prognosis is usually poor. Meningiomas arise from the arachnoid cap cells on the dural surface and occasionally in the lateral ventricles. They are usually benign tumours but may recur if not completely excised. Slow-growing meningiomas may become calcified. Schwannomas most commonly arise from the eighth cranial nerve (occasionally the fifth). The commonly used term 'acoustic neuroma' is really a misnomer as they arise from the nerve sheath not the neurone itself. These tumours are usually benign but they may grow large enough to cause significant pressure on surrounding structures producing a cerebellopontine angle syndrome. Schwannomas are a feature of neurofibromatosis. Craniopharyngioma is a tumour derived from the epithelial cell remnants of the pituitary stalk in the hypothalamus or third ventricle. This tumour may grow quite large and compress the optic nerves, optic chiasm or third ventricle (causing hydrocephalus) or pituitary (causing panhypopituitarism). Medulloblastomas usually occur in children. They most frequently arise in the fourth ventricle or cerebellar vermis. They are highly malignant and may even metastasise outside the central nervous system (eg to lymph nodes, bone marrow or bone). Ependymomas also occur in children, usually in the walls of the fourth or lateral ventricles. They are occasionally malignant and may metastasise throughout the central nervous system via the cerebrospinal fluid.

Q30. RISK FACTORS FOR NEUROPATHY (☆☆☆)

1. D   2. C   3. F   4. A   5. B

Many conditions cause an isolated median nerve palsy because of compression of the nerve in the carpal tunnel. In acromegaly this is probably caused by overgrowth of connective tissue. Less commonly acromegaly may cause a sensorimotor polyneuropathy due to thickening of neural connective tissues. Obturator nerve palsy can be caused by any condition compressing the nerve as it passes through the obturator foramen. The most common causes include obturator hernias and pelvic cancer (eg prostate cancer or cervical cancer). Patients complain of burning paraesthesia on the medial aspect of the thigh and have weakness of adduction of the hip. A third cranial nerve palsy with pupil sparing suggests a vascular cause (eg due to diabetes mellitus or vasculitis). When the pupil is involved (ie dilated), local destruction or compression (eg by posterior communicating artery aneurysm or raised intracranial pressure) of the nerve should be suspected. Diabetes mellitus causes many other neuropathies including mononeuritis multiplex, peripheral sensory neuropathy (can be severe enough to cause Charcot's joints), autonomic neuropathy and proximal amyotrophy. Lead poisoning causes a peripheral neuropathy predominantly affecting the motor fibres. Foot drop is a common feature. Lead poisoning also causes sideroblastic (microcytic) anaemia and a lead line on the gums. Cisplatin commonly causes ototoxicity with deafness and tinnitus. It may also cause a sensory neuropathy as may other anticancer drugs such as vincristine. Vitamin B$_{12}$ deficiency produces a distal sensory neuropathy and a myelopathy known as subacute combined degeneration of the cord.

Q31. RESPIRATORY CONDITIONS (☆☆)

1. B   2. F   3. D   4. E   5. C

The conditions listed all cause pulmonary granulomatous or vasculitic conditions. Churg-Strauss is an uncommon disease causing the triad of asthma, peripheral eosinophilia and systemic vasculitis. Patients may also have rhinitis, transient pulmonary infiltrates, non-cavitating pulmonary nodules, lymphadenopathy and a pleural effusion. On histology eosinophilic infiltrates are found in the lungs and other organs. Wegener's disease causes granulomas in the upper and lower respiratory tracts in association with focal necrotising glomerulonephritis. Patients

develop chest pain, haemoptysis, large cavitating pulmonary nodules, epistaxis, perforation of the nasal septum and saddle nose deformity. Necrotising sarcoid granulomatosis produces multiple non-cavitating small (often miliary) nodules with hilar lymphadenopathy. There is no associated systemic vasculitis or glomerulonephritis. In contrast to sarcoidosis histology shows that necrosis occurs within the giant cell granulomas. Typical features of bronchocentric granulomatosis include alveolar infiltrates involving a single lobe (which is most frequently the upper lobe). Pleural involvement and lymphadenopathy are not usually seen. The clinical features are usually not sufficiently specific to establish the diagnosis, which may not be suspected until histology shows necrotising granulomas surrounding the bronchi. Hughes-Stovin syndrome is an uncommon disease characterised by pulmonary artery aneurysms due to eosinophilic angiitis. It generally presents with haemoptysis following aneurysm rupture. Some patients also have glomerulonephritis. Behçet's syndrome may affect the lungs and this occasionally precedes the typical manifestations of oral and genital ulceration and uveitis. Pulmonary vasculitis leads to haemoptysis, cavitating infiltrates and focal or generalised fibrosis. Vena cava thrombosis may also occur leading to multiple pulmonary emboli.

Q32. HAEMOPTYSIS (☆☆)

1. D   2. A   3. F   4. B   5. C

Goodpasture's syndrome is the triad of pulmonary haemorrhage, glomerulonephritis and autoantibodies to the α3-chain of type IV collagen (antiglomerular basement membrane antibodies). On histology there are red cells and haemosiderin-laden macrophages in the alveoli but no evidence of vasculitis. A linear pattern of antibodies is detectable on the basement membrane of the alveoli and glomeruli but there is no immune complex deposition (in contrast to the systemic vasculitides). Idiopathic pulmonary haemosiderosis usually affects children and young adults. Children often present with acute severe haemoptysis but in adults there are usually recurrent episodes of small volumes of haemoptysis. Recurrent haemorrhage leads to progressive pulmonary fibrosis and iron-deficiency anaemia. The aetiology is uncertain and it seems likely that there may be multiple causes. Mitral stenosis is most commonly due to previous rheumatic fever. In the developed world rheumatic fever is much less common than previously and the majority of patients with mitral stenosis are therefore elderly. Mitral stenosis can lead to pulmonary hypertension. Haemoptysis occurs due to pulmonary oedema, pulmonary infarction or blood vessel rupture. There may be recurrent episodes of cough producing small volumes of blood or acute massive haemoptysis. Other features of mitral stenosis include a malar flush, decreased exercise tolerance, atrial fibrillation and angina. In systemic lupus erythematosus (SLE) acute pulmonary haemorrhage may complicate vasculitis-induced pneumonitis. The butterfly rash and facial telangiectasia are easily recognised features of SLE. Hereditary haemorrhagic telangiectasia is an autosomal dominant condition characterised by telangiectasia of the face, lips and mucus membranes of the nose, mouth, gastrointestinal tract, urinary tract and vagina. These cause recurrent episodes of bleeding particularly epistaxis and gastrointestinal haemorrhage. Patients may have an associated arteriovenous malformation of the lung, which can cause acute severe haemoptysis. A feeding vessel may be seen on CT scan or plain chest X-ray. The haemophilias frequently cause epistaxis but do not usually cause bleeding from the lower respiratory tract. Factor V-Leiden may cause haemoptysis secondary to pulmonary embolism.

Q33. RESPIRATORY DISEASE IN FARMERS (☆☆☆)

1. B   2. E   3. C   4. D   5. F

Extrinsic allergic alveolitis can be caused by many allergens including thermophilic actinomycetes, the cause of farmer's lung. Farmer's lung can present acutely a few hours after exposure to mouldy hay or insidiously where the relation to exposure may not be clear. The clinical presentation of acute farmer's lung is very similar to that of nitrogen dioxide pneumonitis and organic dust toxic syndrome. All three develop within ten hours of exposure to silo material and cause dry cough, breathlessness and general malaise. Acute farmer's lung is rarely life-threatening and responds to steroids. There is usually a history of recurrent attacks. Nitrogen dioxide pneumonitis is strongly correlated with toxic exposure in a confined space. The silo material has usually been stored much more recently than in farmer's lung or organic dust toxic syndrome and has undergone little microbial decomposition. Nitrogen dioxide pneumonitis may be life-threatening, shows little or no response to steroids and methaemoglobinaemia occurs. Organic dust toxic syndrome is caused by exposure to a fungal toxin from silage that has undergone marked microbial decomposition. Fungal hyphae are often found in respiratory secretions or on transbronchial lung biopsy. Steroids have no benefit and may be dangerous as they can occasionally result in invasive fungal pneumonia. Paraquat is a herbicide which is sometimes deliberately ingested in suicide attempts. Six grammes is a rapidly fatal dose causing vomiting, abdominal pain, diarrhoea, circulatory shock, metabolic acidosis, severe pneumonitis, seizures and coma. Death occurs within 48 hours. Lower doses cause progressive breathlessness due to pulmonary fibrosis (often eventually fatal) and painful ulceration of the oropharyngeal mucosa. Q fever is caused by *Coxiella burnetii*, a zoonosis which commonly affects farmers and abattoir workers. The bronchopneumonia is frequently accompanied by gastrointestinal symptoms and severe headache. There is often thrombocytosis and hepatitis. Cryptogenic fibrosing alveolitis may be confused with chronic extrinsic allergic alveolitis but it is usually easy to distinguish from the acute form of the disease.

Q34. RESPIRATORY SIDE-EFFECTS OF DRUGS (☆☆)

1. A   2. E   3. F   4. C   5. D

Hydrochlorothiazide causes acute pulmonary oedema by an idiosyncratic mechanism. Affected patients may be able to take other thiazide diuretics without problems. Other causes of acute pulmonary oedema include salicylates (usually in overdose), low molecular weight dextrans, naloxone and the uterine relaxants used to inhibit premature labour. The probability of alveolitis occurring in patients taking amiodarone depends on the dose and duration of administration. High doses must be avoided if possible as the drug's extremely long half-life makes the condition very difficult to reverse. Diffuse alveolitis can also be caused by high-flow oxygen (in premature neonates), nitrofurantoin and cytotoxic drugs such as busulfan, bleomycin and carmustine. Pulmonary infiltrates with peripheral eosinophilia can be caused by many drugs including sulphonamides, penicillins, aspirin, tetracyclines, naproxen, sulfasalazine and phenytoin. Methysergide causes pleural and retroperitoneal fibrosis. Asthma is commonly exacerbated by the physiological effects of drugs such as β-adrenoceptor blockers or cholinergic agents. This effect also occurs with the so-called cardioselective drugs (eg atenolol) and all β-blockers should therefore be avoided in asthma. Asthma can also be caused by idiosyncratic reactions to many drugs including aspirin, nitrofurantoin, penicillin, N-acetylcysteine and tartrazine-containing preparations. Between 10% and 20% of patients receiving angiotensin-converting enzyme (ACE) inhibitors (such as lisinopril) will develop a dry cough. This is believed to be due to inhibition of

the breakdown of prostaglandins. Less commonly ACE inhibitors may exacerbate asthma.

Q35. VASCULITIDES (☆☆)

1. C   2. D   3. B   4. F   5. E

Takayasu's arteritis and giant cell arteritis affect the large vessels and granulomas are found on histology. Takayasu's arteritis affects the thoracic aorta and can lead to aortic aneurysm formation and aortic dissection. Giant cell arteritis is the cause of temporal arteritis and polymyalgia rheumatica. Temporal arteritis is a serious condition that can cause blindness due to retinal artery infarction. Polyarteritis nodosa and Kawasaki disease affect the medium-sized vessels and granulomas are not seen. In polyarteritis nodosa, aneurysm formation and subsequent thrombosis may cause mesenteric, renal or cerebral infarcts. In Kawasaki disease aneurysms may develop in the coronary vessels predisposing to angina and myocardial infarction. Wegener's disease and Churg-Strauss syndrome affect the small vessels and granulomas are formed. Wegener's disease affects the upper and lower respiratory tracts and the kidneys. Churg-Strauss causes vasculitis with eosinophilia and asthma. Microscopic polyangiitis and Henoch-Schönlein purpura affect small vessels and granulomas are not seen. Microscopic polyangiitis is often a multisystem disease but it may affect a single organ (eg the kidney, gut or skin). Henoch-Schönlein purpura affects the kidney, gut and skin and distinctive immunoglobulin A deposition occurs. Scleroderma is a connective tissue disease rather than a classical vasculitic disorder.

Q36. DRUG THERAPY IN RHEUMATIC DISEASE (☆)

1. B   2. D   3. A   4. E   5. F

The frequency of attacks in chronic gouty arthritis can be reduced by allopurinol, a xanthine oxidase inhibitor that reduces uric acid production. Alternatively a uricosuric drug such as the non-steroidal anti-inflammatory drug azapropazone can be used to increase uric acid excretion. During an acute attack of gout allopurinol should not be used. Treatment with colchicine, a mitotic spindle inhibitor, usually halts the attack. Failure to respond suggests the possibility of an alternative diagnosis. However, improvement with colchicine is not proof of gout as other crystal-associated arthropathies will improve with this therapy. The disease-modifying drugs used in the treatment of rheumatoid arthritis include gold, penicillamine, hydroxychloroquine and sulfasalazine. For severe disease immunosuppressive agents such as methotrexate or azathioprine and cyclophosphamide may be used but corticosteroids should be avoided if possible. Whipple's disease is a systemic disorder characterised by diarrhoea, wasting, inflammatory arthritis and central nervous system disease. Intestinal biopsy reveals PAS-positive macrophages. It is now known that this condition is caused by infection with a Gram-negative bacillus called *Tropheryma whippelii*. Treatment is with penicillin, a tetracycline or a macrolide. Giant cell arteritis (or temporal arteritis) is a serious condition that can rapidly lead to blindness due to retinal infarction. High-dose corticosteroids must be given rapidly to prevent this occurring. Osteoarthritis is treated with analgesics and non-steroidal anti-inflammatory drugs.

Q37. BLISTERING CONDITIONS (☆☆)

1. F   2. D   3. C   4. B   5. A

Chronic blistering diseases can be divided into those that are autoimmune in nature and those that are due to structural disorders. The autoimmune diseases include bullous pemphigoid, pemphigus vulgaris and dermatitis herpetiformis. In bullous pemphigoid, immunoglobulin G autoantibodies are produced against the 180-kDa or 230-kDa hemidesmosomal proteins which anchor basal cells to the basement membrane. This results in a subepidermal split occurring through the basement membrane. Bullous pemphigoid

produces tense, sometimes blood-filled blisters, typically in those over 60 years old. Mucosal involvement is rare. In pemphigus vulgaris, immunoglobulin G autoantibodies are produced against the desmosomal protein dsg3. This produces a superficial intraepidermal split just above the basal layer. The superficial blisters burst easily and rarely remain intact. Mucosal involvement is common. In dermatitis herpetiformis subepidermal blistering occurs with microabscesses in the dermal papillae. Patchy granular immunoglobulin A deposition occurs at the basement membrane. Other autoimmune blistering diseases include pemphigus foliaceus, where the split is in the superficial epidermis, and linear immunoglobulin A disease, where the split is subepidermal. Mechanical bullous disorders are due to inherited defects in anchoring proteins. In epidermolysis bullosa simplex, autosomal dominantly inherited mutations have been found in proteins such as the K5 and K14 keratin filaments and in plectin. These mutations result in a split at the subepidermal level. The diseases are generally mild and do not involve the teeth or nails. In junctional epidermolysis bullosa there is a split in the lamina lucida due to mutations in laminin 5 or $\alpha_6\beta_4$ integrin. These autosomal recessive disorders are severe and many variants are fatal soon after birth. Abnormalities of the nails and teeth are usually seen.

Q38. HISTOLOGY OF SKIN DISEASE (☆)

1. C   2. D   3. F   4. B   5. A

Hyperkeratosis is thickening of the horny layer of the skin due to increased adhesion of epidermal cells. This is most commonly seen in acne vulgaris. In normal skin keratinocytes lose their nuclei as they pass through the horny layer to the skin surface. Parakeratosis refers to the presence of nuclei throughout the cells of the horny layer. This occurs in diseases where there is rapid turnover of skin such as psoriasis. Spongiosis is the separation of prickle cells by oedema. This occurs in cutaneous inflammation such as in eczema. In normal skin prickle cells are held together by desmosomal proteins. In some types of epidermolysis bullosa there are inherited defects in desmosomal proteins and in pemphigus vulgaris there are antibodies produced against desmosomal proteins. These diseases therefore result in loss of adhesion between prickle cells, a phenomenon known as acantholysis. Liquefaction is the degeneration and rupture of basal cells, a feature of several skin diseases including erythema multiforme, lichen planus and lupus erythematosus. Necrobiosis is the presence of macrophages lined up around a central area of collagen necrosis.

Q39. PARAPROTEINAEMIAS (☆☆)

1. E   2. A   3. B   4. F   5. D

Multiple myeloma is the commonest cause of clonal paraproteinaemia, accounting for 60% of cases. This condition is characterised by excess immunoglobulin G (less commonly A or D or light chains) in serum, Bence Jones proteinuria (light chains in urine) and lytic bone lesions, anaemia and a raised ESR. Waldenström's macroglobulinaemia is excess production of monoclonal immunoglobulin M. Marked hyperviscosity results, predisposing to thrombosis, chronic bleeding and retinal haemorrhage. There are no lytic bone lesions in this condition, which makes up approximately 10% of clonal paraproteinaemias. Heavy chain disease is rare, accounting for less than 1% of paraproteinaemias. Excess heavy chains (of which there are α, γ and μ variants) are found in serum and urine but there are no excess light chains. Monoclonal gammopathy of undetermined significance (MGUS) refers to raised serum paraprotein (usually less than 2 g/l) in the absence of Bence Jones proteinuria, anaemia and skeletal lesions. A proportion of subjects will eventually develop multiple myeloma so the older term 'benign monoclonal gammopathy' is not appropriate. MGUS accounts for approximately 20% of clonal paraproteinaemias. Primary

amyloidosis is the presence of excess light chains in the serum and/or urine without an underlying cause being identified. λ light chains are found more commonly than κ. Patients frequently develop nephrotic syndrome. Around 20% of patients have hepatomegaly and 10% have macroglossia. Cryoglobulinaemia refers to excess proteins, which precipitate when cooled and resuspend when warmed. Type I cryoglobulinaemia consists of monoclonal immunoglobulin M or G. Type II is monoclonal immunoglobulin M with polyclonal immunoglobulin G. Type III is polyclonal immunoglobulin only.

Q40. BLOOD DISORDERS (☆☆)

1. F   2. B   3. A   4. C   5. E

The triad of anaemia, thrombocytopenia and haemorrhage can be caused by any of the conditions listed above. Haemolytic uraemic syndrome (HUS) is a microangiopathic haemolytic anaemia with mild thrombocytopenia, which is often associated with *Escherichia coli* O157 infection and generally affects children. Renal failure is a prominent feature and neurological abnormalities are not usually found. Thrombotic thrombocytopaenic purpura (TTP) is a similar condition usually affecting adults. In contrast to HUS, neurological abnormalities are seen in >90% of patients and initial renal impairment is generally mild. In HUS and TTP numerous schistocytes are seen on the blood film. Disseminated intravascular coagulation is a condition that frequently complicates septicaemia, malignancy, obstetric emergencies (eg placenta praevia or amniotic fluid embolus), liver failure and transfusion of incompatible blood. Clotting tests such as APTT are much more abnormal than in the other conditions. In liver failure there is depletion of the vitamin-K-dependent clotting factors (II, VII, IX and X) and failure to remove fibrin and tissue plasminogen activator. Cirrhosis may also lead to thrombocytopenia due to reduced production of thrombopoietin. In renal failure there is anaemia due to failure of erythropoietin production. The bleeding tendency is also increased perhaps because of increased prostacyclin production, decreased thromboxane production and impairment of platelet activation. Evans' syndrome is the combination of autoimmune thrombocytopaenia and Coombs' positive haemolytic anaemia.

Q41. BLOOD FILM ABNORMALITIES (☆☆)

1. E   2. A   3. F   4. C   5. B

Causes of a marked peripheral eosinophilia include the larval migratory stage of helminths (such as *Ascaris lumbricoides*, *Ankylostoma duodenale* and *Strongyloides stercoralis*), *Toxocara* infection, cysticercosis, aspergillosis, polyarteritis nodosa (and Churg-Strauss syndrome) and Löffler's syndrome. Marked basophilia is an uncommon finding which may be seen in urticaria pigmentosa and systemic mastocytosis. Severe allergies and hypothyroidism may cause a less marked basophilia. Acute myeloid leukaemia type M5 is also known as 'acute monocytic leukaemia with differentiation'. Monocytosis also occurs in brucellosis, endocarditis and tuberculosis. A lymphocytosis may also be seen in these conditions. Neutrophilia occurs in bacterial infections (eg pneumococcal pneumonia), malignancy, haemorrhage and with corticosteroid use. Although neutrophilia is the expected finding in acute bacterial infections, if there is overwhelming septicaemia, neutropenia may occur. Neutropenia is also seen in viral infections such as influenza, infectious mononucleosis and viral hepatitis and in some bacterial infections such as typhoid fever and brucellosis.

Q42. HUMAN PATHOGENS (☆☆)

1. A   2. E   3. F   4. C   5. B

Granulomatous amoebic encephalitis can be caused by six species of *Acanthamoeba* and by *Balamuthia mandrillaris*. Unlike *Naegleria fowleri* these free-living amoebae are not associated with swimming. *Acanthamoeba* infects humans through skin ulcers or the lungs and spreads haematogenously to the brain. Treatment is difficult and survival is rare. *Cyclospora cayetanensis* is usually acquired from drinking contaminated water, but outbreaks have also been associated with fresh produce. In 1996, 1465 people in Canada and the USA were infected following importation of infected raspberries from Guatemala. *Leishmania donovani* is a flagellate although its flagellated form, the promastigote, is found in sandflies. The form found in humans is the intracellular amastigote. *Balantidium coli* is the only ciliate to infect humans. The trophozoites are large, occasionally up to 200 μm in length. Many patients are asymptomatic but diarrhoea, colitis and severe dysentery can occur. Extraintestinal invasion has been described but is extremely rare. *Dientamoeba fragilis* is a flagellate without a flagellum. Its presence has been associated with diarrhoea and irritable bowel syndrome but its true significance remains uncertain. *Cryptococcus neoformans* is a yeast that causes meningitis in patients with AIDS.

Q43. HUMAN HERPES VIRUSES (☆☆)

1. C   2. A   3. D   4. B   5. E

The herpes viruses are DNA viruses that can lie dormant in the human body and become reactivated during times of stress, illness or immune suppression. Primary infection with herpes simplex virus 1 usually causes a mild vesicular facial rash with oral stomatitis. However, in children there may be gingivostomatitis that is so severe it is mistaken for Vincent's angina and in adults there may be a severe pharyngitis with fever, lymphadenopathy and splenomegaly. Serious consequences of herpes simplex virus 1 infection include acute necrotising encephalitis and a destructive keratitis with dendritic ulcers. Herpes zoster virus causes chicken pox and shingles. Chicken pox is usually a mild illness but a severe and potentially fatal pneumonia may occur particularly when infection occurs during pregnancy. Encephalitis is not uncommon but it is much less serious than that caused by herpes simplex 1. Recurrence of this virus causes painful vesicular lesions restricted to one or two dermatomes. Herpes zoster of the ophthalmic branch of the trigeminal nerve can cause a destructive keratitis. Herpes zoster is also the commonest viral cause of acute retinal necrosis in the immunocompetent host. This serious condition is not accompanied by cutaneous vesicles. Epstein-Barr virus is the cause of infectious mononucleosis. This virus is also associated with several malignancies including endemic Burkitt's lymphoma (a distinct condition from Burkitt-type acute lymphoblastic leukaemia seen in the developed World), non-Hodgkin's lymphoma seen in the immunocompromised host and nasopharyngeal carcinoma. It is also the cause of oral hairy leukoplakia, which is seen in patients with HIV. Cytomegalovirus causes an infectious mononucleosis-like illness when acquired by adolescents or adults. Perinatal infection causes microcephaly, mental retardation, deafness, jaundice, petechiae and intrauterine growth retardation. Complications of cytomegalovirus infection in the immunocompetent adult include Guillain-Barré syndrome, myocarditis and pneumonitis. In the immunocompromised, particularly HIV patients and transplant recipients, cytomegalovirus may cause pneumonitis, gastrointestinal ulcers and chorioretinitis. Human herpes virus type 6 causes roseola infantum, a common febrile childhood illness. In bone marrow transplant recipients it may reactivate, causing a disease resembling graft-versus-host disease. Human herpes virus type 8 is the cause of Kaposi's sarcoma.

Q44. VIRUSES (✩✩)

1. F   2. A   3. E   4. B   5. D

Viruses are classified by whether they contain RNA or DNA, their capsid structure, size and the presence of an envelope. The following viral families include human pathogens:

RNA-containing viruses

- Picornaviridae, eg polio virus and hepatitis A virus
- Caliciviridae, eg Norwalk virus and hepatitis E virus
- Astroviridae, eg astrovirus
- Togaviridae, eg rubella virus, Ross River virus and the equine encephalitis viruses
- Flaviviridae, eg yellow fever virus, dengue virus, hepatitis C virus, Japanese encephalitis virus, West Nile encephalitis virus, tick-borne encephalitis virus
- Coronaviridae, eg coronavirus
- Rhabdoviridae, eg rabies virus
- Filoviridae, eg Marburg and Ebola viruses
- Paramyxoviruses, eg measles virus, parainfluenza viruses
- Orthomyxoviridae, eg influenza viruses types A, B, C
- Bunyaviridae, eg Congo-Crimea haemorrhagic fever virus, Rift Valley fever virus, Hantavirus
- Arenaviridae, eg lymphocytic choriomeningitis virus, South American haemorrhagic fever viruses
- Reoviridae, eg rotavirus and Colorado tick fever
- Retroviridae, eg HIV, HTLVI and HTLVII

DNA-containing viruses

- Hepadnaviridae, eg hepatitis B virus
- Parvoviridae, eg parvovirus B19
- Papovaviridae, eg human papilloma virus and JC polyoma virus
- Adenoviridae, eg adenovirus
- Herpesviridae, eg herpes simplex viruses, herpes zoster virus, cytomegalovirus, Epstein-Barr virus
- Poxviridae, eg vaccinia or smallpox virus

Q45. ROUTES OF ACQUISITION OF PLATYHELMINTH INFECTION (✩✩✩)

1. C   2. E   3. D   4. F   5. B

At least eight different species of *Paragonimus* infect human lungs, the commonest of which is the oriental lung fluke, *P. westermani*. This parasite is acquired by ingesting the flesh or juice of raw, undercooked or pickled crabs and crayfish in China, South East Asia, India and some Pacific islands. Heavy infections resemble pulmonary tuberculosis with chest pain, cough, night sweats and haemoptysis. *Fasciola hepatica* is a parasite of sheep and is widespread. Human infection occurs after ingestion of watercress that has been contaminated by sheep's faeces. *F. hepatica* lives in the bile ducts and heavy infections may cause obstructive jaundice. Hepatitis may develop during acute infection when parasitic larvae migrate through the liver. *Fasciolopsis buski* is a parasite of the pig and buffalo and is found in China and South East Asia. Eating raw water chestnuts, water caltrop and other edible plants leads to infection developing in the human small intestine. Heavy infection may cause diarrhoea and abdominal pain often accompanied by eosinophilia and allergic skin reactions. *Clonorchis sinensis* is acquired by ingestion of raw or undercooked fish in China, South Korea, Vietnam and other Far Eastern countries. The parasite lives in the bile ducts and can lead to biliary tract obstruction and cholangiocarcinoma. *Schistosoma haematobium* infects humans when the free-swimming cercaria penetrates human skin. After migration to the lungs and along the portal circulation the adult worms eventually develop in the veins surrounding the urinary tract. This leads to haematuria, bladder stone formation, bladder fibrosis and bladder carcinoma. These trematodes are all treated with praziquantel except *F. hepatica*, which is treated with bithionol. Mosquitoes spread *Wuchereria bancrofti* and *Brugia malayi*, the causes of lymphatic filariasis.

Q46. ANTIBIOTIC THERAPY (☆☆)

1. E   2. A   3. C   4. B   5. D

Enterotoxigenic *Escherichia coli* is the commonest identified bacterial cause of traveller's diarrhoea. Empirical treatment with a single dose of ciprofloxacin (1 g) reduces symptom duration. Epididymo-orchitis in those under 35 years old can be due to *Neisseria gonorrhoea* or *Chlamydia trachomatis* and is treated with a single dose of intramuscular ceftriaxone and ten days of doxycycline. If the patient practises anal intercourse or is over 35 years old, coliforms are the most likely cause and treatment with a fluoroquinolone is recommended. The symptoms experienced by the HIV patient are suggestive of *Pneumocystis carinii* pneumonia and first-line therapy is with co-trimoxazole. For severe disease, the addition of steroids reduces mortality. Note that the Committee on Safety of Medicines recommends co-trimoxazole should not be used for urinary tract and other straightforward infections. The patient with a purulent discharge has non-gonococcal urethritis and treatment with doxycycline alone is appropriate. Epiglottitis in a child vaccinated against *Haemophilus influenzae* group B is likely due to *Streptococcus pyogenes* or *S. pneumoniae* and ceftriaxone is suitable treatment. Metronidazole is useful treatment for giardiasis and amoebiasis, but these protozoa do not cause watery diarrhoea.

Q47. TOPICAL EYE PREPARATIONS (☆☆)

1. B   2. A   3. F   4. C   5. E

Pilocarpine is a miotic that causes contraction of the ciliary muscle and promotes drainage in the trabecular meshwork. It is used to reduce intraocular pressure in open-angle glaucoma. Dipivefrine is a pro-drug of adrenaline. It decreases aqueous humour production and increases trabecular drainage. It is used in open-angle glaucoma but as it is a mydriatic it should not be used in closed-angle glaucoma, unless an iridectomy has been performed. Timolol is a β-blocker that reduces the production of aqueous humour. β-blockers are usually the first drugs used in the treatment of open-angle glaucoma. After surgery they are the preferred drugs as miotics may cause formation of posterior synechiae. Topical β-blockers can exert systemic effects that can be potentially hazardous in asthma, heart block, bradycardia or cardiac failure. Atropine is a muscarinic drug used as a mydriatic in the treatment of iridocyclitis to prevent the formation of posterior synechiae. After administration of a single dose, its effects may last up to seven days. It may however precipitate closed-angle glaucoma. Nedocromil sodium is a mast cell stabiliser that is used in the treatment of allergic conjunctivitis. Local anaesthetics used for eye procedures include amethocaine, lignocaine and oxybuprocaine.

Q48. ANTINAUSEA DRUGS (☆☆)

1. E   2. C   3. D   4. B   5. F

Prochlorperazine, like other phenothiazines, acts centrally on the chemoreceptor trigger zone. It is useful for nausea associated with general anaesthetics, neoplastic disease, use of opioids, radiation treatment and cytotoxic drugs. It is not effective in motion sickness. There is a risk of acute dystonic reactions particularly in the very young and very old. It is not appropriate treatment for non-specific symptoms of dizziness in the elderly, although it is unfortunately often prescribed in this situation. Nabilone is a synthetic cannabinoid that is reported to be more effective than prochlorperazine in the relief of nausea. It has a relatively high incidence of side-effects such as difficulty concentrating, dysphoria, behavioural changes and occasionally hallucinations. Ondansetron and the related drugs, granisetron and tropisetron, are selective serotonin inhibitors acting at $5HT_3$ receptors. They are potent antiemetics and are particularly useful for severe nausea induced by cytotoxic chemotherapy. Hyoscine hydrobromide is an antimuscarinic agent that is very effective for prevention of motion sickness. It can be administered transcutaneously by use of a skin patch applied approximately one hour before commencing a journey. Cyclizine is an antihistamine that acts on the emetic centre. It is a useful treatment for motion sickness, nausea associated with vestibular and labyrinthine disorders. Dexamethasone is a potent glucocorticoid used in combination with other antiemetics for cytotoxic drugs that cause severe vomiting.

Q49. HYPNOTIC/ANXIOLYTIC DRUGS (☆☆☆)

1. E   2. B   3. C   4. A   5. D

Short-acting benzodiazepines, such as temazepam, have fewer hangover effects and are more suitable for insomnia. Long-acting drugs, such as diazepam, are useful in patients who have anxiety persisting into the daytime. When benzodiazepines are discontinued, withdrawal symptoms often occur and these are most severe with drugs that have a shorter duration of action. Benzodiazepines should only be used for the short-term treatment of severe insomnia or severe, disabling anxiety. Unfortunately, benzodiazepine dependence is common and drug withdrawal can be difficult. It is best achieved by converting the benzodiazepine used to an equivalent dose of diazepam and reducing the daily dose by 2–2.5 mg every two weeks. It may take up to a year to withdraw the drug in some patients. Chlormethiazole is a hypnotic with a short duration of action which is less likely to cause hangover than most benzodiazepines. It is only licensed for use as a hypnotic in the elderly. Three new hypnotics are now available, zopiclone (a cyclopyrrolone), zolpidem (an imidazopyridine) and zaleplon (a pyrazolopyrimidine). These drugs act at benzodiazepine receptor subtypes and have a short duration of action. Although said to have less dependence potential, withdrawal symptoms have been described. Buspirone is an anxiolytic that acts as a partial agonist at $5HT_1$ receptors. It does not relieve the effects of benzodiazepine withdrawal. Use of barbiturates such as amylobarbitone and sodium amytal should only be prescribed for patients who are already taking them. A withdrawal program should be commenced with specialist help.

Q50. β-ADRENOCEPTOR BLOCKERS (☆☆☆)

1. F   2. A   3. B   4. E   5. C

β-adrenoceptor antagonists are useful in the treatment of acute coronary syndromes, angina, hypertension, tachycardia and many other conditions. They may cause a wide range of side-effects including bronchoconstriction, cold extremities, sleep disturbance, headache and fatigue. Relatively water-soluble β-blockers have fewer central nervous system effects as little drug crosses the blood-brain barrier. Cardioselective drugs, such as atenolol and metoprolol, are less likely to cause bronchoconstriction but they do have some β_2-antagonist activity and are still potentially hazardous in asthma. Propranolol has non-cardioselective action and crosses the blood-brain barrier. It is licensed for a wide range of uses including treatment of thyrotoxicosis, phaeochromocytoma, portal hypertension, anxiety states, palpitations, arrhythmias, essential tremor and prophylaxis against migraine. Oxprenolol and celiprolol have intrinsic sympathomimetic activity and are said to cause less bradycardia and coldness of extremities than other β-blockers. Esmolol has a half-life of only a few minutes and is useful for treatment of narrow complex tachycardias and hypertension especially in the perioperative period or following an acute myocardial infarction. Sotalol has class III antiarrhythmic activity and is used in the prophylaxis of paroxysmal supraventricular tachycardia. Although β-blockers may worsen heart failure, bisoprolol, metoprolol and carvedilol have been shown to be cardioprotective when used to treat this condition. They should only be used under specialist supervision. Labetalol has combined α- and β-adrenoceptor blocking activity and is used to treat malignant hypertension.

Q51. SIDE-EFFECTS OF RESPIRATORY DRUGS (☆☆)

1. B   2. D   3. E   4. F   5. A

Ipratropium is an antimuscarinic agent that can precipitate acute closed-angle glaucoma when administered by nebuliser, particularly if given with salbutamol. A well-fitting mask that prevents leakage of the nebulised drug reduces this risk. Salbutamol can cause severe hypokalaemia particularly if administered

systemically. This risk is increased in those taking theophylline, which can also cause hypokalaemia. Doxapram is a respiratory stimulant that is sometimes used in type II respiratory failure. It often causes a feeling of intense perineal warmth that can be very unpleasant for the patient. Doxapram use can be hazardous, as it stimulates non-respiratory as well as respiratory muscles and can therefore increase oxygen requirements. Monthly nebulised pentamidine is used to prevent *Pneumocystis carinii* pneumonia in HIV patients who are allergic to co-trimoxazole (the first-line choice) with a CD4 count <200×10^6 per litre. It frequently causes bronchoconstriction and administration should therefore be preceded by nebulised salbutamol to prevent this. Hypoglycaemia is a complication of intravenous but not nebulised pentamidine. Montelukast and zafirlukast are leukotriene receptor antagonists. Their place in managing chronic asthma and the timing of their introduction relative to long-acting β_2-agonists is still being investigated. An association between their use and the development of Churg-Strauss syndrome has been found, but whether this is causal is uncertain. The Committee on Safety of Medicines advises that clinicians using these drugs should be alert to the development of eosinophilia, vasculitic rash, peripheral neuropathy, increased pulmonary symptoms and cardiac complications.

Q52. ACUTE POISONING (☆☆)

1. B   2. F   3. D   4. C   5. A

Ingestion of concentrated paraquat causes severe mucosal blistering and several days later a proliferative alveolitis develops. In acute ingestion, absorption can be decreased by the oral administration of Fuller's earth. Ethylene glycol is metabolised to oxalic acid and other organic acids and can cause severe metabolic acidosis. Elimination can be increased by haemodialysis. Carbon monoxide competes with oxygen for binding sites on haemoglobin and therefore inhalational poisoning causes acute hypoxia. The development of cerebral oedema is treated with intravenous mannitol. Hyperbaric oxygen should be considered if the patient has been unconscious or has a carboxyhaemoglobin concentration >20%. Iron poisoning is usually seen in children following accidental ingestion. Abdominal pain, nausea, vomiting, haematemesis and diarrhoea may be followed by hypotension, hepatocellular necrosis and coma. Parenteral desferrioxamine is used to bind excess iron in acute severe poisoning. The antimalarial drug quinine causes cinchonism in overdose. This dangerous condition includes tinnitus, hypoglycaemia, intravascular coagulation, cardiac arrhythmias and blindness. Theophylline overdose causes hypokalaemia, cardiac arrhythmias and seizures.

Q53. BACTERIAL ENDOCARDITIS (☆☆)

1. D   2. F   3. B   4. E   5. A

The diagnosis of endocarditis is made using the Duke criteria, which rely mainly on the observation of vegetations on echocardiography and positive blood cultures. The clinical findings accompanying endocarditis are mostly minor criteria which may sometimes help establish the diagnosis. Roth spots are fundal haemorrhages with a central pale area. They are probably caused by immune-complex deposition and are different from the original lesions described by Roth, which were larger and were due to septicaemia. Osler's nodes are circumscribed, indurated, erythematous, tender nodules that mostly occur on the pulps of the fingers and toes. They are also seen on the thenar and hypothenar eminences and on the sides of the fingers. Janeway lesions are transient, non-tender macules that occur on the palms and soles particularly on the thenar and hypothenar eminences. Petechial haemorrhages may occur on the conjunctiva, skin or under the nails. Subungual haemorrhages are often caused by trauma and are less likely to be significant than those on the conjunctiva. Any increase in the length of the PR interval on the ECG suggests

the development of an aortic root abscess. This serious condition warrants urgent surgical intervention. A new-onset early diastolic murmur indicates aortic valve leakage suggesting there may be a vegetation on this valve. Aortic regurgitation is also one of the principal valve abnormalities that predispose to bacterial endocarditis.

Q54. HEART SOUNDS (☆)

1. D   2. B   3. A   4. E   5. F

The carotid pulse should be felt at the same time as auscultation of the heart is performed to enable identification of the heart sounds and of any added sounds. The first heart sound occurs before systole and is produced by closure of the mitral and tricuspid valves. The mitral valve closes slightly before the tricuspid and in some normal individuals there is a split in the first sound. In mitral stenosis the first heart sound is loud and may even be palpable as a tapping apex. The reason for this is that the valve is still open when systole commences and is therefore forcibly closed during ventricular contraction. In mitral regurgitation or with a long PR interval the first heart sound is soft. In atrial fibrillation the first heart sound has variable intensity. The second heart sound occurs immediately after systole and is due to closure of the aortic and pulmonary valves. The aortic valve closes before the pulmonary producing an audible split. The split is widest on inspiration as the increase in venous return delays right ventricular emptying. Wide splitting of the second heart sound occurs in conditions delaying right ventricular emptying (eg right bundle branch block or pulmonary stenosis). Reversed splitting may occur in conditions delaying left ventricular emptying (eg left bundle branch block or aortic stenosis). In atrial septal defect fixed splitting is heard. The third heart sound occurs immediately after the second and is believed to be due to rapid inflow of blood into the left ventricle. This low-pitched sound is best heard with the bell. It is seen in conditions of fluid overload such as left heart failure. However, it is also seen in any cause of a hyperdynamic circulation (eg pregnancy or thyrotoxicosis) and in healthy, young people. The fourth heart sound occurs just before the first and is caused by atrial contraction against a stiff left ventricle. This sound is heard in left ventricular hypertrophy of any cause. An ejection click occurs shortly after the first heart sound. It is produced by the opening of an abnormal aortic valve and is heard in people with a bicuspid aortic valve or aortic stenosis. An opening snap occurs in early diastole and is caused by the opening of a stenotic mitral valve. Other added sounds such as mid-systolic clicks (mitral valve prolapse), knocks (pericardial disease) and plops (atrial myxoma prolapsing through the mitral valve) may also occasionally be heard.

Q55. PULMONARY OEDEMA (☆☆☆)

1. E   2. A   3. C   4. B   5. D

The Starling hypothesis states that the development of pulmonary oedema is dependent on the balance between the pressures listed in the question. Pulmonary oedema develops if there is an increase in capillary hydrostatic pressure or endothelial permeability or a decrease in interstitial tissue pressure, plasma colloid osmotic pressure or lymphatic drainage. Interstitial colloid osmotic pressure is not generally regarded as an independent factor as it is determined by the plasma osmotic pressure and the endothelial permeability. In many diseases several factors will act together to result in pulmonary oedema. Capillary hydrostatic pressure rises in overvigorous transfusion, cardiac failure, pulmonary embolism, mitral stenosis and exposure to high altitudes. Interstitial pressure decreases when there is upper airways obstruction. This occurs in laryngospasm, epiglottitis, obstructing tumours, head and neck trauma, intrathoracic goitre and obstructive sleep apnoea. Plasma colloid osmotic pressure may be decreased by any cause of hypoproteinaemia (eg cirrhosis, protein-losing enteropathy or nephrotic

syndrome). Endothelial permeability can be increased by inhaled toxins (eg smoke or chlorine), drugs (eg aspirin or opioids), immune-mediated damage (eg Goodpasture's syndrome), infections (eg Gram-negative septicaemia), radiation or metabolic diseases (eg hepatic and renal failure). The lymphatic system acts as an important safety valve to prevent pulmonary oedema. In chronically increased capillary hydrostatic pressure, the lymphatic system can undergo hypertrophy to cope with the increased demands. During lung transplants the lymphatics are severed and this may produce pulmonary oedema in the immediate postoperative period. Decreased lymphatic drainage contributes to the development of pulmonary oedema in other conditions including lymphangitis carcinomatosa and mediastinal obstruction.

Q56. FUNDOSCOPY (☆☆☆)

1. C   2. E   3. F   4. D   5. B

Fundoscopy is essential in patients with hypertension. The presence of grade III or IV hypertensive retinopathy indicates malignant hypertension, which must be treated rapidly to prevent further end organ damage. Grade I hypertension is the presence of an increased light reflex from the thickened arterial walls. When this process is advanced and involves all the retinal arteries it is called 'silver wiring' and indicates grade II retinopathy. Other features of grade II disease include a decrease in the ratio of arterial to venous calibre (ie arteries smaller) and arteriovenous nipping. This latter condition is caused by the thickened arterial wall obscuring visualisation of the column of blood in the vein at the arterial-venous crossing points. Grade III hypertensive retinopathy indicates the presence of one or more of: flame-shaped haemorrhages, dot and blot haemorrhages, hard exudates or cotton-wool spots. Flame-shaped haemorrhages arise in the superficial retina. Their shape is determined by the nerve fibres present in this layer. Dot and blot haemorrhages lie deep to the nerve fibres.

Hard exudates are caused by fluid leakage into the nerve fibre layer. Cotton wool spots (sometimes misleadingly called 'soft exudates') are nerve fibre infarcts caused by vascular occlusion. Grade IV retinopathy indicates the presence of papilloedema. The margins of the optic disk are blurred, the optic cup is lost and venous pulsations are not seen. New vessel formation at the optic disk or elsewhere is a feature of proliferative diabetic retinopathy. In chronic open-angle glaucoma there is cupping of the optic disk.

Q57. SCHIZOPHRENIA (☆☆)

1. D   2. C   3. E   4. B   5. F

Typical features of schizophrenia include delusions of a bizarre nature, prominent third person auditory hallucinations, catatonia, social withdrawal, abnormal behaviour, blunting of emotional responses and breaks in the train of thought. Delusions and hallucinations are called positive symptoms and social withdrawal and abnormal behaviour are described as negative symptoms. Delusions often involve the belief that others can control one's thoughts or actions (called passivity phenomena). Delusions are described as 'bizarre' when they seem particularly irrational and implausible and they cannot be explained by the person's ethnic or cultural background. Depending on the classification system used symptoms must be present for a minimum of between one and six months to make a diagnosis of schizophrenia. In paranoid schizophrenia the thought process and affect are relatively spared but there are prominent delusions often of a paranoid nature. This condition is sometimes difficult to distinguish from delusional paranoid disorder. In the latter condition the delusions are usually non-bizarre and hallucinations are either not present or are not a prominent feature. Believing that aliens are trying to kidnap you would be a bizarre delusion whereas believing that your spouse wants to poison you would be non-bizarre. In hebephrenic schizophrenia, the predominant symptoms are thought disorder and an abnormal affect producing childish and inappropriate behaviour. In catatonic schizophrenia, the motor symptoms are prominent. Patients may exhibit posturing, stereotypy, mannerisms, ambitendence and waxy flexibility. This latter condition is where the limb can be placed in an unusual posture and the patient will then leave it there for much longer than an ordinary subject could without apparent distress. In simple schizophrenia the patient develops an insidious onset of negative symptoms without preceding delusions or hallucinations. This is a difficult diagnosis to establish with confidence and is usually best avoided. In residual schizophrenia the patient has negative symptoms after previous episodes of delusions and hallucinations.

Q58. ANTIDEPRESSANTS (☆☆☆)

1. F   2. D   3. C   4. A   5. E

Amitriptyline and imipramine are well-established, effective and relatively safe tricyclic antidepressants. They are inexpensive and remain widely used. Other more expensive drugs may be useful for selected patients with depression. Amitriptyline has sedating effects and this may be beneficial for anxious patients. Other sedating tricyclics include clomipramine, dosulepin (previously called dothiepin) and doxepin. Imipramine, amoxapine, lofepramine and nortriptyline have fewer sedative effects. The older tricyclics have moderate antimuscarinic effects and may cause a dry mouth, blurred vision, constipation and urine retention. They are also arrhythmogenic and can be hazardous in overdose. The newer tricyclics, such as lofepramine and doxepin, and tricyclic-related drugs, such as mianserin and trazodone, have a lower incidence of cardiac and antimuscarinic side-effects. However, lofepramine can cause hepatotoxicity. Venlafaxine is a serotonin and noradrenaline reuptake inhibitor that lacks the sedative and antimuscarinic side effects of tricyclics. Paroxetine is a selective serotonin reuptake inhibitor (SSRI), which can be used to treat depression, obsessive-compulsive disorder and anxiety-related disorders. Other SSRIs include fluoxetine, sertraline, fluvoxamine and citalopram. Mirtazapine is a presynaptic α_2-antagonist used in the treatment of resistant depression. It may occasionally cause agranulocytosis and patients should be warned to seek medical attention if they develop a sore throat, fever or other signs of infection.

Q59. PSYCHIATRIC PROBLEMS RELATED TO PREGNANCY (✩✩)

1. F   2. A   3. C   4. B   5. D

Pseudocyesis is a rare condition in which a woman believes she is pregnant and develops amenorrhoea, abdominal distension and breast enlargement. This usually occurs in a woman who wants to have children and it may be difficult to convince her that she is not pregnant. In Couvade syndrome a man develops the same symptoms as his pregnant partner (eg morning sickness). The man does not usually believe that he is pregnant! Maternity blues affect more than half of women in the immediate three to four days after delivery. This condition may be due to falling levels of progesterone or other hormones. There are episodes of labile mood, crying and irritability. Puerperal psychosis is a sudden-onset, florid psychiatric illness that presents in the first two weeks after delivery. It occurs in around one in 500 pregnancies and is most common in first pregnancies and in those with a personal or family history of psychiatric illness. Symptoms may be predominantly schizophrenic or affective. The recurrence rate for future pregnancies is around 15–20%. Many affected women will also suffer from non-puerperal psychiatric illness in the future. Puerperal depression affects 10–15% of pregnancies. It usually begins after the first two weeks after delivery, when the support and attention the mother receives is waning. The condition is associated with stressful life events, younger age and lack of support from the husband/partner, relatives and friends. Common complaints include tiredness, irritability, anxiety and phobias. De Clerambault's syndrome is not related to pregnancy. This condition is a variant of paranoid psychosis characterised by morbid jealousy and erotomania.

Q60. URINARY INCONTINENCE (✩)

1. E   2. F   3. B   4. C   5. A

Urge incontinence is the inability to delay passing urine once the feeling of bladder fullness has been experienced. Causes of urge incontinence include urinary tract infection, bladder calculi, bladder diverticuli, prostate enlargement and spinal cord damage. Stress incontinence is the involuntary escape of small amounts of urine when the intra-abdominal pressure rises. This may occur following laughter or coughing, etc. Stress incontinence is much commoner in women because the urethra is shorter and the angle of the bladder outlet is less acute than in men. Common causes of stress incontinence include weakening of pelvic tone after childbirth or genitourinary surgery. Functional incontinence exists when there is no disorder of the physiology or anatomy of the urinary tract. The patient is unable to respond in time to prevent incontinence, despite feeling the urge to urinate. This may occur because of delirium, dementia or immobility, etc. Retention with overflow indicates that the bladder is unable to empty properly. This can occur with bladder outflow obstruction due to prostate enlargement or urethral stricture or because of medicines such as α-blockers or drugs with anticholinergic activity (eg tricyclic antidepressants). Retention with overflow may occur together with urge incontinence due to detrusor instability. Neurogenic urinary incontinence occurs when there is loss of the sensation of bladder fullness and/or control over the voiding reflex. This occurs in autonomic neuropathy (eg in diabetes mellitus), spinal cord compression, multiple sclerosis and Parkinson's disease. Vesico-vaginal fistula can occur as a result of prolonged labour. This condition is uncommon in the developed world but remains a significant problem in areas with poor access to obstetric services.

INDEX

Numbers refer to papers, and questions within each paper

absorption 3.23
acid-base balance disorders 3.13
acute poisoning 1.47, 5.52
b-adrenoceptor blockers 5.50
adverse drug reactions 2.50, 3.47
AIDS, antimicrobial therapy 4.46
amenorrhoea 1.22
aminoaciduria 3.7
anaemia 4.39
antiarrhythmic drugs 4.47
antibiotics 2.44, 3.52
   in AIDS 4.46
   genitourinary medicine 5.46
   mechanism of action 1.52
   prophylaxis 4.49
antidepressants 5.58
antidiabetic agents 3.20
antifungal drugs 4.48
antinausea drugs 5.48
antipsychotic drugs 3.59
apoptosis 3.2
asthma 2.33
atypical pneumonia 4.31
autoantibodies 3.35, 4.36
autonomic nerve supply 4.8

bacteria and toxins 1.43
bacterial taxonomy 4.45
bile 5.10
bilirubin metabolism 4.13
blistering conditions 5.37
blood disorders 5.40
blood film abnormalities 5.41
body water 5.11
bone and joint problems 1.36
bone marrow transplantation 1.42
bone, physiology 5.13
bowel disease 3.25
brain lesions 5.28
brain tumours 5.29
broad complex tachyarrhythmia 2.55
bronchial carcinoma staging 1.33

calcium and bone metabolism disorders 3.22
calcium metabolism disorders 4.21
carbohydrate metabolism 3.1
cardiac arrhythmia 3.53
cardiovascular clinical signs 1.54
cardiovascular medicine
   American Heart Association classifications 3.56
   bacterial endocarditis 5.53
   broad complex tachyarrhythmia 2.55
   cardiac arrhythmia 3.53
   cardiac problems associated with other conditions 2.56
   chest pain 1.55
   clinical signs 1.54
   congenital heart disease in adults 4.55
   ECG 1.56, 2.53
   fundoscopy 5.56
   heart murmurs 2.54
   heart sounds 5.54
   hypertension 4.53
   infective endocarditis 4.56
   investigations 3.55
   jugular venous pressure 1.53
   narrow complex tachyarrhythmia 3.54
   pulmonary oedema 5.55
   risk factors for cardiac conditions 4.54
cellular and molecular biology
   apoptosis 3.2
   carbohydrate metabolism 3.1
   DNA regions 1.1
   enzymes 1.2
   intercellular adhesion molecules 5.1
   intracellular organelles 2.2
   nitric oxide 4.1
   oncogenes 2.1
   receptor types 5.2
   tissue inflammation and repair 4.2
cerebral cortex 5.9
cerebral visual function disorders 1.29
chest pain 1.55
chest X-rays 4.33
cirrhosis 5.26

clinical genetics
    aminoaciduria 3.7
    familial patterns of inheritance 4.7
    genetic abnormalities 2.7
    genetic inheritance patterns 1.7
    genetic syndromes 4.6
    inborn errors of metabolism 5.7
    inherited disease 5.6
    patterns of inheritance 2.6
    syndromes and associated abnormalities 3.6
    syndromes and genetic mutations 1.6
clinical pharmacology
    acute poisoning 1.47, 5.52
    b-adrenoceptor blockers 5.50
    adverse drug reactions 2.50, 3.47
    antiarrhythmic drugs 4.47
    antibiotic prophylaxis 4.49
    antibiotics 3.52
    antifungal agents 4.48
    antinausea drugs 5.48
    conditions and drugs to avoid 2.49
    corticosteroid potency 2.52
    cytotoxic drugs 2.51, 4.51
    drug interactions 1.48
    drug side-effects 4.50
    drugs in pregnancy 3.48
    enzymes and drug metabolism 1.51
    general anaesthesia 3.50
    hyponotic/anxiolytic drugs 5.49
    inflammatory bowel disease 4.52
    laxative drugs 3.51
    mechanism of antibiotic action 1.52
    Parkinson's disease 3.49
    pharmacokinetic interactions 2.48
    prescribing for infectious diseases 2.47
    recreational drugs 1.49
    route of drug administration 1.50
    side-effects of respiratory drugs 5.51
    topical eye preparations 5.47
clotting 2.39, 3.14
clotting factors 4.41
collagen vascular disease 4.34
complement 4.4
complement receptors 4.5
congenital heart disease 4.55
congenital problems in gastroenterology 4.23
connective tissue disease 4.36
coronary blood flow regulation 5.14
corticosteroids
    potency 2.52
    production 2.20
cranial artery occlusions 1.27
cranial nerve lesions 2.29
cranial nerves 1.8, 2.8

Cushing's syndrome 5.20
cutaneous drug eruptions 2.38
cutaneous lesions 3.37
cytokines 2.5
cytotoxic drugs 2.51, 4.51

dementia 4.29
dermatology
    blistering conditions 5.37
    cutaneous drug eruptions 2.38
    cutaneous lesions 3.37
    facial eruptions 2.37
    histology of skin disease 5.38
    nail abnormality 1.38
    photodermatoses 4.37
    pregnancy-associated dermatoses 3.38
    skin lesions 1.37
    skin tumours 4.38
dermatomes 3.8
diabetes, aetiology 1.20
diabetic coma 2.12
diabetic neuropathy 3.21
disease transmission vectors 1.42
DNA, regions 1.1
drugs
    adverse reactions 2.50, 3.47
    antiarrhythmic 4.47
    antifungal 4.48
    antinausea 5.48
    antipsychotic 3.59
    cutaneous eruptions 2.38
    cytotoxic 2.51
    and endocrine problems 5.21
    hypnotic/anxiolytic 5.49
    inhaled 2.34
    interactions 1.48
    laxatives 3.51
    metabolism 1.51
    in pregnancy 3.48
    psychiatric 4.59
    recreational 1.49
    renal excretion 4.18
    respiratory 5.51
    in rheumatic disease 5.36
    route of administration 1.50
    side-effects 4.50
        respiratory system 5.34
    to avoid 2.49
dyskinesia 3.27
dysphagia 1.24

ECG 1.56, 2.53
electrolyte abnormalities 4.12
endocarditis

bacterial 5.53
infective 4.56
endocrine conditions, treatment of 1.19
endocrine disease 5.19
endocrine disorders 4.22
endocrinology and diabetes
  aetiology of diabetes 1.20
  amenorrhoea 1.22
  antidiabetic agents 3.20
  calcium and bone metabolism disorders 3.22
  calcium metabolism disorders 4.21
  corticosteroid production regulation 2.20
  Cushing's syndrome 5.20
  diabetic neuropathy 3.21
  diagnosis and test results 3.19
  drug-induced problems 5.21
  endocrine disease 5.19
  endocrine disorders 4.22
  inherited abnormality 2.19
  intersex disorders 5.22
  pituitary function tests 2.21
  pituitary tumours 2.22
  thyroid cancer 4.20
  thyroid disorders 4.19
  thyroid function test 1.21
  treatment of endocrine conditions 1.19
enzymes 1.2, 1.51, 4.11
error reduction 1.3
excretion 3.23

facial eruptions 2.37
faecal incontinence 4.60
familial patterns of inheritance 4.7
farmers, respiratory disease in 5.33
fundoscopy 5.56
fungi 1.44

gait abnormality 2.30
gastroenterology
  absorption and excretion 3.23
  blood tests for hepatitis B virus 1.25
  bowel disease 3.25
  cirrhosis 5.26
  congenital problems 4.23
  dysphagia 1.24
  gastrointestinal cancer 3.24
  gastrointestinal disease 2.23, 2.24
  gastrointestinal disorders 4.24, 5.23
  gastrointestinal hormones 1.23
  gut motility 3.26
  hormone-secreting tumours 2.25
  infections 4.25
  investigations 2.26
  jaundice 5.24

  oral lesions 1.26
  systemic conditions 5.25
  viral hepatitis 4.25
gastrointestinal cancer 3.24
gastrointestinal disease 2.23, 2.24
gastrointestinal disorders 4.24, 5.23
gastrointestinal hormones 1.23
genetic abnormalities 2.7
genetic inheritance patterns 1.7
genetic syndromes 4.6
genitourinary medicine
  antibiotic therapy 5.46
  antimicrobial therapy in AIDS 4.46
  genitourinary conditions 2.46
  HIV-associated infections 3.46
  syphilis 1.46
Glasgow Coma Scale 4.29
glomerular filtration measurement 4.15
glomerulonephritis 1.16
  treatment 1.17
gut motility 3.26

haematology
  anaemia 4.39
  blood disorders 5.40
  blood film abnormalities 5.41
  bone marrow transplantation 1.41
  clotting 2.39
  clotting factors 4.41
  haematological abnormality 3.41
  haemoglobin 4.40
  haemolysis 2.41
  iron status 3.39
  leukaemia 1.40, 3.40
  paraproteinaemias 5.39
  red blood cell abnormality 1.39
  white blood cell abnormalities 2.40
haemoglobin 4.40
haemolysis 2.41
haemoptysis 5.32
headache 3.29
hearing loss 1.60
heart murmurs 2.54
heart sounds 5.54
helminth infection 1.45
hepatitis B virus, blood tests for 1.25
herpes virus 5.43
histology
  renal disease 2.17
  restrictive lung disease 2.31
HIV-associated infections 3.46
hormone production 1.9
hormone-secreting tumours 2.25
human leukocyte antigens 1.4

human pathogens 5.42
hypersensitivity reaction 3.4
hypertension 4.53
hypnotic/anxiolytic drugs 5.49
hyponatraemia 4.10

immunodeficiency syndromes 3.5
immunoglobulin isotypes 2.4
immunology
   complement 4.4
   complement receptors 4.5
   cytokines 2.5
   human leukocyte antigens 1.4
   hypersensitivity reaction 3.4
   immunodeficiency syndromes 3.5
   immunoglobulin isotypes 2.4
   macrophage membrane receptors 5.5
   monocyte-derived cells 5.4
   T cell differentiation antigens 1.5
impaired decision-making capacity 2.60
inborn errors of metabolism 5.7
infection
   diagnosis 2.42
   gastrointestinal 4.25
   risk factors 4.44
   transmission of 2.43
infectious diseases and tropical medicine
   antibiotics 2.44
   bacteria and toxins 1.43
   bacterial taxonomy 4.45
   clinical presentation 3.42
   diagnosis of infection 2.42
   disease vectors 1.42
   drug regimes 3.45
   fungi 1.44
   helminth infections 1.45
   human herpes viruses 5.43
   human pathogens 5.42
   infectious organism transmission 2.43
   malignancy associated with microorganisms 2.45
   platyhelminth infection 5.45
   prescribing for 2.47
   rickettsiae 3.43
   risk factors for infection 4.44
   streptococci 4.43
   viruses 4.42, 5.44
   zoonotic infection 3.44
infective endocarditis 4.56
inflammatory bowel disease 4.52
inhaled drugs 2.34
inherited abnormality 2.19
inherited disease 5.6
intercellular adhesion molecules 5.1
intersex disorders 5.22

intracellular organelles 2.2
intravenous urography 3.17
iron status 3.39

jaundice 5.24
jugular venous pressure 1.53

laxatives 3.51
leukaemia 1.40, 3.40
lipids 1.13
loss of consciousness 1.30
lung function tests 1.34
lung tumours 4.32
lung volume measures 1.14

macrophage membrane receptors 5.5
maladaptive behaviours 1.58
monocyte-derived cells 5.4

nail abnormality 1.38
narcolepsy 4.28
narrow complex tachyarrhythmia 3.54
nerve injury and signs 1.9
nerve roots 2.9, 3.8, 4.9
nerve supply 5.8
neuroanatomy
   autonomic nerve supply 4.8
   cerebral cortex 5.9
   cranial nerves 1.8, 2.8
   dermatomes and nerve root supply 3.8
   nerve injury and signs 1.9
   nerve roots 2.9, 3.8, 4.9
   nerve supply 5.8
   spinal cord tracts 3.9
neurological findings 4.27
neurology
   cranial artery occlusions 1.27
   cranial nerve lesions 2.29
   dementia 4.29
   disorders of higher cerebral visual functions 1.29
   dyskinesia 3.27
   gait abnormality 2.30
   Glasgow Coma Scale 4.29
   headache 3.29
   hereditary conditions 5.27
   intracranial brain tumours 5.29
   loss of consciousness 1.30
   narcolepsy 4.28
   neurological findings 4.27
   nystagmus 2.27
   optic disc swelling 3.30
   pathology 2.28
   risk factors for neuropathy 5.30
   signs of brain lesions 5.28

speech disorders 3.28
vertigo 1.28
neuropathy, risk factors 5.30
neuroses, classification of 1.57
nitric oxide 4.1
nystagmus 2.27

oncogenes 2.1
optic disc swelling 3.30
oral conditions 3.60
oral lesions 1.26

paraproteinaemias 5.39
Parkinson's disease 3.49
patterns of inheritance 2.6
    familial 4.7
personality disorders 1.59
pharmacokinetic interactions 2.48
photodermatoses 4.37
physiology, biochemistry and metabolism
    abnormalities of porphyrin metabolism 3.12
    acid-base balance disorders 3.13
    bile 5.10
    bilirubin metabolic pathway 4.13
    body water 5.11
    clotting 3.14
    crystals in synovial fluid 2.11
    diabetic coma 2.12
    electrolyte abnormalities 4.12
    hormonal regulation of salt and water
        homeostasis 5.12
    hormone production 1.10
    hyponatraemia 4.10
    lipids 1.13
    lung volume measures 1.14
    physiology of bone 5.13
    pleural effusion 3.10
    regulation of coronary blood flow 5.14
    serum electrophoresis pattern 1.12
    serum enzymes 4.11
    serum proteins 1.11
    signal pathways 3.11
    sites of compound production 4.14
    thyroid hormone production 2.13
    tumour markers 2.10
    vitamins 2.14
pituitary function tests 2.21
pituitary tumours 2.22
platyhelminth infection 5.45
pleural effusion 3.10
pneumonia
    aetiology 3.33
    atypical 4.31
porphyrin metabolism disorders 3.12

pregnancy
    drugs in 3.48
    psychiatric problems in 5.59
pregnancy-associated dermatoses 3.38
psychiatric therapy 4.59
psychiatry
    antidepressants 5.58
    antipsychotic drugs 3.59
    classification 2.57
    classification of neuroses 1.57
    definition of terms 4.57
    maladaptive behaviours 1.58
    personality disorders 1.59
    psychiatric diagnosis 3.58
    psychiatric problems in pregnancy 5.59
    psychiatric therapy 4.59
    psychological defence mechanisms 3.57
    schizophrenia 2.59, 5.57
    symptoms 2.58
    UK Mental Health Act (1983) 4.58
psychological defence mechanisms 3.57
pulmonary oedema 5.55

receptor types 5.2
recreational drugs 1.49
red blood cell abnormality 1.39
red eye 1.35
renal disease classification 2.18
renal disease histology 2.17
renal failure
    first-time presentation 5.15
    reversible 5.18
    risk factors 5.16
renal impairment 3.18
renal medicine
    drug characteristics 4.18
    first-time presentation of renal failure 5.15
    glomerular filtration measurement 4.15
    glomerulonephritis 1.16, 1.17
    inherited kidney disease 3.15
    intravenous urography 3.17
    renal disease classification 2.18
    renal disease histology 2.17
    renal impairment 3.18
    renal replacement therapy 5.17
    renal stones 4.16
    renal toxicity 4.17
    renal tract investigations 1.15, 2.15
    renal transport defects 1.18
    reversible renal failure 5.18
    risk factors for acute renal failure 5.16
    risk factors in kidney disease 3.16
    urinary protein excretion 2.16
renal replacement therapy 5.17

renal stones 4.16
renal toxicity 4.17
renal tract investigations 1.15, 2.15
renal transport defects 1.18
respiratory conditions 5.31
respiratory medicine
    aetiology of pneumonia 3.33
    asthma 2.33
    atypical pneumonia 4.31
    bronchial carcinoma staging 1.33
    chest X-rays 4.33
    collagen vascular disease 4.34
    haemoptysis 5.32
    histology of restrictive lung disease 2.31
    inhaled drugs 2.34
    investigations 2.32
    lung function tests 1.34
    lung tumours 4.32
    respiratory conditions 5.31
    respiratory disease in farmers 5.33
    respiratory side-effects of drugs 5.34
    respiratory support 3.34
    risk factors for respiratory disease 3.31
    signs of respiratory disease 3.32
    upper airway obstruction 1.32
    X-ray findings 1.31
respiratory support 3.34
restrictive lung disease 2.31
rheumatology
    autoantibodies 3.35, 4.36
    bone or joint problems 1.36
    clinical presentation 3.36
    connective tissue disease/vasculitides 4.36
    drug therapy in rheumatic disease 5.36
    infectious aetiology of rheumatic disease 4.35
    lesions and nodes 2.36
    red eye 1.35
    rheumatological disease risk factors 2.35
    vasculitides 5.35
rickettsiae 3.43
route of drug administration 1.50

salt and water homeostasis 5.12
schizophrenia 2.59, 5.57
screening tests 5.3
serum electrophoresis pattern 1.12
serum enzymes 4.11
serum proteins 1.11
signal pathways 3.11
sites of compound production 4.14
skin lesions, description of 1.37
skin tumours 4.38

speech disorders 3.28
spinal cord tracts 3.9
statistical terms 4.3
statistics and epidemiology
    definitions 2.3
    error reduction 1.3
    screening tests 5.3
    statistical terms 4.3
    study designs 3.3
streptococci 4.43
syndromes and genetic mutations 1.6
synovial fluid crystals 2.11
syphilis 1.46

T cell differentiation antigens 1.5
tachyarrhythmia
    broad complex 2.55
    narrow complex 3.54
thyroid cancer 4.20
thyroid disorders 4.19
thyroid function test 1.21
thyroid hormone production 2.13
tissue inflammation and repair 4.2
topical eye preparations 5.47

UK Mental Health Act (1983) 4.58
upper airway obstruction 1.32
urinary incontinence 5.60
urinary protein excretion 2.16

vasculitides 4.36, 5.35
vertigo 1.28
viral hepatitis 4.25
    blood tests for 1.25
viruses 4.42, 5.44
vitamins 2.14

white blood cell abnormalities 2.40

X-ray findings
    chest 4.33
    respiratory system 1.31

zoonotic infection 3.44